CONSCIOUS IN A VEGETATIVE STATE?
A CRITIQUE OF THE PVS CONCEPT

INTERNATIONAL LIBRARY OF ETHICS, LAW, AND THE NEW MEDICINE

VOLUME 23

The titles published in this series are listed at the end of this volume.

CONSCIOUS IN A VEGETATIVE STATE?
A CRITIQUE OF THE PVS CONCEPT

by

Peter McCullagh

KLUWER ACADEMIC PUBLISHERS
DORDRECHT / BOSTON / LONDON

A C.I.P. Catalogue record for this book is available from the Library of Congress.

ISBN 1-4020-2629-3 (HB)
ISBN 1-4020-2630-7 (e-book)

Published by Kluwer Academic Publishers,
P.O. Box 17, 3300 AA Dordrecht, The Netherlands.

Sold and distributed in North, Central and South America
by Kluwer Academic Publishers,
101 Philip Drive, Norwell, MA 02061, U.S.A.

In all other countries, sold and distributed
by Kluwer Academic Publishers,
P.O. Box 322, 3300 AH Dordrecht, The Netherlands.

Printed on acid-free paper

Printed in the Netherlands.

For Ted Freeman

CONTENTS

ACKNOWLEDGEMENTS

I am indebted to many friends who have assisted with suggestions and comments on drafts during the preparation of this manuscript, but the contributions of several stand out. Two people, Alison Davis and Warwick Neville, provided me with a constant stream of references and, to the extent that I have succeeded in extending my investigation of vegetative states beyond basic biomedical aspects, this is largely a reflection of their enthusiasm. That enthusiasm left me with no alternative but to complete the exercise when other commitments militated against this. Ros Robertson undertook a very detailed critical examination of a draft of the manuscript which resulted in considerable reshaping of subsequent drafts. An anonymous North American Kluwer referee committed much time to the manuscript at a later stage to produce a comprehensive critique. I have taken account of all of this referee's points and I believe that the final manuscript has benefited from a viewpoint disparate both geographically and in discipline. Transformation of a mass of handwritten abstracts of references, through a succession of drafts into a completed camera-ready manuscript has been accomplished from first to last by Maria Tankosic – an example of real persistence. My wife, Mary, committed many hours to reading and checking drafts in the final stages of preparation. My sincere thanks go to those I have mentioned and to the many others who have helped me.

Peter McCullagh,
Bungendore, April 2004

INTRODUCTION

My awareness of use of the term "vegetative" to describe patients has been aroused in the course of a number of year's association with the National Brain Injury Foundation, a community based organisation providing support for Australians living with acquired brain injury and for their families. People coming to the Foundation often recounted a story of being told that their family member was "vegetative'. This was regularly converted, presumably in the retelling, to the proposition that he or she was "a vegetable". Virtually all of these patients had been deemed to be "unsuitable for rehabilitation" within a health care system but had participated in community based rehabilitation programs under the guidance of Dr Ted Freeman.

It is not possible to assure oneself that all of the patients who had been categorised at some stage as "vegetative" had been diagnosed in accordance with world's best practice. Nevertheless, it is not feasible to dismiss the use of the 'v' word as exuberant licence on the part of interns. All of these people had been examined by consultants on one or more occasions. Notwithstanding the use of the verb "to veg out" in vernacular Australian, much in the same way as the referee at a football game is regarded as "brain dead" by half of the spectators, it stretches one's credulity to source the "vegetative" description of these patients other than to their medical attendants. With this background, it became of interest to enquire more thoroughly into the *real* vegetative states, their scientific basis and their wider influence. This book is the result.

The book has two closely associated aims. The first is to trace the origins of prevailing perceptions about patients who remain unconscious after brain injury and are diagnosed as being in a vegetative state. In doing so, I intend to submit to critical examination many claims that have been made in development of these perceptions of vegetative states. My second aim is to formulate an assessment of the current status of vegetative states in the light of the evidence underpinning them.

My approach to examination of vegetative states will be basically epistemological, namely what are the origins of knowledge of the subject? how was that knowledge obtained? and what are its limitations? This will entail the retrieval of original reports on the subject coupled to an assessment of their evidentiary worth. Anyone who has read even a limited amount of the extensive literature on the subject is likely to have been struck by the mix of data and assumption and, perhaps, by the frequent blurring of the distinction between them. Of its nature, the subject of prolonged loss of consciousness by a patient who appears to retain other functional capacities is likely to raise many questions to which it is not feasible to provide clear answers. However, there has commonly been a failure to retain an adequate awareness of the limitations inherent in much of the primary data when value-based interpretations have been applied to it. The claims have been persistent, but the original limitations to them have generally not been so following their first citation.

The subject of patients in a vegetative state reeks of semantics and examples are discussed at several places in the book. However, in order to write about a subject, it is necessary to operate within the constraints of the commonly used vocabulary, irrespective of one's assessment of its value. The original introduction of the phrase "persistent vegetative state" was intended to facilitate discussion of a group of patients and comparison of clinical data. However, during the ensuing 30 years, the terms "vegetative state" and "persistent vegetative state" have not been applied consistently by different authors. Furthermore, the definitional requirements for their application, for example the interval that must elapse before "vegetative state" has "persistent" prefixed to it, has both varied between institutions and changed over time. The convenient acronym of "PVS" for "persistent vegetative state" has become much less convenient as many authors have used it to denote "permanent vegetative state". In this book, "vegetative state" (while I doubt that the term describes a single condition) will be used as a term descriptive of a set of clinical features, irrespective of their duration. There has been considerable variation and interchange in the use of "vegetative state" and "PVS". In referring to a published report, the terminology of the original is used, unless indicated otherwise. "PVS" will be used exclusively with its original connotation and references to reports concerned with a "permanent vegetative state" will describe it as such.

PVS has bulked large in the discussion, and sometimes in the evolution, of other quite disparate subjects. Examples include decision-making on behalf of incompetent patients, the use of advance directives, determination of a patient's best interests by others, the right to die, euthanasia, resource allocation, personhood and many others. Any one of these topics could be the subject of a book, and all have previously been the subject of many. This book is about people who remain unresponsive for extended periods after brain injury, not primarily about any of the subjects in the preceding list. It is, however, necessary to include some consideration of all of them insofar as they relate to this group of patients.

Each Chapter includes presentation of the prevailing "orthodox" position on its subject together with the background to its development. When I am unconvinced about the validity of the "orthodox" position, my reasons for dissenting are presented in detail. Each of Chapters 2 to 15 will conclude with a short recapitulation which will emphasise the points that I have sought to make in that Chapter. Frequently used names, for example those of professional bodies, are abbreviated when repeatedly used, although generally spelt out in full on the first occasion of use in a Chapter.

The first Chapter considers the origins of the PVS, semantic considerations underlying it and the manner in which the use of terminology has evolved in the course of 30 years. Attention is drawn to the ongoing interrelationship between the concepts of PVS and brain death. The impact of thinking, writing and acting about PVS on other, apparently discrete, issues is also discussed.

The second Chapter summarises the available information on the neuropathological changes observed at autopsy in patients who have been clinically vegetative. In doing this, limitations inherent in the conclusions which have been drawn about the neuropathology of PVS will be identified. The pathological heterogeneity underlying the uniform clinical classification has impeded the establishment of reliable clinicopathological correlations with the confidence possible for many other medical conditions.

Chapter 3 retraces the sequence of statements and guidelines on PVS which have been issued, predominantly in the U.S. These have frequently had the effect of converting primary data, shorn of any qualifications, into authoritative pronouncements. This re-examination entails critical examination of the data citation in some of the most influential statements.

Chapters 4 and 5 deal with two neurophysiological subjects, consciousness and sentience. Both are deemed, by definition, to be lacking in vegetative patients. Their absence has provided the basis for classifying and managing these patients. I believe that information about conscious and sentient status in neurologically intact subjects may be relevant for developing a better understanding of the nature of the disability, and of its management, in vegetative patients.

The variety of technological approaches that have been used in investigation of patients in vegetative states are reviewed in Chapter 6. Whilst their value in diagnosis is usually not considered to be great, some of them offer opportunities for future research to improve understanding of the nature of vegetative states. Notwithstanding their acknowledged diagnostic limitations, the results of some technological procedures have been repeatedly claimed to provide proof of complete unawareness in affected patients. This Chapter questions the scientific validity of claims such as that for a similarity between the levels of unawareness in vegetative states and deep general anaesthesia which has been accorded the status of dogma. This issue is further considered in Chapter 7 when the question of awareness during deep anaesthesia is examined. If, as is claimed, there is a comparable degree of unconsciousness in the two states, information about the nature of one may assist in interpreting the other.

Chapter 8 and 9 are concerned with the diagnosis of vegetative states and the recognition of emergence from them, that is the regaining of consciousness. The reliability with which diagnoses of vegetative states can be made has been called into question in the last decade by reports of a high frequency of misdiagnosis. In some cases, the distinction of initial misdiagnosis from accurate diagnosis followed by emergence can be very difficult. The subsequent course of patients who have regained consciousness and the capacity to communicate with others may provide information that otherwise remains unavailable.

Vegetative patients are regarded as one class of disabled individual in Chapter 10 which examines the question of evaluation of their quality of life by others. In doing so, it runs counter to the strongly expressed opinions of some authors that these patients are "beyond disability" and so cannot validly be compared with those with lesser levels of disability. This is followed in Chapter 11 by an account of the measures which are available in attempting rehabilitation of vegetative patients. The second part of the Chapter outlines the case which is often presented to dismiss any attempts at rehabilitation of vegetative patients as futile.

Chapter 12 presents the evidence, predominantly derived from animal experimentation, which calls into question the common contention that a vegetative patient cannot experience thirst. It is proposed that this contention runs counter to a substantial body of physiological data which implies that the brain lesions commonly found at autopsy of patients who were clinically vegetative do not exclude retention of a capacity for thirst. Chapter 13 extends the subject of the preceding Chapter with an examination of the theoretical and practical issues raised by the practice of withdrawal of food and fluids from vegetative patients.

The issue of health care resource allocation for patients who are in a PVS or who have severe neurological disability with retention of varying degrees of consciousness is the subject of Chapter 14. The reported cost of the care provided to vegetative patients varies as widely as does the associated neuropathology. The difficulties of estimating overall costs to a health care system introduced by this diversity are further compounded by lack of reliable prevalence data relating to these patients.

Compilation of reviews of legal decisions about patients in, and close to, PVS has become a self-sustaining industry. Chapter 15 does not attempt to duplicate the many accounts which have been published on this subject. It will use court proceedings and decisions from some U.K. cases to illustrate what appear to me to be some of the outstanding ambiguities in the manner in which medical aspects of the patients concerned have been dealt with in a legal context.

Finally, Chapter 16 contains some positive suggestions about future management of patients who remain unresponsive for prolonged periods as an outcome of brain injury.

This book is dedicated to a remarkable medical practitioner who learnt from his patients, while bringing hope to them and their families. He sought to teach his colleagues by example, challenged the prevailing paradigms about recovery from brain injury and paid a heavy price for doing so.

CHAPTER 1

HISTORY AND CONTEXT OF THE PERSISTENT VEGETATIVE STATE

1.1 TWENTY-FIVE YEARS ON: AN IDEA

On November 1, 1997, the English medical periodical *The Lancet* published an article from a distinguished international group of 10 authors (Hoffenberg *et al.* 1997) titled: *Should organs from patients in permanent vegetative state be used for transplantation?*. This article appeared a quarter of a century after publication in the same journal of the original article which had launched the *persistent* vegetative state. Between 1972 and 1997, a name suggested to describe a set of clinical features not only changed itself whilst preserving its acronym (PVS) but came to assume a life of its own and influence medical practice well beyond that concerned with affected patients.

The authorship list for the 1997 Lancet article of Hoffenberg *et al.* was collectively described as *The International Forum for Transplant Ethics*. The *International Forum* paper dealt with possible advantages and disadvantages of the course of action queried in its title. Two obstacles to the use of permanent vegetative state patients in organ donation were identified, namely the risk of misdiagnosis and the possibility of late emergence of a patient who had been correctly diagnosed. Hoffenberg *et al.* disposed of these by restricting subsequent discussion to the use of

> "those patients in whom a decision has already been taken to withdraw treatment and allow them to die".

In these circumstances they maintained

> "the actual cause of their unresponsive condition is not in this sense relevant" (ibid: 1320).

Presumably, any mistake in diagnosis or prognosis was to remain the responsibility of an earlier medical attendant.

A major impediment identified by Hoffenberg *et al.* to the use of the organs or, more accurately, to the use of the patients to whom the organs belong was the illegality of causing death by organ removal rather than by withholding fluids and food. Recalling earlier arguments about the practicality of using anencephalic infants as organ donors, Hoffenberg *et al.*, made the point that tissues and organs would no longer be suitable for transplantation if patients were allowed to deteriorate as a consequence of dehydration and starvation and then to die from "natural causes". Three rhetorical questions were asked.

The first question posed by Hoffenberg *et al.* was whether patients should continue to receive fluids and food, until they died naturally? The *International Forum* concurred with the endorsement by many authoritative groups of the practice of withdrawal of hydration and nutrition from PVS patients. Secondly, once a decision has been taken to end the life of a patient, how should this be done? The authors presented a case for "a more speedy termination" than can be accomplished by dehydration and starvation. While acknowledging that patients in a vegetative state are considered to be non-sentient and so unlikely to

> "experience distressing thirst or hunger when food and fluids are withdrawn"

the point was made that, were this to occur,

> "such distress would be a strong argument in favour of a more expeditious mode of death, for example, administration of a lethal drug".

This was followed by the conditional:

> "If patients in a permanent vegetative state are thought to be sentient"

(never mind that, if sentient, they are definitionally *not* in a vegetative state)

> "a strong case would exist for routine analgesic or psychotropic medication" (ibid: 1321).

The third question concerned the legal, moral and practical possibilities of using organs from permanent vegetative state patients for transplantation. Their response to this ran as follows:

> "We believe that, though the means by which death is attained has legal implications, there is no clear moral distinction between allowing to die by omission of treatment and more actively ending life" (ibid: 1321).

In concluding, Hoffenberg *et al.* returned to the issue of use of anencephalic infants as organ donors, and noted that the American Medical Association (A.M.A.) Council on Ethical and Judicial Affairs had stated in 1995 that it was ethically permissible for a newborn anencephalic infant to be used as an organ donor, although still legally alive according to the definition of death.

Illustrating the vagaries of publication, the paper cited by the *International Forum* to document the A.M.A. position was from the American *Neurological* Association and, furthermore, did not include the word "anencephalic" in its text. Wrong authors, wrong page, wrong volume, wrong year and wrong journal: score 0 out of 5. Ten authors with the distinction of the *International Forum* should have been able to do better. The article to which, presumably, it was their intention to refer was published in the *Journal of the American Medical Association* (American

Medical Association Council on Ethical and Judicial Affairs 1995). As a postscript, Hoffenberg *et al.* could have noted that the A.M.A. revisited the issue and, having undertaken

> "review of additional submitted scientific evidence on the condition of anencephaly"

decided to suspend its opinion which had deemed the use of anencephalic organs prior to legal death of the infant ethically permissible (Plows 1996).

1.2 RESPONSES TO AN IDEA

The paper from the *International Forum for Transplant Ethics* evoked some lively responses. The first response in *The Lancet* was from Karlheinz Engelhardt in Kiel, who expressed surprise that a highly contentious article was not accompanied by either an editorial or a commentary. The writer pointed out that, as a German, he was sensitive to promotion of euthanasia (1998). Hoffenberg's response to Engelhardt on behalf of the *International Forum* was first to call for the discussion of issues like this "in a liberal open society" and then to suggest that such debate could still not take place in Germany (Hoffenberg 1998).

A retired neurosurgeon noted Hoffenberg's denial in a newspaper article that, contrary to the impression which many readers had gained from *The Lancet* article, he was not proposing that PVS patients be killed for their organs (King 1998). Reference was made to the case of Anthony Bland, who had remained in a vegetative state for a period in excess of 4 years following a stampede at an English football stadium. A House of Lords, decision had endorsed the withdrawal of hydration and nutrition with the intention of ending his life. Noting that Hoffenberg *et al.* had laid responsibility for sanctioning the ending of Bland's life with the Law Lords with the express implication that "the transplant surgeons would be simply making practical use of the opportunity", this correspondent stressed that legality and morality were separate (and, by inference, that the expertise of their Lordships was confined to the former) (ibid).

A third correspondent from the same Liverpool renal transplant unit as a member of the *International Forum* maintained that Hoffenberg *et al.* held no official positions within the British Transplant Society or the International Transplantation Society. This correspondent considered that the *Lancet* article would "bring transplantation into disrepute" (Bakran 1998). Hoffenberg responded in the following terms:

> "Most of us are not connected with transplantation and it is this multidisciplinary approach that allows us to venture into an area of public and social interest which more closed professional societies might find it difficult to address" (Hoffenberg 1998).

Finally, a letter from David Evans pointed out an inaccuracy in the article from the *International Forum*. In describing the removal of organs from brain dead individuals the article had stated:

> "When cardio-pulmonary support is withdrawn, spontaneous function of the heart and lungs rapidly ceases, the circulation stops and immediate organ retrieval is allowed" (Hoffenberg *et al.* 1997).

This is an accurate description of practice in relation to "cardiac arrest" donors. However, the use of such donors for transplantation of kidney or liver has been abandoned by most transplantation clinics for a quarter of a century in favour of "beating heart" donors whose organs are removed *before* cardiopulmonary support is withdrawn. Procurement of organs from "beating heart" donors entails organ removal *followed* by withdrawal of support, in this instance the disconnection of the ventilator. The significance of this misrepresentation being pointed out by Evans is that he had retired prematurely as a cardiologist working in association with a very high profile British transplant unit precisely because of his concerns about the propriety of the use of "beating heart" donors. In pointing out that people

> "who have signed organ donor register forms in the belief that they are assenting to removal of their organs after circulation has finally ceased…have made their generous offer on a false premise" (Evans 1998),

Evans attracted personal criticism from Hoffenberg.

> "David Evans, who for many years has criticised the brain death criteria, makes a point about the method of retrieval of organs in ventilated patients which does not alter the sense of what we were saying and we do not see why this knowledge should affect those who wish to be donors" (Hoffenberg 1998).

I believe it should have been the accuracy, or otherwise, of what Evans was claiming rather than his persistence with the claim which required a response. Furthermore, incorporation of a patently misleading and inaccurate statement in an article of which at least two of the co-authors claimed transplantation as their medical specialty might occasion concern about the accuracy of the article as a whole.

An administrative approach that could facilitate the use of patients diagnosed as in a PVS as organ donors would be to adjust the definition of brain death to conform with a "higher brain" standard. If this was done, any patient in whom those functions commonly attributed to the cerebral cortex were considered to have been irreversibly lost would satisfy the brain death criteria. Another approach which could, at least theoretically, enable a patient diagnosed as in a PVS, who had previously expressed a wish to become a donor, to accomplish this has been described by Veatch (1999). This would entail the refusal of life support until cardiac function ceased at which time protocols applicable to the "non-heart-beating cadaver" would come into operation. The practical obstacle to this course of action, noted above, would be the deterioration in transplantable organs following withdrawal of fluids and food.

Whilst Hoffenberg *et al.* did not attempt to estimate the possible logistic impact of inclusion of permanent vegetative state patients in the donor pool for transplantation, an earlier article by Youngner and Arnold (1993) calculated that collection of organs from patients who had sustained severe brain damage and were currently ventilator-dependent, but did not meet brain death criteria, could increase the available pool by 25-30%.

1.3 THE NAMING OF PVS

The article *Persistent vegetative state after brain damage. A syndrome in search of a name* was published in *The Lancet* in April, 1972 under the category heading *Points of view*. The critical features of the condition as described by Jennett and Plum were that, after emerging from coma as indicated by opening of their eyes, these patients

> "lie for periods with their eyes open; at other times they seem to sleep.... The eyes are open and may blink to menace, but they are not attentive; although roving movements may briefly seem to follow moving objects, careful observation does not confirm any consistency in this optimistic interpretation. It seems that there is wakefulness without awareness" (Jennett and Plum 1972: 734).

In explaining their reasons for proposing the new name, the authors quoted the advice of an earlier, distinguished neurologist, that one should not be inhibited from applying a name to a concept in order to facilitate its discussion. While not questioning the original validity of their aim, allocation of a memorable descriptive name has served to entrench the perception of a discrete, well demarcated condition. This perception has often been more effective in stifling than in promoting discussion. (As indicated in the Introduction, I will use the acronym 'PVS' only to connote *persistent* vegetative state. The substituted term *permanent* vegetative state will not be so abbreviated).

Jennett and Plum were at pains in their original paper to stress four points. These were that the concept denoted by the term PVS related to behavioural features that could only be observed by clinical means, that its central feature was lack of evidence of a functioning conscious mind, that there was unlikely to be a consistent neuropathological basis for the condition and that the PVS was likely to represent part of a continuum of neurological disability. However, these four caveats, along with other reservations expressed at that time, have frequently been casualties of subsequent discussion of PVS.

The issue of communication, and its inadequacies, has impacted on development and understanding of the concept of vegetative states in more than one way. First, communication in relation both to the definition of a PVS and to its diagnostic recognition in the individual patient was an essential feature of its establishment as an entity. Its naming conferred the capacity to discuss the condition:

> "There is clearly need for an acceptable term to describe their (the patients), state in order to facilitate communication, between doctors or with patients' relatives or intelligent laymen, about its implications" (ibid: 734).

Secondly, the entire concept of a vegetative state has been predicated on equating the inability of the patient to communicate with attending medical personnel with a total lack of any consciousness. The original paper of Jennett and Plum which named PVS referred to:

> "The absence of any evidence of a functioning mind which is either receiving or projecting information" (ibid: 736)

(a statement that has often subsequently been abbreviated to *the absence of a functioning mind*) and to patients' inability to speak or to signal appropriately by eye movements with the attending medical personnel (subsequently equated with a total lack of any consciousness). The presumption that lack of capacity for detectable communication with others is synonymous with total loss of cognition lacks a logical basis. Inability to communicate of itself need not connote complete loss of cognitive capacity in a "vegetative" patient any more than it does in one who is regarded as representing a "total locked-in syndrome". As the first syllable of the word suggests, *co*mmunication is a process which requires participation by two parties and consequently it would seem imprudent on general grounds automatically to attribute its failure to one party.

The disappearance of some of the original caveats of Jennett and Plum concerning the interpretation of clinically observable features has been noted above. The varying connotation attached to the first letter of the acronym "PVS" and the manner in which I propose to use the PVS terminology has been spelt out in the Introduction. However, as policy decisions affecting groups of patients are increasingly being taken on the assured basis that PVS patients are "permanently unconscious", it is necessary to address the question at this stage of whether *everyone* who is diagnosed as in a PVS can be considered with reasonable certainty to be unconscious.

The replacement of the original proposition of "no evidence of a functioning mind" by an unchallenged presumption of "no functioning mind" has been emphasised already. This substitution requires that anyone meeting the clinical criteria for diagnosis as in a PVS, *must* therefore be unconscious. However, a sound basis for this change in interpretation of "PVS" is lacking. New evidence has not been forthcoming to replace the guarded interpretation of conscious status of patients diagnosed as in a PVS that was originally formulated by Jennett and Plum. The interpretation has changed: the data on which it is based has not. In the absence of additional evidence, I find the evolving interpretation unconvincing. However, the entrenchment of a concept of what "PVS" represents has been such that, when presenting the basis for my scepticism in this monograph, it remains necessary to employ the nomenclature that is in common use.

As will be emphasised at a number of places, especially in Chapter 4, consciousness remains a poorly defined entity, the absence of which in another individual can be inferred, but never directly confirmed, by an observer. Apart from the impossibility of formal documentation of permanent absence of consciousness, evidence from several sources leads me to question the invariable reliability of the nexus between vegetative states and unconsciousness. These sources include neurological observations derived from subjects not in a PVS (Chapter 4), the reported frequency of retention of consciousness by people diagnosed as in a PVS (Chapter 8) and the accounts of patients who have emerged from a PVS (Chapter 9).

One consequence of the widespread acceptance of the proposition that there is an entity "PVS", patients in which must always be unconscious, has been to dismiss every account of retention of consciousness by a patient diagnosed as in a PVS as an instance of misdiagnosis. The alternative response, namely of challenging the validity of the concept of an established and recognisable entity "PVS", characterised by lack of a functioning mind, is rarely aired. Is a case of PVS, diagnosed in accord with all clinical criteria, invariably accompanied by unconsciousness?

The question of the level of certainty that should be attained before a clinical decision to withhold fluids and food on the basis of irreversible unconsciousness may be made arises in individual cases. The frequent use of sedative and analgesic agents in management of patients deemed to be unconscious after diagnosis of PVS (Chapter 13) sits rather uneasily beside claims that a high degree of certainty of irreversible loss of a functioning mind follows from that diagnosis. However, responses to it in individual cases inevitably influence the development of general policy. Such policy is likely to affect not only patients diagnosed as being in a PVS but any others who are considered to be "sufficiently close" to that condition. In an analogous situation, the perception that certain specified diagnostic criteria must be satisfied before specified procedures may be discontinued has undoubtedly been fostered by the widespread conviction that a definite diagnosis of brain death is a necessary prerequisite to ventilator disconnection. In reality, long before the notion of "brain death" as a formal entity came into existence it was accepted that one could cease treatment (including ventilation) which was not benefiting a patient. The arrival of the brain death concept, and the associated diagnostic criteria, on the scene should not have altered this principle. In the same way, management decisions about any patient (whether diagnosed as in a PVS or not) ought to be made on the merits of the individual case, including efficacy and benefits of any procedures in use. However, the recent trend to attaching the cessation of tube feeding (at least in the first instance) to a diagnosis of PVS *per se*, equated with irreversible unconsciousness, appears to be discarding clinical judgement in favour of a trite formulation. I believe that the precedent of brain death as an instance of making a clinical withdrawal decision conditional upon satisfaction of a set of diagnostic criteria owed much more to affording legal endorsement for organ harvesting than to providing guidance on patient management.

Reflecting my scepticism about the presumptions inherent both in conceptualising the PVS and in deriving policies from that concept, my references to the condition will necessarily be more qualified, and accordingly longer, than would otherwise be necessary. I will use the phrase "diagnosed as in a vegetative state (or a PVS)" rather than simply stating "in a vegetative state" with its connotation of assured unconsciousness. A contention, linked to that of unconsciousness, is that any patient diagnosed as in a PVS will therefore lack capacity for appreciation of sensation, whether generated externally (pain in response to a noxious stimulus) or internally (thirst during dehydration). However, it will be suggested, in Chapters 5 and 12 respectively, that sufficient evidence exists to question whether *all* individuals diagnosed as in a PVS lack these capacities. The retention of sentient capacity in some subjects who, for all intents and purposes, have been regarded as fully anaesthetised and therefore unconscious (Chapter 7) may be relevant to understanding the capacities of some patients diagnosed as in a PVS. Anaesthetised patients have the opportunity subsequently to describe their experience whilst unconscious.

Patients who have been diagnosed as in a "minimally responsive state", that is who evince some detectable signs of consciousness, are often asserted to be more in need of withdrawal of fluids and food, as a means of effecting their death, than others actually diagnosed as being in a PVS. In practice, this proposition leads to another, namely that the retention of some level of consciousness by a patient who has been diagnosed as in a PVS is not significant when withdrawal management decisions are to be made. In contrast with this approach, I do not consider that a tendency to the implementation of a common management strategy for "PVS" and "minimally responsive" patients renders moot the question of whether patients, accurately diagnosed as in a PVS, could retain consciousness.

1.4 PRE-EXISTING NAMES

Any attempt to summarise the evolution of the terminology applied to vegetative states is inevitably bedevilled by the use of the common initial "p" to denote both "persistent" and "permanent". Two articles discussed to this point, namely those of Jennett and Plum and of Hoffenberg *et al.*, illustrate these variant uses. To place the naming of PVS in context, I will consider briefly the situation which existed at that time and the effect of that naming upon the subsequent recognition and diagnosis of previously recognised clinical syndromes. Jennett and Plum noted that existing terms were based either on clinical description of patients or on a neuropathological basis inferred from their clinical features. Whilst brain death and the locked-in syndrome survived the naming of PVS, several other terms subsequently became casualties and ceased to be recognised. Confusion, argument and advocacy concerning the relationship of brain death to PVS have persisted to the time of writing and will be considered below. Whilst the locked-in syndrome, which was first named by Plum and Posner in 1966, will be considered in Chapter 8, occurrence of a "total locked-in syndrome," in which *all* means of communication detectable by an observer have been lost, raises issues of differentiation from PVS, both conceptually and diagnostically.

Several terms describing patients with severe neurological damage were examined by Jennett and Plum in 1972 but considered not to be useful in naming the group of patients about whom they wrote. "Coma" was excluded because of the implication that the eyes were closed, "stupor" on account of its established use in psychiatric practice and "dementia" in view of its connotation of a progressive, rather than a static, condition. The clarity of distinction between dementia and PVS has been slightly blurred with the subsequent description of the latter as a late stage of dementia and by reports of the high risk of misdiagnosis of demented patients as being in a PVS. The distinction has not been materially assisted by Wikler's (1988) reference to PVS as "amentia".

Other descriptive terms which Jennett and Plum considered not to be useful in referring to patients with features defined as PVS included "decerebrate" and "decorticate" states. As the clinical features to which they referred are of motor dysfunction, rather than conscious status and, as variable combinations of neurological abnormality, including motor dysfunction, could be present or absent in patients with the cognitive features specified as the basis for a PVS diagnosis, the terms were of no discriminatory value. Those cognitive features incorporated into its definition, have greatly assisted in the entrenchment and defence of the concept of PVS itself. Thus, in the event that any patient considered by experienced neurologists to be in a vegetative state is shown to have cognitive capacity, he or she is by the common definition *not* vegetative. Irrespective of the frequency with which such patients are detected, the integrity of the state of persistent vegetation remains secure. "Wrong diagnosis" serves to protect the concept.

Two terms for disorders which had been described prior to 1972, namely akinetic mutism (or coma vigil) and apallic syndrome, were considered but excluded by Jennett and Plum when devising the PVS nomenclature. The former condition typically entailed inability to speak or to move by an individual who, nevertheless, appeared to remain attentive. It was regarded as "rather loosely defined and potentially recoverable" and as having variability in its combination of symptoms (ibid: 735). The term "apallic syndrome" referred to patients who were open-eyed, uncommunicative and unresponsive. This term was considered by Jennett and Plum to be likely to cause confusion both because the word apallic (inferring interference with function of the cerebral cortex) was unfamiliar to most clinicians and also because it implied that an unproved neuropathology was responsible for its clinical features.

Reports of further cases described as akinetic mutism appear to have become rare with the introduction of PVS as a diagnosis. Whilst the term "apallic syndrome" has disappeared from the English literature being referred to as "archaic" by the Multi-Society Task Force (M.S.T.F.) on PVS (1994a), its translation has continued to describe PVS in German medical literature. It seems reasonable to conclude that patients who would formerly have been diagnosed as examples of akinetic mutism, or as apallic syndrome (outside Germany) have been thereafter considered to be in a PVS. A 1960 description of patients diagnosed as in akinetic mutism resembled subsequent descriptions of patients in a PVS in their lack of capacity to communicate. However, the *interpretation* of their condition differed markedly from the *concept* of PVS in the inferred retention of awareness:

> "They appeared motionless and speechless as if in coma but their eyes remained open for long periods, moving in all directions.... Although they

> seemed aware of their surroundings, communication through visual and auditory commands could not be established" (Cravioto *et al.* 1960: 20).

The virtual disappearance of case reports of akinetic mutism has been queried by one commentator in 1996 on the basis that, having cognitive features intermediate between the locked-in syndrome and a vegetative state, akinetic mutism might be expected to be diagnosed with an incidence comparable with that of these two conditions (Howsepian 1996). The explanation proposed for the paucity of diagnosis was that, being in a continuum between the locked-in syndrome and a vegetative state, cases of akinetic mutism were likely to be reclassified as the latter. The availability of a neat descriptive title may have led to the artificial imposition of sharp, but illusory, cut-off boundaries on a continuous distribution of clinical disability. Perhaps analyses suggesting that PVS is a "growth stock" which is proliferating in response to refinements in intensive care practice have encouraged the reassignment of other, clinically similar conditions which antedated the introduction of the PVS nomenclature.

Naming and definition of a group of clinical features as a syndrome may have a number of effects. The description of clinical features inherent in the process of definition will clearly assist its further identification. The impact that the naming of the locked-in syndrome had on its ascertainment and reporting has been remarked by neurologists reviewing *that* condition. Thus, Bauer *et al.* (1979) observed that despite several quite extensive reports in the medical literature, the condition "did not become popular among neurologists until Plum and Posner introduced the term" (ibid: 77). It is likely that the naming of PVS 6 years later effected a similar boost in *its* ascertainment. It is difficult to write an account of a series of cases if there is not some common terminology that can be applied to them. It is likely to be even more difficult to have such an account accepted for publication by an editor. In addition to describing *what a condition is*, a definition will probably go some way towards demarcating it from other conditions, that is, to describing *what it is not*. However, if sharply defined categories of classification are imposed on a biological situation, such as a disease state, in order to facilitate description, that classification may engender a misguided sense of precision.

1.5 PERCEPTIONS ENGENDERED BY A NAME

Apart from the possibility that the term PVS may have imposed a sharp distinction where in reality none exists, the actual words selected have attracted considerable unfavourable comment on the grounds that they are likely to generate adverse perceptions of affected individuals. Anticipating the criticism that judgement about a patient's mental activity could not be made solely on observation of behaviour (in a person incapable of communication) as required in the definition and diagnosis of PVS, Jennett and Plum pointed out that no alternative approach was available at the bedside where decisions were required. They also emphasised the desirability of avoiding "the mystique of highly specialized medical jargon". Additionally, the basis for selection of the words "persistent" and "vegetative", but not of "state" was discussed (1972).

In selecting "persistent", Jennett and Plum pointed out that it was safer than "permanent" or "irreversible" until criteria required to support either of the latter terms had been validated. "Prolonged" was not considered to be strong enough. Subsequent events have not validated the appropriate criteria. Nevertheless, "permanent" has been introduced as a category additional to "persistent" and, by the late 1990s, was replacing it. Whilst the medical literature tends to be shaped by the experience of English-speaking practitioners, a significant variation with language exists in the qualifying adjective attached to "vegetative state". For example, the term PVS is replaced in France by "état vegetatif chronique" (O'Connell 1992).

In proposing the adjective "vegetative" as part of their new term, Jennett and Plum cited the Oxford English Dictionary definition of "an organic body capable of growth and development but devoid of sensation and thought". They also noted that this adjective was used to describe functions of the autonomic nervous system (such as temperature and blood pressure regulation) in physiological writing. Application of the term "vegetative" to patients with features similar to those contained in their paper had already occurred. For instance, Shalit *et al.* anticipated that paper by some 3 months in using the heading "chronic vegetative state" to classify a group of patients who were described as having features typical of the yet to be named PVS (Shalit *et al.* 1972). Reasons for the success of the Jennett and Plum term rather than that of Shalit *et al.* in achieving recognition are not clear but may include its incorporation in the title of an article in a widely circulated non-specialised medical journal. Somewhat surprisingly, Jennett and Plum failed to comment upon the predictable effects of application of the adjective to *individuals* diagnosed as being in a vegetative state, as distinct from its use in defining a medical condition. Allowing for the attitudes prevailing in 1972 towards people with disabilities, failure to take account of the probability of transference of the term, and its pejorative implications, from a medical diagnosis to an affected individual may not have been unreasonable. Nevertheless, the demeaning aspects of attaching the word to an individual have caused increasing concern among the families of PVS patients and medical specialists responsible for their longer term care since then.

The full emotive impact that can be extracted from "vegetative", by its conversion to the noun, has been well illustrated by Dworkin (1993) probably not unintentionally:

> "We also dread – some of us dread it more – life as an unthinking yet scrupulously tended vegetable" (ibid: 180),

or again, his reference to "living as a manicured vegetable" (ibid: 192). Some of the most vigorous criticism of "vegetative", has come from Keith Andrews, medical director of the Royal Hospital for Neuro-disability, Putney the major referral centre for patients diagnosed as vegetative in the U.K. In addressing the question of whether PVS patients should be treated, Andrews drew attention to two alternatives to "vegetative" which were less pejorative, namely "post-comatose unawareness" and "reflexive state" (1993c). To date, neither alternative appears likely to supplant the snappy single term "vegetative". Interviewed 3 years later about some of the patients in his care, Andrews was emphatic:

> "I would like to ban the label, along with prevailing prejudices about PVS patients and their prospects. The moment you utter the word 'vegetative' you are in a negative frame of mind which will colour all your attitudes. And the word 'persistent' gives the impression of permanence, which also sets up negative expectations" (Cornwell 1996).

Andrews suggested that the term "PVS" had become a stumbling block in the treatment of brain damage rather than part of the solution.

A review by Jennett, published 25 years after launching of the term "PVS" acknowledged that concern had been expressed about the use of "vegetative" (1997). He noted that an alternative name "the wakeful unconscious state" had been suggested in response to concerns of some commentators that the term "vegetative" could suggest that a patient is a vegetable or is in some way subhuman (this certainly appears to have been precisely what it suggested to Dworkin (1993)). Jennett and Andrews agreed that the term "vegetative" had only been introduced into the medical literature as a descriptive term for some patients with brain injury in the years immediately preceding the naming of the condition. However, earlier transfer of its use from description of the *condition* of patients to description of the patients *themselves*, had generated some remarkably demeaning comments about affected individuals. For example, in a 1949 report entitled: *Operant conditioning of a vegetative human organism* (revealed in the subsequent account to be a child), Fuller noted that:

> "While of normal human parentage, this organism was, behaviourally speaking, considerably lower in the scale than the majority of infra-human organisms used in conditioning experiments – dogs, rats, cats" (Fuller 1949: 590).

Two further articles in which psychological "research" was undertaken on "vegetative subjects" (aka children with mental retardation) (Rice and McDaniel 1966; Rice *et al.* 1967) could be mistaken, in their attitudes towards their subjects, for part and parcel of some of the recent literature characterising PVS patients as "non-persons".

The last word in the term "PVS", although its selection was not discussed by Jennett and Plum, merits more than a passing comment. Reference to "state" rather than terms, such as "syndrome", more commonly used to describe an assembly of medical signs and symptoms, has undoubtedly enhanced the status of the name when it has appeared in non-medical situations, especially courts of law and legal and philosophical commentaries. One presumes that the original intention of using "state" was that it would be taken by a medical readership as little more than a nondescript noun to which the two specific adjectives could be anchored. However, once the PVS attracted the attention of moral and legal philosophers, the potential of the third word has blossomed. I suspect that one of the other connotations of "state", namely that of the "mode of existence of a spiritual being" (again the Oxford English

Dictionary) would convey considerably more to these readers than it did to medical practitioners in 1972. Its inclusion may have helped to fuel some of the debate over PVS in relation to personhood. Apart from implying the existence of a discrete condition rather than a salad of attributes shared with other collations, the use of "state" could be viewed as having "imparted artistic verisimilitude to an otherwise bald and unconvincing narrative" (Gilbert 1885). Syndromes may come and go; states are perceived to have some permanence.

1.6 THE INTERFACE BETWEEN PVS AND BRAIN DEATH

A relationship between brain death and PVS has been maintained at varying levels – semantic, conceptual and advocatory – from the time of definition of each until the present. As recently as 2002, Bernat referred, in an editorial in *Neurology*, to brain death as lying at the most extreme end of "the continuum of brain damage" (Bernat 2002). Having been categorised as absolutely separate and separable two decades ago, the two concepts seem destined soon to collide head-on. If so, it is likely that the immediate future of the two terms may be as inter-related as was their origin. It should be recalled that the opening sentence of the report of the *Ad Hoc Committee of the Harvard Medical School to Examine the Definition of Brain Death* established the connection by declaring its primary purpose to be the definition of irreversible coma as a new criterion of death. Several lines later, the report referred to "permanent loss of intellect" (Beecher 1968). If the source were to be concealed from a reader, many of the viewpoints in the report could readily be mistaken for what was to be written a quarter of a century later about individuals diagnosed as vegetative. The issue of whether the distinction between the two conditions is no more than quantitative has been raised by calls for extension of the definition of brain death to embrace PVS, and for the course of patient management in PVS to approach that adopted for the brain dead. Recent historical analyses of the influences underlying the gestation of the brain death concept 30 years previously also reveal some striking background similarities. Attention has been drawn to the trend at the time of the early debate on brain death for the emergence of "other claimants to authority" (Pernick 1999) who disputed the convention of leaving decisions to the discretion of medical practitioners.

The potential for ongoing confusion between brain death and PVS, at least at a semantic level, was well established before the introduction of the latter term. Following introduction of the brain death concept, it was commonly referred to as "cerebral death" rather than "brain death". A large series of patients were described in 1971 as being in irreversible coma and exhibiting "cerebral" death. Reference was made to a large Collaborative Study of Cerebral Death, in progress at that time, and to a four volume collection of reprints, *Bibliography on cerebral death* (Korein and Maccario 1971). Patient descriptions indicated unequivocally that they met the criteria which were to be adopted in defining brain death, in particular the absence of any return of spontaneous respiration (ibid). Clearly, the designation "cerebral" was intended to be an adjective for "brain", perhaps as a means of avoiding the ambiguity subsequently introduced by recruiting that noun for use as an adjective (The expression "brain death" has remained open to interpretation either as *death of the brain* (noun) or as death that is *indicated by brain* (adjective) *criteria*, and this has provided ample fuel for later debate).

Use of "cerebral death" as an alternative to "brain death" eliminated one source of semantic confusion but implanted another, more enduring one based on the specific meaning of cerebral as referring to the cortex, rather than to the brain as a whole. Jennett and Plum specifically identified PVS, in their original description, as a condition in which the cerebral cortex is out of action either as a result of direct injury to it or following damage to other parts of the brain (Jennett and Plum 1972). Fortuitously, the 1971 paper to which Jennett and Plum referred in making the preceding point described two (PVS) patients who had regained spontaneous respiration, but had been found to have generalised necrosis of the neocortex at autopsy (not mandatory for PVS) and who were described in the original report as having sustained "neocortical death" (Brierley *et al.* 1971). This cluster of semantic overlaps could have been the end of the matter. However, persisting confusion concerning the neuropathological correlates of PVS and repeated advocacy for adoption of a *higher brain* standard of death has ensured that this did not occur. "Neocortical death" could fall within the definition of "higher brain death", but death of the entire cortex would not necessarily be required in order for a patient to meet "higher brain" criteria for death, as advocates of the latter would accept the survival of some cortical cells. On the other hand, depending upon the extent to which consciousness could be achieved subcortically in the thalamus, all of the cortex might be destroyed without a patient meeting the "higher brain" criteria.

An additional source of confusion, at the philosophical if not at the clinical level, arises from the different concepts of the intended meaning of the term "brain death" as applied in the U.K. and the U.S. As reviewed by Plum, an American neurologist, the U.S. definition, as embodied in the 1981 U.S. President's Commission report, was concerned with loss of all functions of the entire brain whereas the U.K. Royal Colleges definition confined itself to loss of brainstem function (Plum 1999). Additionally, the U.K. criteria have been concerned exclusively with signs of brain death which are clinically ascertainable, whereas U.S. practice has often included the use of technological procedures. Although the clinical guidelines operative in the U.K. and the U.S. for the diagnosis of brain death are, in practical terms, interchangeable, concern has been expressed by American commentators that, theoretically, it could be possible to retain a functioning cerebral cortex linked to a dead brainstem the function of which had been replaced by a life support system.

As recently as June 1999, an article in the *British Medical Journal* stressed that:

> "Confusion among the public over the difference between brain stem death and a persistent vegetative state can make it difficult to obtain consent to withdraw ventilation"

(from patients diagnosed as brain dead) (Swinburn *et al.* 1999: 1753). Substitution of the term "brain stem death" for "brain death", with retention of the existing diagnostic criteria was recommended by a British working party in 1995 (Royal College of Physicians 1995). In two commentaries appended to the 1999 *British Medical Journal* article, the two clinicians most published on the subject of PVS over the last two decades enlarged on the basis for confusion. Ronald Cranford (1999) referred to the failure of the concept of brain death to be recognized as equivalent to death as traditionally envisaged:

> "The ethical and legal concept of brain stem death is still in transition in the United States, the United Kingdom and elsewhere. It has not yet been fully accepted by practitioners by the general public, or by patients and their families".

Bryan Jennett (1999) expressed concern that families might

> "doubt the reliability of the diagnosis of brain death because of reports of the misdiagnosis of patients in a persistent vegetative state and of the few vegetative patients who make a partial recovery".

Clinical distinction between PVS and brainstem death should certainly be within the competence of any neurologist but distinction between the two *concepts* and what the two clinically distinguishable conditions actually represent is a more complicated issue as will be discussed below.

In 1989, the *Journal of the American Medical Association* ran an editorial titled *Appropriate confusion over brain death* (Wikler and Weisbard 1989) in order to highlight the publication of the results of a survey suggesting that many specialists working in intensive care facilities still had an imperfect understanding of the *concept* of brain death (Youngner *et al.* 1989). While it was emphasised that the survey did not suggest that brain death was being misdiagnosed, it was concluded that "most respondents (58%) did not use a coherent concept of death consistently". In particular, the concept of brain death held by 19% of physicians and nurses likely to be involved in organ procurement for transplantation was logically consistent with the classification of PVS patients as dead (ibid: 2205). A co-author of the report added further thoughts about the confusion in relation to brain death several years later. Stuart Youngner referred to a "fragile and superficial consensus" in the definition of death in this 1992 article (Youngner 1992). Commenting on the persistence of the term "brain death" in medical use, he remarked that:

> "This type of paradoxical speech is also the rule among health professionals, who, in my experience, almost never refer to patients who have lost all brain function as 'dead' but consistently and insistently call them 'brain dead'" (ibid: 571).

Whilst clinicians dealing on a day-to-day basis with patients diagnosed as brain dead or in a PVS may have no difficulty in distinguishing between the two categories, their writing on the subject may nevertheless have confused others. For instance, in the course of a 1979 article outlining critical distinctions between brain death and the PVS, Cranford and Smith referred to:

> "Neocortical death, a variant of the persistent vegetative state in which the EEG shows no electrical activity".

To illustrate the manner in which terminology has been used to devastating effect in confusing the subject, Cranford and Smith cited a 1978 editorial written by a member of the Harvard *Ad Hoc* Committee which had pioneered brain death. This asserted that electrocerebral silence, measured according to the specified standards, was a sure indication that "the cerebral hemispheres are dead" and that such patients are as certainly dead as those with a dead brainstem (Sweet 1978). A patient with "dead" cerebral hemispheres but a functioning brainstem may continue to breath spontaneously whereas another with a "dead" brainstem will require connection to a ventilator and, in its absence, will immediately meet all the conventional criteria for diagnosis of death based upon cessation of circulation.

The relative reliability of diagnosing brain death and a vegetative state has been cited as a basis for separating them. Thus, attention has been drawn by Gormally to a statement in a 1988 report of the British Medical Association (B.M.A.) Working Party on Euthanasia which appeared to imply that the primary ground for exclusion of PVS patients from the scope of any brain death definition was uncertainty in establishing a prognosis in PVS:

> "At present we cannot move from brain death to neocortical death because there is no way to establish that irreversible and complete loss of all neocortical function has occurred" (Gormally 1993: 45).

A further stimulus to continuing discussion of the relevance of understanding of brain death for PVS was provided by a 1994 autopsy report that called into question the conventional view of the location of brain damage responsible for PVS. At the time of its publication, Youngner and O'Toole, the former of whom had been senior author on the 1989 survey report on familiarity with the concept of brain death among professionals canvassed the inclusion of PVS within the framework of brain death in the following terms:

> "We have had to select a time of death when many signs of life do, in fact, remain. For patients in a persistent vegetative state, the most disturbing sign of life is spontaneous respiration. The signs of life in brain-dead patients, though less dramatic, are nonetheless very real and cannot be discounted in human terms, even if we have done so in public policy. *The critical philosophical question remains controversial: when do the signs of life no longer represent the life of a human being?*" (my emphasis) (Youngner and O'Toole 1994).

1.7 REVISING BRAIN DEATH: IMPLICATIONS FOR PVS

Notwithstanding its general use during the last quarter of the twentieth century, the concept of brain death was under sustained attack from two opposing directions as the century ended. Some considered its definition to be too restrictive: others considered the entire concept to be invalid. Both types of attack have major implications for PVS patients. Veatch has, for many years, advocated the introduction of a "higher brain" standard of death. In an article provocatively entitled *The impending collapse of the whole brain definition of death*, he predicted that the requirement for irreversible loss of brain stem function in diagnosing brain death would be replaced by another for loss only of cortical function, effectively encompassing PVS (Veatch 1993).

A fundamental objection to any system under which the retention of a certain specified level of brain function has been identified as essential for an individual to be regarded as "alive" was spelled out by an ethicist:

> "So it becomes a matter of choice what degree of which abilities are required in someone if he is to have a claim to be treated justly. But to base one's behaviour towards other human beings on such choices is to act in an unavoidably *arbitrary* fashion" (emphasis in original) (Gormally 1993: 46).

A similar conclusion was reached by a neurologist responding to the question, posed in the title of his article, of "*How much of the brain must die in brain death?*" (Bernat 1992a). He stressed the potential for a slippery-slope situation created by the *continuum* of PVS cases ranging from complete neocortical destruction to more variable degrees of brain damage.

An Australian philosopher, Peter Singer, has advocated replacement of the existing conventions on brain death by a system in which a doctor may intentionally end the life of a patient who is considered not to have a life worth living, thereby casting the net considerably wider than PVS. Singer (1995) set out to dispose of the existing concept of brain death maintaining that "people have enough common sense to see that the brain dead are not really dead". He then panned the brain death criterion as "nothing other than convenient fiction". In support of this position, Singer cited unpublished 1967 correspondence between Henry Beecher, chair of a Harvard human experimentation ethics committee (and subsequently of the *Ad Hoc* Committee responsible for developing the criteria for brain death) and Robert Ebert, Dean of the Harvard Medical School, suggesting that the primary purpose of defining brain death criteria was to facilitate organ transplantation.

An approach similar to that of Singer has been proposed by Robert Truog. Having dismissed brain death as an incoherent, confused means of facilitating procurement of organs, he suggested that this end be achieved by abandoning a requirement that death (in some form) precede organ removal in favour of one in which legitimated killing was available with PVS patients being prime candidates (Truog 1997). In defending the concept of brain death prevailing in the United States which requires inactivation of the whole of the brain, Bernat (1998: 14) asserted that:

> "The higher brain argument has gone nowhere outside of scholarly journal pages and college seminar rooms".

Bernat accorded more weight to the second attack currently underway on the whole brain concept of brain death. This has been mounted most notably by Alan Shewmon, an American paediatric neurologist who was originally a strong advocate of brain death formulations but who, by 1997, was vigorously rejecting any diagnosis of death that had been based exclusively on brain-determined criteria. Shewmon has specifically contradicted the proposition that death of the brain constitutes death because it is the body's central integrating organ. He argues that it would be necessary to re-define "death" as the loss of personhood as a result of the permanent loss of consciousness if brain death is to become the equivalent of death. While stressing that brain death is not death, Shewmon (1997) has concurred with Karen Gervais, a supporter of the "higher-brain" criterion of death, namely:

> "If the brain dead patient is dead, then so is the PVS patient, because the only *coherent* argument that brain death is death logically applies to PVS as well" (emphasis in original) (ibid: 84).

Whereas Gervais regards both "brain death" and PVS as "death", Shewmon considers that neither is.

Discussion of the title subject in a monograph on *The definition of death* has implications for patients diagnosed as in a PVS. In a contribution to that discussion, Veatch (1999) proposed that the question which should be addressed is not that of whether there can be only one true definition of death but whether a public policy which accepts different beliefs about that definition can be viable:

> "We are asking whether society can treat people as dead, based on their own beliefs rather than whether people are really dead, really conform to some metaphysically correct concept of what it means to be dead, in such circumstances" (ibid: 149).

Following the approach espoused by Veatch over many years, Miles (1999) has suggested that it could be possible to "offer individuals a choice from a menu of socially acceptable definitions of death". The alternative was to "decouple a variety of perimortal medical acts from a declaration of death" ("perimortal" apparently referred to events closely preceding or following death). Adoption of the first option would, according to Miles, make possible a situation in which:

> "The value *choice* (my emphasis) that a loved one is 'dead' in the condition of PVS would permit that person to be an organ donor without the family regarding organ procurement as a form of killing" (ibid: 315).

The option of becoming an organ donor as a result of implementation of their previous selection of a preferred definition of death is likely to be attractive to some people. Nevertheless, the possible impact upon participating medical and nursing staff and the implications for patients diagnosed as in a PVS, as a group, may not be so simply discounted.

1.8 SEMANTIC IMPLICATIONS

> "Judgements are peppered with semantic distinctions, which are dubiously founded, lend nothing to clarity and, indeed, the very need to invoke such distinctions is a telling criticism in itself".

This comment, by Andrea Fenwick (1998: 91) a lawyer from the University of Edinburgh writing on the issue of "best interests" of PVS patients as determined in U.K. courts up to 1998 would be appropriate as a description of the evolution of PVS terminology in general. In a commentary by Molinari (1991) accompanying a review of PVS by another U.S. neurologist (Spudis 1991) and challengingly titled *Persistent vegetative state, do not resuscitate... and still more words doctors use*, attention was drawn to the frequent need, in medical writing on vegetative states, to resort to the use of quotation marks when attaching specialised meanings to specific words. At the cost of introducing further quotation marks, I suggest that this practice represents a medical example of the "Humpty Dumpty syndrome", namely "when I use a word, it means exactly what I choose it to mean- neither more nor less" (Carroll 1872: 75). Molinari's commentary drew attention in particular to the popularisation, in medical and legal parlance, of non-clinical terms such as cognition, self-awareness and humanhood. Whilst the practicability of precise, agreed definition of such terms is highly arguable, they have often come to be used in a manner previously reserved for words with clear, scientifically founded, clinical meanings. One suggestion from a medical ethicist discussing PVS, which would itself be a certainty to qualify for any short list of the most felicitous euphemisms, was for "careful retraining of speech habits" (Wikler 1988: 46).

1.9 EVOLUTION OF THE TITLE

The original description of PVS, and many subsequent accounts, have been at pains to stress that "persistent" was being applied in a descriptive sense and was not intended to have the prognostic implications that might be read into "permanent". The question of *permanence* of a vegetative state, as distinct from its *persistence*, has been a feature of some of the authoritative statements that have characterised the condition. Whilst some of these statements will be examined in more detail in Chapter 3, attention can be drawn now to the semantic issues raised by them. Both the 1990 A.M.A. report (American Medical Association Councils 1990) and the 1994 M.S.T.F. consensus statement (Multi-Society Task Force 1994a; 1994b) discussed permanence extensively whilst retaining "persistent" exclusively as the adjective abbreviated in the title of PVS. Both report and statement were criticised by Howsepian (1996), on the grounds that they addressed the question of a vegetative patient's state *becoming* permanent. As Howsepian pointed out, designation of a case of vegetative state as permanent represents a change in the physician's assessment, not a change in the patient's status. The disability which may always have been permanent at last comes to be *recognised* as such.

A change from discussing permanence of PVS to specifically designating an additional condition as the *permanent* vegetative state became apparent in 1995 in the practice parameters of the American Academy of Neurology (Quality Standards Committee 1995). The permanent vegetative state was defined by its irreversibility, so conflating permanence and irreversibility. An irreversible condition will *always* be permanent: a condition which will be permanent, in the absence of successful intervention, need not be irreversible (Howsepian 1996). Having been introduced as an *additional* category, the permanent vegetative state has progressed to become a *replacement*. Designation as permanent rather than persistent required no modification of a well established acronym. The 1996 statement of the U.K. Medical Royal Colleges abandoned "persistent" vegetative state in favour of "permanent" vegetative state, with this description to be applied "when the diagnosis of irreversibility can be established with a high degree of certainty" (Royal College of Physicians 1996). By 1998, an influential text *Principles of medical law*, edited by Kennedy and Grubb, could refer, in its section 4.205 on futility to "a permanent (formerly called persistent) vegetative state". The author of this section of the text, J. Munby Q.C., had appeared for the Official Solicitor in most of the PVS cases brought to English courts (Munby 1998: 274).

1.10 ALIVE OR DEAD?

Apart from neurologically based relationships between PVS and brain death already discussed, the question of conceptual and semantic relationships between a vegetative state and death has attracted attention. Attitudes towards the management of individuals in PVS have altered significantly since the condition was first described, most notably evidenced by an increased readiness to cease feeding. However the questioning of the vital status of affected individuals, which may have encouraged management changes, is certainly not new. Several years after the first description of PVS, Jennett and Bond (1975) concluded that the question of whether death and the vegetative state should be regarded as a single category was a philosophical issue. They suggested that vegetative states could be envisaged as "death anticipated". Continuing ambivalence was reflected by another neurosurgeon, Grant Gillett. After a discussion, which flitted between the metaphysical and the anatomical, about whether the soul had departed from a vegetative patient he suggested that "we can make the decision that this patient is no longer, in any ethically interesting sense, alive" (Gillett 1986: 85). Uncertainty was similarly reflected by Wikler (1988) in an article headed *Not dead, not dying*? He suggested that PVS could be viewed either as the lowest-functioning phase of life, or as the highest-functioning phase of death.

1.11 DYING FOR HOW LONG? AN EXERCISE IN TERMINAL SEMANTICS

Courts have often been remarkably generous in classifying patients in a PVS "as terminally ill" and approving forms of treatment (or lack of treatment) that would be uncontentious in more conventional examples of terminal illness. The application of a "terminal" classification to a patient has not been seen, by some commentators, to be incompatible with continuing survival over many years. One quasi-medical U.K source which explicitly expanded the catchment of "terminal" was the Institute of Medical Ethics (1990). Its working party on the ethics of prolonging life and assisting death redefined the word in the following terms:

> "The word terminal here implies a progressive illness whose distressing symptoms cannot be eased by any alteration of treatment. Such patients are usually close to death but there are some, such as those with disabling breathlessness or paralysis, who may have to face months or even years of increasing distress" (ibid: 611).

Medical common sense might be expected clearly to indicate that (excluding complications) patients in a PVS are *not* terminally ill. However, common sense has failed to prevent medical discussion of PVS patients from being framed *as though* they were terminally ill. The Council on Ethical and Judicial Affairs of the A.M.A. (1999) initially placed PVS and terminal illness in a disjunctive relationship but then proceeded to negate the separation:

> "Use of life-sustaining or invasive interventions in patients in a persistent vegetative state or who are terminally ill may only prolong the dying process".

The duration for which the "dying process" may reasonably be expected to continue (outside some notable operatic performances) was not canvassed. Cessation of hydration and nutrition would be guaranteed to facilitate entry into the "dying process" irrespective of the extent to which one was in PVS.

Redefinition by the courts has resulted in considerable broadening of the meaning of "terminal illness". In the Greenspan case, for example, the Supreme Court of Illinois excluded any extension of life resulting from medical treatment from consideration in determining whether death was sufficiently imminent for an individual's state to be designated as "terminal". "Imminence must be judged as if the death delaying procedures were absent" (*re Estate of Sidney Greenspan* 1990). The Court regarded tube feeding as such a procedure. It remains unclear whether it maintained a consistent position in relation to the use of insulin by a patient with diabetes or of home dialysis by another with chronic renal failure, two instances in which early death could be guaranteed if those specific death-delaying procedures were absent. The B.M.A. Guidance on Withholding and Withdrawing Life-Prolonging Medical Treatment, having acknowledged that withdrawal of treatments such as provision of insulin to an insulin-dependent diabetic will lead to the patient's death as inevitably as will deprivation of food and fluids, identified a need for "procedural safeguards" applicable in both situations (British Medical Association Medical Ethics Committee 2001).

1.12 ARTIFICIAL HYDRATION, NUTRITION AND SEMANTICS

> "The Law Lords' ruling referred to 'artificial' nutrition and hydration and there is no consensus on what this is".

This April 1999 comment in an interview with the chair of the B.M.A. medical ethics committee may well be one of the most accurate statements made on the subject of provision of food and fluids to PVS patients (Hallows 1999). The ruling referred to was that of the U.K. case of *Airedale NHS Trust v Bland*. This case, which will be discussed in Chapter 15, concerned an application seeking a declaration that withdrawal of tube feeding from a PVS patient would not be illegal. Withdrawal of hydration and nutrition from PVS patients will be considered in Chapter 13 but the extent to which semantic twists have affected this subject justifies some earlier mention. Considerable objection has been raised by some authors to the use of expressions which might be considered unexceptionable by many others. An article by Ahronheim and Gasner (1990) considered the word "starvation" when applied to PVS patients dying following the withdrawal of hydration and nutrition to be "especially provocative".

Armstrong and Colen (1988) found it necessary to refer to food, water and feeding in quotation marks:

> "Because artificial support is referred to as feeding…. The very idea of withdrawing such basic humane support goes against the grain not only of most physicians, but of many lay persons as well".

Truly an amazing insight!

An objection to what might previously have been regarded as reasonable and unexceptionable terminology has not inhibited some of those who raised it from themselves opting for some creative use of other terms. For example Ahronheim & Gasner, while objecting to the use of "starvation" to describe the course of PVS individuals dying following withdrawal of hydration and nutrition (or fluids and food), repeatedly referred to the process as "allowing to die". In providing reasons for his decision in favour of withdrawing artificial (or artificially-administered) hydration and nutrition from the Hillsborough stadium victim Tony Bland, one of the Law Lords appeared not to restrict his reasoning to *artificial* means. The tendency to adopt the abbreviated form of "hydration and nutrition" in place of the earlier "artificial hydration and nutrition" (which was originally regarded itself as an abbreviation for "artificially administered hydration and nutrition") has not been confined to courtrooms. Howsepian's comprehensive critique of the M.S.T.F. statement observed that it

> "was initially careful to note that the American Academy of Neurology classified artificial nutrition and hydration as forms of 'medical treatment".

However, he noted:

> "Later the M.S.T.F. states that 'hydration and nutrition' *simpliciter* are forms of medical treatment" (1996: 28).

As Howsepian remarked, presumably breast-feeding of an infant by its mother now represents 'medical treatment'. A 1992 recommendation from the B.M.A. medical ethics committee referred to artificial means of feeding as "invasive", hardly a neutral term (Dyer 1996a). The semantic diversity which has characterised description of the management of PVS patients has been paralleled by the variety of descriptions of causes of death following cessation of feeding.

Before leaving the question of the impact of semantic stratagems on perceptions of PVS patients, it is appropriate to take account of the explanations presented for the events which follow withdrawal of hydration and nutrition. The *underlying* cause of death is commonly attributed to the pre-existing disease which prevented self-feeding rather than to the withdrawal of fluids and food (Cranford 1984). The *immediate* cause of death has usually been dissected off as a separate issue. Writing in general terms in a *British Medical Journal* commentary the title of which asserted that *Withdrawing artificial feeding from children with brain damage is not the same as assisted suicide or euthanasia*, Cranford indicated that "the immediate cause of death is dehydration" (1995: 464). Furthermore he stressed that "the patients do not show any of the terrible signs of starvation described by pro-life supporters". Whilst deferring to Ronald Cranford's experience of the subject of the characteristics of patients following withdrawal of food and fluids, some divergent observations will be discussed in Chapter 13. In a Scottish court case seeking withdrawal from a PVS patient, the medical director of the hospital concerned reassured the media that

> "the patient would not starve to death but would gradually slip away, probably because of a kidney infection" (Clancy 1995).

1.13 PVS AND THE RIGHT TO DIE MOVEMENT

The case of Karen Ann Quinlan has been credited with being the trigger that initiated the right to die movement. The Quinlan case revolved around disconnection of a ventilator from a PVS patient. This case was *not* about cessation of feeding. Karen Ann's capacity for spontaneous respiration had been retained and she did not die after ventilator disconnection. While the Quinlan case is often equated with the claim by the right to die movement to have hydration and nutrition withdrawn from PVS patients, it is paradoxical that Karen Ann's father, while seeking ventilator disconnection, expressed opposition to withdrawal of food and fluids (Campbell 1984). PVS has provided the basis for one of the scenarios most commonly presented in advocating recognition of the right to die. There is a continuing absence of any reliable early predictors that PVS will subsequently develop which are detectable at the time when patients are ventilator dependent (as future PVS patients have commonly been when initially comatose) and when ventilator disconnection will lead to death. Consequently, the only aspect of management that can be modified, so as reliably to lead to death of the patient, is that of provision of food and fluids. The withholding of antibiotics for infections is of limited applicability in achieving death unless the individual is subject to repeated life threatening infections. Cardiac arrest is uncommon in PVS patients and so the withholding of cardiopulmonary resuscitation in response to it is unlikely to become an issue.

Whilst the reasons which have been advanced for achieving legislative changes to assist dying will be considered in Chapter 15, attention may be drawn to a particularly obvious point made by a London newspaper editorial. This was that to speak in terms of release from pain or suffering as a reason for facilitating death of these individuals flatly conflicts with the numerous medical statements that PVS patients "cannot feel anything" (Editorial, *The Daily Telegraph* 1997). The relief of suffering by the *family* of the PVS patient, may be closer to the mark. Two American rehabilitation specialists, writing about severely disabled individuals and the introduction of right to die legislation quoted a disabled person asserting that:

> "Only a handful of disabled people have publicly sought death. Yet... laws are being passed at record speed to ease the way to our demise" (Bach and Barnett 1994: 135).

Although cases of people in PVS have been in the forefront of advocacy for legislative recognition of the right to die, the changes that have been achieved in their name appear to be in the process of being extended to other people, who are *not* in a PVS. For example, an Irish court ruled in 1995 that a woman who it considered had been terminally ill whilst she had been in a *near-PVS* for 23 years qualified for withdrawal of food and fluids (Wall 1995). The Chief Justice of the Irish Supreme Court concluded that: "Her right to life necessarily implies the right to die a natural death" (Irish Correspondent, *The Catholic Times* 1995). Two years later, when the English High Court sanctioned the cessation of feeding of "Miss D", who again was described as not in a PVS, because she did not comply with the guidelines of the Royal College of Physicians, the editor of the *Bulletin of Medical Ethics* was reported as referring to "constant attempts to quietly push back the frontiers" (Macdonald 1997b).

Apart from extension of the right to die concept to patients who are not in a PVS, there has been an increasing level of discussion about the possible existence of a *duty to die*. An affidavit filed in a U.S. District Court in 1994 in relation to the *Death with Dignity Act* of the U.S. State of Oregon by a clinical psychologist who was also wheelchair and ventilator dependent queried when the *right to die* that was recognised in the Act would become a *duty to die* (*Affidavit of C.J. Gill*). The phrase *duty to die* was introduced by Richard Lamm in 1984 when Governor of Colorado. Addressing a group of elderly listeners, and citing economic reasons, he stressed that elderly people with terminal illness had a duty to die and get out of the way (Lamm, *New York Times* 1984). Exploration of the phrase by John Hardwig (1997) based the *duty* primarily on the burden (economic and other) that an elderly person could impose on his or her family. Whilst Hardwig did not consider that incompetent patients retained a duty to die, he suggested that a person could have such a duty when incompetence was approaching. This position was more conservative than that of the Institute of Medical Ethics (1990), a paper from which on the subject of "assisted death" noted that "disapproval of involuntary termination of patients' lives is strongly entrenched in the concepts of most doctors and layman" with the qualification "except in the case of irreversible unconsciousness". It is interesting to juxtapose this viewpoint with that of Charles Baron, a self-acknowledged long-time advocate of the right to die. Discussing legal proceedings concerned with the withdrawal of hydration and nutrition from a PVS patient, Nancy Cruzan, Baron referred to the "mere lip service" afforded to substituted judgements (that is decisions as to what an incompetent patient's wishes would have been that are formulated by a substitute for the patient) advanced in court proceedings in distinctly unflattering terms:

> "Almost any evidence is deemed sufficient to establish a preference for death over PVS" (Baron 1990: 8).

How is a right to die to be exercised if an individual does not anticipate possible entry into a PVS and indicate a wish to exercise a right to die, specifically if this occurred, or is not considerate enough to conform to a duty to die in anticipation of it? The use of some general form of words requesting the withholding of food and fluids if an individual becomes unable to consume these unaided could certainly cover those who are in a PVS, or in the actual process of dying but could equally well be applied in other, less extreme situations. In a commentary, at the time of the Cruzan case, on the exercise of an incapacitated patient's right to die, Ellman drew a sharp distinction between the *right of the patient* and *the entitlement of his or her family* with respect to that right. He maintained that:

> "The family's claim to decide cannot be piggybacked on the *patient's* right of self determination" (emphasis in original).

Specific to the case under consideration, Ellman emphasised that:

> "The Cruzans can no more exercise Nancy's right to choose her treatment than they can exercise her right to vote" (1990: 48).

(At issue in the case of Nancy Cruzan, a young woman diagnosed as being in a PVS, was the question of the extent to which a patient's previous wishes could be construed in the absence of a formal advance directive).

Whilst the impact which semantics has had on evolution of the PVS as a discrete condition, and on general perceptions of PVS patients, has been discussed above, it remains relevant to the present topic to draw attention to some associated semantic aspects of the right to die issue. Carol Gill, an American psychologist living with disability, has written of the inequality of effort expended in suicide intervention on behalf of physically normal people compared with that expended on behalf of others who have disabilities. She has pointed out that the desire of a non-disabled person to die is likely to be classified as "suicidal". However, a similar desire by a person with severe disabilities (perhaps requiring a ventilator and/or feeding assistance) is much more likely to be described as

> "refusal of treatment .... a wish to avoid prolonged suffering" or "a desire to let a terminal disease take its natural course"

(often, it could be added, with *terminal* being applied in very liberal fashion). Gill concluded that:

> "The implication is that there is something natural, reasonable, or proper about a disabled person's dying as opposed to a nondisabled person's dying" (1992: 39).

Examples of the attitude to which Gill objected appear in the writings of Ronald Dworkin. On the one hand, Dworkin maintained that: "Every day, rational people all over the world plead to be allowed to die" (1993: 179). On the other, some 40 pages later, he denies the exercise of such autonomy, expressed as a wish to live, to seriously incapacitated individuals who had previously expressed a wish for future withholding of treatment. Discussion of the relationship of a "right to die" to a "right to suicide" has infrequently been directly addressed in discussion of the former right. However, in probing the distinction between the two, Siegel suggested that changes in societal attitudes about acceptable grounds for not prolonging life, "what some would call passive euthanasia", are likely to presage some extension of the reasons presented for "rational suicide" (1986: 411).

The demarcation between advocacy of a "right to die" and "euthanasia" may be difficult to define. I understand the term euthanasia to encompass the accomplishment of the death of one individual by one or more others with an expressed intention of thereby helping the first individual. The decisions by English courts (most notably the House of Lords) in relation to withdrawal of hydration and nutrition from PVS patients have tended to stress that the course of action that is being sanctioned is not euthanasia. Certainly, the literature relating to "allowing nature to take its course" following withdrawal of food and fluids from PVS patients rarely alludes to "euthanasia". In one relatively early exception to this, an article on PVS concluded with the advice to

> "*explore the legalisation* and ethical acceptance of euthanasia as an act of ultimate kindness to terminate suffering and subhuman existence using the argument that society and the *law should give PVS patients the right to die with dignity*" (emphasis in original) (Ivan 1990: 994).

A more specific exhortation to consider euthanasia for PVS patients was provided in 1997 by a lawyer from the University of Dundee. Ferguson (1997) compared and contrasted a recent case in which a doctor was convicted of attempted murder of one of his patients, who was said to be in considerable pain, with two PVS cases (*Bland* and *Johnstone*) in which courts (English and Scottish respectively) sanctioned cessation of feeding. Having drawn attention to the conviction of one doctor for administering lethal treatment to a patient described as terminal and in pain and the exoneration of others responsible for proposing to allow patients "to be starved to death", when they were neither terminal nor in pain, she queried whether there was not a moral obligation "to procure death more humanely by a lethal injection".

Whereas most of those advocating withdrawal of food and fluids from PVS patients have gone to some lengths to distinguish their actions from euthanasia, other commentators with an explicit commitment to promoting acceptance of euthanasia have claimed proposals for the withdrawal of hydration and nutrition as their own on the basis of a right to die. For example, an article entitled *Euthanasia by stages*, co-authored by a member of the Voluntary Euthanasia Society of Scotland, hailed the House of Lords' decision in the Bland case as a step in the right direction. In advocating the introduction of a Medical Futility Bill which would take care of PVS or, more precisely, of PVS patients, Mason and Mulligan expounded some debatable views on PVS. The condition was said to be "relatively common" and also to be "the most obvious candidate for isolation" (presumably because it was believed that it could be clearly diagnosed and separated from other conditions) (Mason and Mulligan 1996). Both assertions are suspect. The proposed Medical Futility Bill, it was said, "by its name, would eliminate many of the emotional responses to euthanasia". Exemplifying the trend, already noted, for substitution of nomenclature under cover of a retained acronym, the Bill was to refer to a *permanent* rather than a *persistent* vegetative state.

Pieter Admiraal, one of the most active and articulate practitioners of euthanasia in the Netherlands, in discussion with a group of physicians and bioethicists in Minneapolis in 1989, was reported (Dolan 1994: 64) as unequivocally placing withdrawal of hydration and nutrition in the euthanasia category. In reference to the withdrawal of hydration and nutrition, Admiraal's opinion was:

> "You're doing the same thing I am; you're just playing games with words when you describe what you're doing".

He added that he personally would never kill a patient by withdrawal of hydration and nutrition.

1.14 UTILISATION OF PVS PATIENTS

The question of the utilisation of PVS patients by incorporation into research or therapeutic (for others) procedures has generally remained off limits until quite recently. The possibility of using *brain dead* individuals in experiments has evoked many unfavourable responses with the actual use of a brain dead patient in an experiment by a French anaesthetist being widely condemned (McCullagh 1993: 77-78). Writing about the distinctions between brain death and PVS, Cranford and Smith (1979) were adamant that the latter group could not be considered as organ donors.

The *Lancet* paper of Hoffenberg *et al* discussed at the beginning of this chapter may have permanently reset the conventions for discussion of possible use of PVS patients although there had been some suggestions for their experimental use preceding it. David Morton, Professor of Bio-ethics and Veterinary Science at the University of Birmingham (U.K.) told a seminar on animal experimentation ethics at the 1996 Edinburgh International Science Festival that experiments on PVS people

> "would give more accurate results than those on chimpanzees and would reduce the number of animal experiments carried out" (Anon. *The Independent* 1996).

Underpinning the issue of whether they could be utilised, Morton raised the question of whether humans in coma were people: "In the actual sense of the word 'person', they are no longer people, they are individuals" (O'Neill 1996). He indicated that, as a prerequisite to experimental use, consent would have had to be obtained from the individual before he or she became comatose or entered PVS. When interviewed after his seminar, Professor Morton suggested that a decision to use a PVS individual in an experiment would only be taken after it had been decided to withdraw food and water. (This would place the starting point for intervention at the time suggested by Hoffenberg *et al.*). Any decisions concerning subsequent use were to be regarded as quarantined from the preceding decision to withdraw food and water. Proposals for entry of a subject into experimentation once a decision had been taken to initiate a course of action certain to lead to death of that subject are reminiscent of the lively bioethical debates of the late 1970s on experimentation on the fetus in the course of abortion (Ramsey 1975). In that situation, a requirement was established that the decision to abort must be irrevocable before experimentation could be considered.

The issue of avoiding experimentation on animals has underpinned much of the advocacy of human experimentation, be it on embryos, fetuses, the disabled or convicted criminals. Material prepared for an undergraduate course at an Australian university and strongly criticised in a bioethics journal presented the case as follows:

> "Take on the one hand, a massively retarded, physically disabled human being, unable to maintain *itself* (my emphasis) alone in life... Take on the other hand, a fully grown ape, alert, apparently intelligent... Why would you use the alert, aware, communicative, responsive ape as a subject for medical research rather than using the unalert, unaware, uncommunicative, unresponsive disabled human?" (Borthwick 1998: 33).

A different slant on the question which, perhaps because it did not come from an academic commentator, did not automatically accept that animal and human use had necessarily to be placed in an adversarial context, came from the mother of a comatose English youth in response to David Morton's proposal:

> "I don't even believe in testing on live animals so how could I agree with it on my own son?" (Anon. *The Independent* 1996).

In April, 1997, the Council of Europe Convention on Human Rights and Biomedicine was signed by 21 countries (not including the U.K.). The convention permitted research on individuals unable to give consent, provided the research was into their own "condition, disease or disorder" (Berger 1997). Whilst the convention would restrict research to that which entailed minimal risk and burden, a number of groups representing people with handicaps expressed considerable alarm. David Morton once again identified PVS patients as an appropriate candidate group of subjects (ibid).

1.15 PERSONHOOD AND PVS

Reference has already been made to the popularisation, and incorporation into medical literature, of poorly defined terms. PVS has engendered a preoccupation of some medical practitioners with "personhood". This is not new. An article by Cranford and Smith (1987) in the *American Journal of Law and Medicine* presented its central argument in its title *Consciousness: the most critical moral (constitutional) standard for human personhood.* Its introduction identified the definition of death with loss of personhood. The article, which dealt principally with the status of PVS patients, stated as a fact not requiring further consideration that the level of consciousness is similar in PVS and in death. Coupled with the position, asserted in the title, that consciousness was a *sine qua non* of "personhood", the authors concluded that "permanently unconscious patients lack personhood". They called for vigorous dialogue and debate about the "actual medical reality". In view of the persisting obstacles (to be summarised in Chapter 4) that exist to the definition and understanding, not to mention the diagnosis, of consciousness, it would seem a little presumptuous to refer to the medical reality of an entity of personhood that is, on any assessment, much more complex.

CHAPTER 2

THE PATHOLOGICAL BASIS OF VEGETATIVE STATES

Two features underpinning the scientific basis of medicine have been, first, the establishment of a consistent relationship between the fine structure of a normal organ or tissue and its function and, then, the delineation of the nature of any abnormal structural features and *their* precise relationship to abnormal function. Adequate information about the normal structure : function relationship is mandatory in order to understand the physiological operation of any organ system. Deviations from the established normal structure lead to the disordered function, or pathophysiology, that is expressed clinically as the symptoms of disease. Delineation of the nature of pathological deviations from normality, either after biopsy undertaken on the living patient or at autopsy, is one of the most common approaches to diagnosis of clinical abnormalities. When seeking to understand any disease condition, information about its underlying pathophysiology is likely to be essential. The extent of the confidence one can have in the validity of any proposed *causative* association between pathological and clinically observable features will be dependent upon the extent to which two requirements can be met. First, are the typical pathological characteristics always accompanied by the clinical features? Second, are those clinical features ever observed in the absence of the pathological features?

Description of its pathological features should, logically, be given at an early stage in any account of a medical condition in order that other features of that condition can subsequently be described and interpreted in relation to the structural abnormalities underlying them. Attempts to follow this course in relation to PVS encounter a number of difficulties. In the first place, as emphasised by Jennett and Plum, the term relates to a grouping of clinical features and a clear underlying pathology is lacking. Whilst PVS is hypothesised to result from destruction of the cerebral cortex or its disconnection from the remainder of the nervous system, consistent neuropathological indications of this, attaining the evidentiary standards required in many other fields of medicine, are incompletely developed. Furthermore, patients in a PVS almost invariably have additional clinical neurological abnormalities reflecting neuropathological lesions other than those responsible for interference with consciousness. As Jennett and Plum observed:

> "Whilst it is usual for the mental state which we are defining to be associated with severe motor disorders, the pattern of this is by no means consistent" (1972: 735).

Consequently, it becomes necessary to discriminate between those pathological features responsible for the accompanying neurological disabilities and those which are specifically causative of PVS if the latter are to be accurately characterised. Finally, the nature and extent of any neuropathological changes which have occurred *after* the initial damage responsible for PVS are likely to vary between patients with the duration of their survival in PVS and their management and so further to complicate reliable correlation of previous clinical features with neuropathological findings at autopsy.

Whilst some accounts of the PVS may leave the impression that the condition represents a recent development which had not existed for any significant period before its description in 1972, this is not an accurate representation. Comprehensive accounts of the neuropathology subsequently described in patients diagnosed as in a vegetative state were published two decades before the actual naming of the condition. Whilst Jennett and Plum referred to these earlier reports in their paper, popular presentations of the relationship of the pathological features underlying the PVS to the clinical features and status of patients, have generally paid scant attention to them.

The PVS was defined in 1972 on the basis of clinical features summarised in Chapter 1. It was acknowledged then that different combinations of pathological features were likely to be associated with the specified set of clinical features. Notwithstanding this initial prediction of pathological heterogeneity, subsequent writing on PVS in legal and philosophical contexts suggests that later authors not only believed, but also sought to convince others, that it should be regarded as a consistent, well defined pathological condition. This belief has not been confined to non-medical authorities. For example, a spokeswoman for the British Medical Association (B.M.A.) revealed at a conference on PVS jointly organized by the B.M.A., the U.K. Official Solicitor's office and the Centre for Medical Law and Ethics, King's College, London that:

> "When we looked at vegetative patients, we thought that it was a discrete condition and it wouldn't have applications for other cases" (Dyer 1996c).

This belief in the unique and distinctive character of PVS was exemplified by the ethicist Daniel Callahan in stressing that supportive attitudes towards those disabled by severe dementia should not extend to PVS as this was a condition *sui generis* (Callahan 1995). Many others have claimed that any rules which common decency might impose on dealings with individuals subject to extreme disability could reasonably be suspended in the case of those who have been diagnosed as in a PVS.

Many philosophers and courts, and some physicians, have subscribed to the existence of reliably consistent neuropathological characteristics for PVS on the basis of which there has been irreversible inactivation of the cerebral cortex with resulting loss, not only of recognisable cortical function, but also of any entitlement to personhood. Arguments linking loss of cortex, consciousness and personhood have been notable for their circularity. Thus, the major supporting data for the contention that patients diagnosed as in a PVS lack any *capacity* for consciousness or cognition has been the frequent, clinically based assertion that their cerebral cortices are no longer functional. However the strongest basis for asserting that the cortex is no longer functional has been the attachment of a clinical diagnosis of PVS coupled to the requirement that they must *by definition* be unconscious and incapable of cognition and so, inferentially, lack a functioning cortex.

As described in Chapter 1, not only the evolution of the PVS concept, but also its subsequent development, have been inextricably linked with the refinement and popularisation of the concept of brain death and with the description and characterisation of minimally responsive states. The close relationship, both clinically and semantically, between the original delineation of brain death as a discrete condition and the (at that time unnamed) PVS was exemplified in a report by Korein and Maccario (1971). Its title *On the diagnosis of cerebral death* appeared from the substance of the report to be using "cerebral" as an adjective synonymous with "brain", rather than referring exclusively to destruction restricted to the cerebral cortex as intended in the article on "neocortical death" published in the same year by Brierley *et al.*, (1971) which described two patients with the clinical features of a vegetative state. Whilst Korein and Maccario considered "cerebral death" to be equivalent to systemic death, the resumption of spontaneous respiration in 10 out of 55 of those patients clearly demarcated at least that subgroup from any patient who would meet the current, required criteria for brain death. It is of more than passing interest that the authors, nevertheless, stated that all 55 patients met the "Harvard criteria" for brain death at the time of entry to their study. From the clinical descriptions provided in the report, none of the 10 patients who resumed spontaneous respiration appeared to exhibit the characteristics of a vegetative state. All of these patients died within a month of the onset of their illness.

2.1 INTERPRETATION OF THE PATHOLOGICAL FEATURES OF PATIENTS IN VEGETATIVE STATES

The extent to which factual considerations have been reflected in descriptions of PVS has varied with the anticipated readership of many articles. For instance, a 1987 article by Cranford and Smith in the *American Journal of Law and Medicine* stated that:

> "In all PVS patients studied to date, post-mortem examination reveals overwhelming bilateral damage to the cerebral hemispheres to a degree incompatible with consciousness or the capacity to experience pain or suffering" (1987: 240).

This description with its categorical assertions on neuropathology, consciousness and sentience could be juxtaposed with a paper from Fred Plum's Department at Cornell in the *Annals of Neurology* in the same year which acknowledged that:

> "The distribution and severity of postmortem anatomical damage to the cerebral hemispheres can vary considerably in vegetative patients making it

> difficult to infer on pathological grounds alone whether or not all self-awareness was lost during life" (Levy *et al.* 1987: 673).

Quite apart from problems introduced by the heterogeneity of neuropathological features in people diagnosed as in a PVS, it is self-evidently impossible to infer on pathological grounds *what is* the minimum severity of damage required for loss of self awareness. Once a severely brain-injured individual has lost the capacity to communicate vocally with others (or to undertake motor activity recognisable as an attempt at communication), there is no way in which self awareness can be detected, or confirmed. In the absence of any objectively certifiable parameter which can be independently validated as correlating reliably with awareness, any attempt to specify *what degree* of severity of damage to *which* combination of structures in the brain (as documented at autopsy) is equivalent to previous loss of awareness must fail. The paper by Cranford and Smith is typical of many of the descriptions to be found in non-medical and quasi-medical literature. The designation of a particular location and level of brain damage as excluding consciousness appears invariably to have been an arbitrary choice.

A good example of the manner in which interpretation of the linkage between underlying pathological changes and clinical features could be complicated was provided by Shalit *et al.* (1972). They raised the possibility that reduced levels of cerebral blood flow, which could lead one to infer a reduced cerebral metabolic rate, could, alternatively, reflect the lack of contribution to total brain blood flow of irreversibly damaged or scarred regions of brain tissue. Viable regions of brain might regain normal metabolic activity but this could be masked because of inclusion of the reduced level of blood flow to the scarred regions in achieving the aggregated calculation.

2.2 EARLY NEUROPATHOLOGICAL REPORTS OF PATIENTS IN A VEGETATIVE STATE

Jennett and Plum referred to the possible diversity of the neuropathological condition underlying PVS in the following terms:

> "The lesion may be in the cortex itself, in subcortical structures of the hemisphere, or in the brain-stem, or in all of these sites" (1972: 734).

They stressed that the *common* feature of all of their patients was the absence of function in the cerebral cortex, as judged clinically, rather than a common neuropathology. (Perhaps a more precise description would have been the absence of *detectable* function). They drew attention to two earlier clinicopathological reports which, in retrospect, may have described patients in vegetative states. A report by French (1952) which had anticipated the naming of PVS by twenty years, described five patients who had survived for periods of from four to nine months, following vascular lesions or trauma, in a state of inattentiveness characterised by intermittent periods in which their eyes were open.

It is not intended as a criticism of any of the neuropathological reports describing changes in the brains of patients with disorders of consciousness to observe that they have generally been driven by specific hypotheses about what types of lesions might be anticipated. Any research-motivated set of observations not planned to test a specific idea runs the risk of collecting a mass of data which defies interpretation. This risk will be especially high if one is examining the brain, an organ unique in the multiplicity of different structures and the complexity of their connections. In searching at autopsy for abnormal structural correlates specific for loss of capacity for consciousness in the absence of some working hypothesis that directs attention to localised regions of brain tissue, it is probable that an enormous data collection over a prolonged period would be necessary even to examine a small group of patients. The focus of French's investigation was the reticular activating system, which occupies the upper, central brain stem and the region below the thalamus and which had been shown by a collaborator of French, H.W. Magoun, to be responsible for arousal in animals.

Apart from one patient with tertiary syphilis, it was noted that the cerebral cortex was "singularly uninvolved" or showed "minimal evidence of injury to the hemispheres" or "surprisingly little alteration". The lesions in these four patients occurred predominantly in the upper brain stem or thalamus and corresponded with the localisation by Magoun of the activating system which is demonstrable in cats and monkeys. The patients described by French had been observed in the period 1946-1951 and the similarity of their clinical features to those described as PVS two decades later suggests that vegetative states did not suddenly emerge from nowhere as a new condition due to the introduction of intensive care, but had occurred previously as unaggregated, and variously categorised, cases. The increasing incidence of PVS has been identified frequently as a looming issue in resource allocation. The absence of reliable data on current prevalence makes it difficult either to support or refute this proposition, but the 1952 report of French directs attention to the distinction between changes in *ascertainment* of vegetative states and changes in their *prevalence*.

The second comprehensive clinicopathological account of patients in vegetative states, noted by Jennett and Plum and published some 16 years before formal naming of the condition, came from Strich in Oxford. The five patients described in this report survived for 5-15 months following head injuries and were described as having "severe dementia" (Strich 1956). They showed apparent sleep/awake cycles and periods during which, although their eyes were open, they appeared to be unaware. All patients were "almost completely unresponsive though they lay awake for most of the day" (ibid: 178) and showed "extreme indifference to the environment" (ibid: 182). Some were said to have a limited capacity for speech. At autopsy, the cerebral cortices of these patients again appeared to be "remarkably normal" (ibid: 166). There was severe degeneration of white matter throughout the cerebral hemispheres and the thalamus was markedly shrunken in two patients. It was suggested that traumatic interruption of connections between different areas of the cortex and between the cortex and lower parts of the nervous system had led to secondary atrophy of the thalamus.

2.3 NEUROPATHOLOGICAL FEATURES OF TWO DEFINING CASES OF PERSISTENT VEGETATIVE STATE

A widely known case of a specific medical condition in an identifiable person often has more impact on attitudes to that condition than a published series of unidentified patients. Case reports, are invariably published in a deidentified form but PVS has been a prominent exception to this generalisation. Widespread awareness in the community about both the identity and the story of a number of patients has resulted from media attention in response either to their unexpected emergence from a vegetative state or to court proceedings intended to release them from it by withdrawing hydration and nutrition. The frequency with which PVS patients, and their medical history, have been identifiable was the subject of an editorial comment in the *British Medical Journal* in which the reasons and justification for this apparent breach were explored (Smith 1996). The point was made that the doctor-patient relationship is built on trust, especially the trust of patients that information about them will remain confidential. Recognising the media attention that some patients had already received, it was considered likely that any individual whose personal clinical details were subsequently described, albeit in deidentified form, in medical journals might be readily identifiable. The editor's conclusion, on the commendable basis that expediency is not a good reason to override ethical issues, was that consent for publication of clinical details should be obtained from patients or their relatives.

The two most prominent cases of PVS in the U.S. and U.K. respectively, so defined because of the high profile of legal proceedings relating to them, were those of Karen Ann Quinlan in the U.S. and Tony Bland in the U.K. In both cases, their families gave permission for identified publication of the outcomes of autopsies. In view of the very common perception of the anatomical basis of PVS, which has remained prevalent among legal and philosophical commentators, namely that it represents destruction of the cerebral cortex, it is instructive to review the pathological findings in these two cases the legal proceedings associated with which have had such a substantial influence on later court hearings.

Karen Ann Quinlan suffered a cardiac arrest in 1975 and, following resuscitation, passed into a vegetative state. Her parents sought court permission for the discontinuation of "extraordinary treatment", in particular the use of a ventilator, in the expectation that this would allow her to die. In the course of the court hearing, Fred Plum testified that she might resume spontaneous respiration following ventilator disconnection, dependence on such support not being a typical feature of patients in a PVS (Beresford 1997). (A requirement for mechanical ventilation is not a feature of patients in vegetative states, other than in the early stages before the diagnosis becomes possible). In the event, Karen Ann Quinlan breathed spontaneously once the ventilator was disconnected. The court case generated an unprecedented level of discussion of the issue of maintaining the life of patients in a PVS and has been credited with initiating the right to die movement. She died in 1985 and an autopsy was performed 13 hours later. Its results, however, were not presented until 9 years later, coincidentally in the same issue of the *New England Journal of Medicine* which carried the report of the Multi-Society Task Force on PVS (M.S.T.F.). Whilst the delay between death and reporting of the autopsy has occasioned much comment, especially because of the intense debate on all aspects of PVS in the interim, I am not aware that any explanation for it has been provided. However, in the absence of its publication, the popular perception of an invariable correlation between loss of the cortex and PVS certainly became firmly entrenched.

The Quinlan pathology report revealed:

> "Contrary to expectation, the most severe damage was not in the cortex but in the thalamus, and the brain stem was relatively intact" (Kinney *et al.* 1994: 1472).

Cortical damage was observed primarily in the occipital region. The authors of the report concluded that the case raised fundamental questions about the neuroanatomical basis of human consciousness (and, presumably, about the basis for PVS). While noting that some earlier reports of the neuropathological basis of PVS had reinforced "the accepted role of the cerebral cortex in cognition and awareness" (ibid: 1469), they noted that the extent of cortical damage in the case of Quinlan and some other patients seemed insufficient to explain the clinical features. The nexus between cerebral cortical destruction and PVS had become sufficiently entrenched (in particular in the courts) during the 9 years which elapsed between Karen Ann Quinlan's autopsy and its reporting that the latter event had a much weakened impact on beliefs and firmly held convictions about the structural basis for PVS. Reappraisal of the pathological basis for vegetative states in the wake of the Quinlan report emphasised the interpretation that the cortex could be functionally inactivated in the absence of direct damage to it. The reasoning which was accepted to explain the Quinlan findings ran on the lines that the cortex is essential for consciousness, the patient had a relatively intact cortex but was unresponsive, therefore her cortex *must have been* disconnected by her injury. However, precise examination of specific tracts or pathways from the cortex was not undertaken. One essential component of the logic invoked in reconciling PVS clinical features and pathology, namely that consciousness is absolutely dependent on normal cortical functioning, will be discussed in Chapter 4. While not contesting cortical disconnection in the Quinlan case, the possibility of continuing activity in the "disconnected" cortex might have been considered worthy of comment.

Publication of the Quinlan autopsy report evoked a description of a similar Viennese case of PVS in which there was disproportionately severe damage to the thalamus rather than to the cerebral cortex (Jellinger 1994). Another comment, applicable to virtually all reported examinations of the cerebral cortex in PVS, queried the validity of non-quantitative studies in assessing the extent of damage (Hawton and Ohara 1994). Four years before the Quinlan report, Fred Plum's group had referred to increasing evidence for a critical role for the thalamus in consciousness and cognition on the basis of four autopsies of PVS patients in whom damage to brain structures other than the thalamus was described as mild (Relkin *et al.* 1990). This report of four patients with features apparently similar to those of Quinlan, however, had failed to have the high impact of the paper based on the nationally known patient, despite its earlier release and more extensive set of observations.

The case of Tony Bland in the English courts almost two decades after the Quinlan case had been decided in the United States, probably had a comparable impact on perceptions of, and legal management of, patients in PVS in this second jurisdiction. Tony Bland was diagnosed as being in a PVS following traumatic asphyxia sustained when crushed in a football stadium disaster in 1989. Whilst the Quinlan case had concerned the disconnection of a ventilator, the issue in his case was the withdrawal of food and water. Withdrawal was approved in 1993 and his death followed. Autopsy revealed a significant degree of cerebral atrophy together with considerable loss of cells from the cortex. There was also marked loss of axons (the extensions of neurones by means of which outgoing impulses are transmitted to other neurones) in the white matter of the brain whereas the thalamus was relatively well preserved (Jarmulowicz 1995). The report of the Bland autopsy drew particular attention to the differences in neuropathology from Quinlan stressing differences in the degree of damage and its main location and commented that this variability highlighted the limitations to our understanding of human brain function.

2.4 NEUROPATHOLOGICAL REPORTS OF SERIES OF PATIENTS IN VEGETATIVE STATES

Autopsy reports of patients diagnosed as "PVS" have described severe damage to the cerebral cortex in some patients but substantial sparing of this structure in others. A paper correlating clinical and pathological features of affected patients was published by a group of authors, including Fred Plum, in 1981 (Dougherty *et al.* 1981). All 10 patients had experienced prolonged periods of interruption of blood circulation to the brain, in the majority of cases following cardiac arrest, and all met the clinical requirements of Jennett and Plum for the diagnosis of vegetative state. All had substantial damage to the cerebral cortex. A report of 35 patients who had been either vegetative or severely disabled following traumatic head injury was published two years later from the Institute of Neurological Sciences at Glasgow. Sixteen of these patients had extensive cortical damage while others showed diffuse axonal injury (that is, damage to the cellular extensions by means of which nerve cells are interconnected) (Graham *et al.* 1983).

A comprehensive account of the relative frequency of the different pathological accompaniments based on examination of the brains of a series of 49 patients who had been in a vegetative state for periods ranging from one month to 8 years was published in 2000 (Adams *et al.* 2000). Adams *et al.* reported in this that diffuse damage to the white matter (the "diffuse axonal injury" referred to above) was the most common abnormality, together with thalamic damage. Cortical damage was less frequent. They concluded that these lesions would

> "render any structurally intact cortex unable to function because connections between different cortical areas via the thalamic nuclei are no longer functional" (ibid: 1336).

As already noted, the conclusion that the cortex was non-functional, rather than directly damaged, was necessarily based on the absence of any detectable clinical signs of consciousness in these patients, accompanied by direct observation at autopsy of cortical preservation. Direct clinical observation that cortical output was lacking would not be feasible in any case in the absence of connections. However, Adams *et al.* mentioned in this paper that the autopsy results obtained from some severely disabled, *but non-vegetative* patients whom they had examined were not readily distinguishable from those of the vegetative patients described in the report.

The closest approach to achieving the goal of differentiating, on pathological grounds, between patients in a PVS and those who have regained consciousness has been a clinicopathological study by Jennett *et al.* (2001). It found that diffuse axonal injury and thalamic damage were both less common in severely disabled, but conscious, individuals than in vegetative patients. Whereas half of the severely disabled groups had only focal lesions, this feature was not found in any of those in a PVS. Nevertheless, some of the severely disabled, but conscious, group had lesions similar to those in the vegetative patients. Two major limitations to concluding from this study that lesions essential for loss of consciousness had been identified were this overlap and the semi-quantitative assessment that was applied. The overlap is entirely consistent with the existence of a continuous spectrum of disability as originally implied by Jennett and Plum. It remains the case that consistent identification of any pathological feature, accurate measurement of which reliably separates severely brain-injured, but non-vegetative, patients from others considered to be vegetative, has yet to be achieved.

There are limitations, inherent in autopsy examination of the brains of patients, to identifying structures which are critically involved in consciousness. When compared with approaches to structure : function correlations in experimental pathology studies of *other* organ systems, the methodology applied to distinguish vegetative from conscious subjects appears rather limited. In the first place, an appropriate *control* group is required for comparison with the group manifesting the feature of interest. In the case of PVS, a normal brain is certainly not an adequate control if one is seeking to define which lesions are responsible for unresponsiveness (and of the unawareness this is taken to reflect). The required control group of patients should have had neurological damage, similar to that of the PVS group *except for loss of consciousness*. Secondly, some attempts at *quantitative measurement* of relevant features, such as loss of specific classes of neurones, should be made. Given the repetition of the mantra that a particular patient could not have remained aware because of the magnitude of brain injury, some measurement with a greater degree of sophistication than the weight of the organ at autopsy is highly desirable. Computer assisted image analysis has now been introduced into morphometric examination in many other fields of experimental pathology and could have something to offer in achieving this. A third essential prerequisite for validation of qualitative comparisons of organs from two groups of patients is the collection of data on a "blinded" basis – that is the assessor *must not* know the origin of any sample.

The variability observed in neuropathological findings among series of patients all of whom met the clinical criteria for classification as being in a PVS prompts the question of the extent to which PVS can ever be demarcated from other conditions of severe damage to the nervous system in which retention of a range from impaired to full consciousness has been recognised. Demonstration of this point would require that, in pathological studies such as those of Adams *et al.* (2000) and Jennett *et al.* (2001) it was possible reproducibly to differentiate "blinded" specimens obtained from patients clinically in a vegetative state from specimens taken from other patients dying with very severe brain injury who had retained consciousness. Given the limited quantity of tissue which could be examined in considerable detail in a reasonable time, from such a large and heterogeneously structured organ as the brain, the risk of sampling errors would also have to be considered in any attempt to attain certainty.

2.5 NEUROPATHOLOGICAL DELINEATION OF THE PVS FROM THE LOCKED-IN SYNDROME

The paper of Jennett and Plum in which PVS was first named as such acknowledged the likelihood that a variety of pathological lesions could produce a similar clinical syndrome. It also suggested "that a continuum must exist between this vegetative state and some of the others described" (1972: 737). Both of these entirely reasonable points have tended to be progressively omitted from subsequent "simplified" accounts of PVS. In view of the loose correlation between structure and function in predicting consciousness in the damaged brain and the repeatedly emphasised importance of differentiating PVS from a locked-in condition in which a person remains fully conscious but with limited or no capacity to communicate with others, the degree of precision attained in pathological and clinical correlation in the locked-in syndrome (LiS) may be questioned.

The LiS is defined by a range of neurological disabilities comparable with those occurring in PVS but with retention of consciousness. Unfortunately, a clinical description as "locked-in" is equally applicable to patients whose features may closely resemble those of a vegetative state, except for detectable retained consciousness accompanied by limited or absent ability to communicate, as it is to those who exhibit the "typical" clinical features of LiS as originally described by Plum and Posner (1966). Even more unfortunately, automatically requiring that all instances of *being locked-in* accord with that original clinical description may retard or prevent recognition of cases who do not conform to the "typical" features. The practical distinction between PVS and the typical LiS, as the syndrome was originally described, is made on the basis of retention of eye movements that can be used by the LiS patient to convey responses to questions. The most striking difference between patients in a PVS and a LiS relates to their management. Whilst calls for the withdrawal of hydration and nutrition from PVS patients have become increasingly frequent, the general response to the LiS has been to extend the greatest consideration to the maintenance of support unless a patient exercises his or her retained cognitive and communicative capacities specifically to request otherwise.

Historically, the conventional presentations of the two conditions, PVS and LiS, have ascribed quite discrete pathologies. Thus, it is usually spelt out that there has been severe damage to, or inactivation of, the cerebral cortex in the former and damage to the ventral part of the pons (in the brainstem) with complete preservation of the cortex in the latter. Reports of the pathological basis of the "typical" LiS suggest that this may not be as neatly definable as the conventional description of a pontine lesion suggests. One early case report described an "*essentially intact*" ventral pons but necrosis of both cerebral peduncles. It noted that:

> "The pathological correlate of this clinical syndrome is more variable in location and vascular anatomy than the homogenous literature on the subject suggests" (Karp and Hurtig 1974).

This assessment referred to those patients showing the clinical features of the LiS as originally described by Plum and Posner. If the "pathological correlate" of others who are effectively "locked in" but who do not show those clinical features is considered, it would be even more variable. Nevertheless, the reassuring distinction between the pathology of the PVS and that of the LiS remains quite firmly entrenched. While acknowledging that the understanding of different clinical syndromes resulting from brain damage cannot be based on individual cases, it is relevant to recall that much of the accepted understanding of conditions related to PVS *has*, in reality, been so based. Logically, it should remain unarguable that even a single well documented case that deviates significantly from the accepted paradigm which purports to explain the pathological basis of a clinical syndrome, requires modification of that paradigm. It is of some interest that the question was asked, during the hearing of the Bland case in the House of Lords, whether it was possible to be in LiS, in the absence of a retained capacity for eye movement and, if so, how is the attending clinician to distinguish it from PVS? No answer was forthcoming.

2.6 EFFECTS OF MEDICAL MANAGEMENT ON PVS PATHOLOGY

By definition, PVS only becomes *apparent* with the passage of time. However, as stressed by Howsepian in his critique of the M.S.T.F. on PVS and will be discussed in Chapter 3, a PVS (depending upon the meaning attributed to the acronym) does not *become* persistent or permanent (Howsepian 1996). The *recognition* of its nature only *becomes evident* as time elapses. As its recognition and the death of the patient are necessarily delayed, it is not possible to identify the neuropathological features of such cases at the outset. Some of the changes observed at autopsy may be direct consequences of early damage whereas others reflect later, superimposed events (Adams *et al.* 2000). It is likely that some of the neuropathological features observed in longstanding cases of PVS are secondary to other factors, for example chronic nutritional impairment, a common feature of individuals in a PVS. Subnutrition impairs brain development (Winick *et al.* 1970) and is also likely to compromise any capacity of central nervous system tissue for repair (see Chapter 6). The extreme cachexia, as documented by the body weights of Quinlan (27kg) and Bland (36kg), may be highly relevant in this context. Surprisingly, reference in case reports to the possible complicity of impaired nutrition in producing neuropathological changes has been rare. Whereas the autopsy report on Quinlan referred to the possible significance of her poor nutritional status, including vitamin deficiency, in producing wasting of the posterior columns of the spinal cord, the possibility of similarly produced changes in the brain was ignored (Kinney *et al.* 1994).

2.7 DEAFFERENTATION AS A FACTOR IMPEDING ASSESSMENT OF CONSCIOUS STATUS

As any attempt to communicate with a patient with a brain injury will be dependent upon the integrity of inward (afferent) nerve pathways, neuropathological evidence of interruption of these pathways (deafferentation) in any individual requires reassessment of interpreting lack of responsiveness as evidence for lack of consciousness. A negative outcome in response to attempts at communication could indicate either the absence of consciousness, or its retention accompanied by impairment of the individual's capacity to receive sensory input from an observer or, alternatively, to produce a detectable response to it. Consequently, the presence of neuropathological lesions that affect either afferent or outward (efferent) pathways in the nervous system of suspected PVS patients, should constitute an insurmountable obstacle to making that diagnosis. The archetypal example of complete loss of afferent and efferent peripheral pathways despite the presumed retention of brain function is the Guillain Barré syndrome, a disease which inactivates peripheral nerves. Efferent (motor) pathways may remain intact in individuals diagnosed as vegetative although any degree and distribution of paralysis remains consistent with diagnosis of the condition. However, preservation of efferent or motor pathways may not reliably guarantee that a conscious individual remains able to respond to an observer. This is because co-ordination of peripheral motor function, in order to produce recognisable responses, will require an additional contribution from other structures in the nervous system. If afferent pathways have been interrupted, a conscious individual will have no more capacity to receive input from an observer, and so to respond, than another who is completely unconscious. A most striking example of the results of interruption of an afferent pathway, which has been reported in some patients misdiagnosed as in a PVS, is the "cortical" blindness that can occur if a patient has sustained damage to the visual (occipital) cortex.

Deafferentation, or loss of sensory input, can theoretically affect any of the sensations, for example touch, hearing or vision. Vision appears to be more likely to be impaired than other forms of sensation in patients diagnosed as in a PVS. A 1996 report describing a high frequency of positive misdiagnosis of PVS noted that 65% of the patients who had been wrongly diagnosed were either blind or subject to very severe visual impairment (Andrews *et al.* 1996). Maximum damage to the cerebral cortex in the occipital region, where vision is represented has often been observed at autopsy of PVS patients. Dougherty *et al.* (1981) noted that, in 4 out of their 10 PVS cases, the most severe cortical damage was located at the occipital pole. Whilst the authors of this report were prepared to speculate on the level of curtailment of capacity for consciousness that could be anticipated from the extent of the pathological changes, they did not consider the possibility that loss of visual capacity with cortical blindness as a result of occipital lesions could have thwarted attempts to detect any conscious capacity. On the contrary, the occipital cortical damage was interpreted solely as an indication that any of the eye movements observed in these patients need not be taken to "imply return of cortical integrative function". The cortex of Karen Ann Quinlan was likewise described as being relatively well preserved apart from the occipital region (Kinney *at al.* 1994).

2.8 FROM THE INDIVIDUAL TO THE GENERAL: PERCEPTIONS OF TYPICAL PVS NEUROPATHOLOGY AND PERSONHOOD

The statement of Cranford and Smith (1987) referred to above about the consistency of cerebral damage as the basis for PVS is an example of the popular perception equating this clinical condition with destruction of the cerebral cortex and, increasingly, with loss of personhood. A physical lesion, albeit one still incompletely understood, is assumed to explain loss of an attribute, consciousness, that remains undefined, inadequately understood and, inherently unobservable by another individual. The impact that a simplistic presentation on the neurological basis of personhood from an authoritative source can have is well illustrated in the account by given Pete Busalacchi, the father of Chris, a 20 years old Missouri woman in a PVS. In explaining his attitude towards his daughter, Mr Busalacchi described a television program which had influenced him:

> "In a PVS special aired last December, Dr Fred Plum, a well-known neurologist, held a model of the brain and pointed out those areas that make us human beings, and those that merely control the reflexive actions that still exist in Nancy (Cruzan, another PVS patient) and Chris" (1990).

A 1998 volume, *Companion to bioethics* neatly encapsulated the situation for the benefit of philosophers:

> "It is in the 'higher brain', and in particular the cerebral cortex, which is the outer layer of the cerebrum, that consciousness and mental activity are realized" (McMahan 1998: 251).

2.9 RECAPITULATION

What can an understanding of the underlying pathology of PVS contribute to understanding the clinical condition? Ultimately, any medical condition should be definable on the basis of its underlying pathology in addition to the clinical features. That this goal remains yet to be attained in extensive areas of medicine, for example in psychiatry, as well as in some common conditions frequently diagnosed on clinical grounds alone, such as repetition strain injury, does not negate its significance. A prerequisite to explaining a disease state in terms of its underlying pathology is the availability of an accurate and comprehensive description of the relationship of *normal* function to *normal* structure. The PVS was first identified (as was brain death) as an exclusively clinical diagnosis and its underlying pathological features were imputed secondarily from this. The proposition that the cortex is destroyed has not been consistently supported by the results of autopsy examination of the brains of PVS patients. Attempts to link loss of personhood to PVS on the basis of locating an anatomical lesion which ablates structures required for personhood appear destined to fall at the first hurdle, namely the lack of uniform structural pathological features. The lack of a reliable distinction, based on pathology, separating vegetative patients from others with very severe disability *but retaining consciousness* is a further impediment to attempts to establish some objective basis for consciousness, let alone for personhood, and for its withdrawal. Both groups of patients, namely those diagnosed as in a PVS and those with major neurological disability, but with retention of consciousness, have brains characterised by widespread pathological changes. However, examination of brains from both groups by observers unaware of their origin has yet to identify pathological lesions that are present in PVS patients but lacking in any of those who have regained some level of consciousness. The interpretation that unconsciousness of patients, who apparently have an intact cortex but who have extensive white matter damage, results from cortical disconnection is plausible. However, it appears to depend on the circular argument that, as an intact cortex is considered to be essential for consciousness, its loss must signify interference with that structure. To the extent that structures additional to the cortex are increasingly regarded as involved in consciousness, the interpretation remains susceptible to disproof.

CHAPTER 3

AUTHORITATIVE STATEMENTS

3.1 AUTHORITATIVE STATEMENTS AND GUIDELINES

Three prominent features in the history of PVS have been a number of highly publicised cases of emergence, some equally high profile legal proceedings involving the withdrawal of hydration and nutrition from PVS patients and the succession of statements and position papers on the subject from authoritative bodies. Instances of emergence will be considered in Chapter 9 and of court cases concerned with PVS in Chapter 15. The present Chapter will examine a number of the statements and guidelines that have been issued on the subject of PVS. In introducing this topic, it is appropriate to observe that instances of emergence of individuals from PVS and court proceedings relating to PVS patients have commonly served as the catalyst for the preparation of these statements.

It is highly unlikely that any other medical condition as uncommon as PVS has generated as many authoritative or expert pronouncements. Perhaps the uncertainty inherent in the pathophysiology, the diagnosis and, as a consequence of these two features, in the prognosis of the condition PVS has led to the formulation of sets of rules that provide reassurance in their certainty with language often verging on that usually associated with infallible doctrine. PVS has tended to be adopted as an example with which to illustrate and argue the case for making decisions about withdrawing support from *other* groups of patients whose quality of existence is judged to be sufficiently poor not to justify its continuation. Court proceedings in many cases concerned with the withdrawal of food and water, most notably that of Tony Bland to be discussed in Chapter 15, reveal that their explicit intention was to end life (*Airedale NHS Trust v Bland* 1993).

Whilst the aspect of most statements and guidelines on PVS that has had the most widespread impact has been that dealing with the issue of withdrawal of hydration and nutrition, unequivocal pronouncements on topics such as the neuropathological features of the condition, the neurological capacities (or, more accurately, the lack thereof) of PVS patients and the diagnosis and prognosis of the condition, have often acquired the status of primary sources, especially in the courts. PVS statements and guidelines have certainly had the effect of firmly entrenching acceptance of the widespread perception of PVS as a single, clear cut condition with a set of well defined features and prognosis which can be reliably diagnosed and for which a generally accepted management approach is applicable.

Some claims about PVS, originally based on rather limited data, have with repeated citation but no additional data been accorded a deference usually reserved for fundamental truths. Accompanying this, with repeated citation, claims have varied increasingly from their original form. The composition of expert groups or working parties responsible for producing statements, and their differing experience has also had a discernible influence on the outcome when a report or statement is released. Comparison of the attitudes towards PVS of neurologists and neurosurgeons, accustomed to dealing with the acutely ill, with those of rehabilitation specialists responsible for management of similar patients one or two years later illustrates this difference. The age of patients may also substantially influence attitudes. As indicated by the report of the U.S. Child Neurology Society to be considered below, the outlook of medical practitioners caring for adult and paediatric patients in PVS appears to differ substantially. A number of reports, mostly prepared by U.S. groups, will be considered and compared with each other in this Chapter as a means of illustrating the manner in which they have shaped general perceptions about PVS.

3.2 THE AMERICAN ACADEMY OF NEUROLOGY (A.A.N.) GUIDELINES

The A.A.N. issued guidelines on the vegetative state in 1989. This paper was prepared, in the first instance, by the Academy's Ethics and Humanities Subcommittee chaired by Ronald Cranford. The points raised by a number of the statements in the paper, and in its accompanying commentary, merit comment.

> - "The capacity to chew and swallow in a normal manner is lost because these functions are voluntary, requiring intact cerebral hemispheres" (American Academy of Neurology 1989: 125).

This statement is at odds with other reports of PVS patients to the effect that a capacity to swallow is retained by some patients in vegetative states. For instance, Higashi *et al.* (1977) reported that 26% of a series of 110 patients in a PVS could be fed orally.

> - "Persistent vegetative state patients do not have the capacity to experience pain or suffering. Pain and suffering are attributes of consciousness requiring cerebral cortical functioning" (American Academy of Neurology 1989: 125).

This statement contains two assumptions. First, that the cortex is the only part of the brain capable of mediating pain and suffering. Second, that no part of the cortex is functioning in a PVS patient. Three independent bases for the conclusion were presented, the first of which was the lack of "behavioural indication of awareness of pain or suffering" (ibid: 125). In response to this, it would seem self-evident that any reaction capable of interpretation as a "behavioural indication" requires retention by the patient of the capacity for some degree of co-ordinated motor reaction. Secondly, it was stated that all PVS patients studied (up until 1988) had "overwhelming bilateral damage to the cerebral hemispheres to a degree incompatible with consciousness or the capacity to experience pain or suffering" (ibid: 125).

Two qualifications come to mind, the first being that the variable distribution of neuropathological changes in PVS patients (sometimes almost entirely sparing the cortex) had already been emphasised in other reports dealing specifically with that subject. The report of Levy *et al.* (1987) published two years before the A.A.N. guidelines, stressed the considerable variation that had been found in the distribution and severity of damage to the hemispheres in PVS patients. A second qualification is required given the absence of any indication of *how* the degree of damage known to be incompatible with capacity for suffering was (or, for that matter, *could* be) ascertained. The third basis for the Academy's conclusion was that positron emission tomography (PET) had indicated a degree of reduction of cerebral glucose metabolism "incompatible with consciousness" in PVS patients. Paradoxically, the report cited to support this point was that of Levy *et al.* which also stressed the variability in hemisphere damage in PVS. The question of *how* the degree of metabolic reduction required to extinguish consciousness was to be determined was not addressed.

- "Only a neurological organization can make a definite statement on the neurological facts as the Academy does ... only a neurological society can categorically state, with sufficient expertise and credibility, that persistent vegetative state patients cannot experience (consciously perceive) pain and suffering" (American Academy of Neurology 1989: 124).

This statement, in the commentary accompanying the guidelines, if read by anyone other than the A.A.N. Ethics and Humanities Subcommittee, could be seen as saying more about the Subcommittee than about PVS.

Finally, it could be noted that this 1989 paper considered that PVS could reliably be considered "permanent" after it had lasted for 1 – 3 months, a perception which itself came to be quite *im*permanent during the following decade in the aftermath of a series of reports of late arousal. The self confidence of the executive of the Academy was not shared by all of its members. A batch of correspondence generated by the paper was published in *Neurology* a year later, alongside responses to them from Ronald Cranford. One correspondent commented that it was inappropriate for the personal ethical beliefs of one group in the Academy to be portrayed as the position of all Academy members (Burke 1990). He made the additional points that the absence of self-awareness in a patient could not be determined with certainty, that the stated lack of capacity to experience pain was only an opinion, that nasogastric tube placement was as frequently done by nursing as by medical staff and that the pattern of regulation of breathing in PVS patients suggested that some higher control of this function remained intact. The response was that:

"Every medical organization, every learned medical-ethical organization and every major court decision disagrees with most of his views and I see no great value in addressing each point at this time" (Cranford 1990: 385).

A second correspondent fared equally badly at the pen of Ronald Cranford. This correspondent's assertion that "our goal should be to preserve life, even of vegetative patients or fetuses" (Crisci 1990: 384) attracted the rejoinder that "the Academy statement rejects this absolutist vitalist view" (Cranford 1990: 385).

3.3 THE AMERICAN MEDICAL ASSOCIATION (A.M.A.) REPORT

The A.M.A. represented by its Councils on Scientific Affairs and on Ethical and Judicial Affairs, issued a report on vegetative states in 1990 (American Medical Association Councils 1990). Its susceptibility to slippage in terminology was apparent with descriptions of the *persistent* vegetative state and of *permanent* unconsciousness in the absence of any clear demarcation between them. Language in the report could reasonably be criticised as overly emotive. For example, reference is made to

> "the family's suffering and the heavy social and economic costs of maintaining a residual collection of systemic body organs" (ibid: 426)

(the latter being presumably a form of longhand for "patient"). Any possibility that sensation of pain could be retained by a patient in a PVS was defined away. If a patient was experiencing (undetected) pain then, according to the A.M.A., she or he would, by definition, not be in a PVS, so quarantining the concept of PVS from potentially conflicting observations. A subsequent A.M.A. Council Report extended the arguments. Titled *Medical futility in end-of-life care*, this 1999 report immediately bracketed patients in a PVS together with others who were terminally ill on the basis that any intervention on behalf of either only served to prolong the dying process, a considerable advance on the earlier report in sanctioning withdrawal of care from PVS patients (American Medical Association Council 1999).

An informative commentary specifically directed to the A.A.N. and 1990 A.M.A. PVS statements was provided from inside the system by an American neurology professor, James Bernat, in the *Journal of Clinical Ethics*. He noted and questioned the implication that the boundaries of PVS are "relatively distinct" and that, consequently, diagnosis can be made "with a high level of confidence" and illustrated his point by summarising the divergent reports of the 4 neurologists who had been retained to provide an opinion on whether Nancy Jobes, was in a PVS (Bernat 1992b). Nancy Jobes, a 29 year old woman, had suffered a cardiac arrest during surgery 5 years before her case was brought to a New Jersey court. In the course of litigation to determine whether her gastrostomy tube should be removed, Ms Jobes was examined by 4 neurologists each of whom was said by Bernat (ibid: 176) to be "a widely regarded expert in the evaluation of patients with altered consciousness". A split 2-all decision on whether she was in PVS was resolved by the judge who, after examining the patient, concluded that the two "non-PVS" neurologists had made an incorrect diagnosis.

Bernat nominated four factors constraining the certainty of diagnosis of PVS. The first was the subjective nature of consciousness:

> "The ultimately subjective nature of conscious experience produces an irreducible level of diagnostic uncertainty in the PVS patient that will not be eliminated by future technological advances" (ibid: 178).

Secondly, he emphasised the consequences, for an observer's detection of awareness, of minor stresses or medication affecting the patient. These could

> "sever the patient's last thread of awareness and temporarily lunge him into an unaware vegetative state" (ibid: 178).

Bernat's third qualification concerned the non-specificity of confirmatory laboratory tests for PVS, whilst the fourth noted the manner in which the diagnosis of PVS was being applied to a wide spectrum of conditions.

3.4 THE AMERICAN NEUROLOGICAL ASSOCIATION (A.N.A.) STATEMENT

Apparently in response to the fracas evoked by the A.A.N. guidelines, another authoritative body, the Committee on Ethical Affairs of the A.N.A., weighed in, with what was described by its Chairperson as a "clarifying statement" (American Neurological Association 1993). In an accompanying editorial, he noted that whilst the 1989 position paper of the A.A.N. had been endorsed by most neurologists some had disagreed with it and consequently the A.N.A. Committee had, after 2 years of deliberation, concluded that there was "sufficient confusion and controversy on the medical and ethical aspects of PVS" to warrant clarification. It further noted "the need for the neurosciences to speak with a single voice" (Celesia 1993) and, to this end, supported the establishment of a multi-society task force on PVS. The proposition in the introduction to the A.N.A. statement that:

> "The public must be assured that the PVS can be diagnosed with a high degree of certainty by well-defined clinical criteria"

explicitly identified the need for ensuring general acceptance of the diagnostic competence of neurologists, *not* for examining the basis for the concept of PVS or its diagnosis. Subsequent reports, such as that of Andrews *et al.* (1996), of the occurrence of a high frequency of misdiagnosis of PVS by neurologists might now lead one to question the soundness of the assurance in the A.N.A. Statement.

The A.N.A. statement suggested that the occurrence of visual tracking is not inconsistent with a diagnosis of vegetative state. While conceding, in a more open-minded approach than the A.A.N., that the question of the capacity of patients in a vegetative state to feel pain and undergo suffering "may not be resolved scientifically to everyone's complete satisfaction" (American Neurological Association 1993: 387), the statement follows with the contention that "later postmortem examinations support the belief that they lack awareness of self and surroundings" (ibid: 387). This reassuring statement was not referenced nor was it indicated precisely *how* such examination could provide evidence for loss of self-awareness. It raised an unacknowledged and unanswered question of *exactly how* one determines precisely *what* proportion of *which* parts of the brain must be preserved if some awareness of self or surroundings is to remain possible. In concluding, the statement placed the magnitude of the PVS problem in the United States at 10,000 to 50,000 affected individuals without referencing. It did acknowledge that this estimate "may or may not be accurate", perhaps its most reliable conclusion.

3.5 THE MULTI-SOCIETY TASK FORCE (M.S.T.F.) ON PVS CONSENSUS STATEMENT

As a response to the A.N.A. plea, the neurosciences at last spoke "with a single voice" in 1994. While "authoritative statements" on PVS have appeared in profusion during the last decade, the two part article on *Medical aspects of the persistent vegetative state* published in the *New England Journal of Medicine* in 1994 under the authorship of the M.S.T.F. has undoubtedly been the most frequently cited (M.S.T.F. 1994 a & b). Under co-chairmen Stephen Ashwal and Ronald Cranford, the M.S.T.F. represented five U.S. medical groups. These were the A.A.N., the A.N.A., the Child Neurology Society, the American Association of Neurological Surgeons and the American Academy of Paediatrics. Since its publication, the statement has been cited on 80 occasions in medical journals and many more times in legal and philosophical publications. Given the deference accorded it, I believe that the M.S.T.F. consensus statement requires thorough scrutiny of the content of its claims and the referenced sources on which claims were based. As a means of assessing the quality of the M.S.T.F. statement, I intend to examine its handling of three topics in the light of information published by 1994 and to examine the background to another, namely evidence for unawareness of PVS patients, in later Chapters.

When considering objective evidence for unawareness, the statement concludes, that the low levels of metabolism reported in PVS patients were

> "comparable to those reported during deep general anaesthesia in normal subjects whom all would agree are unaware and insensate" (M.S.T.F. 1994a: 1502).

Of two questions raised by this claim, the first concerning the soundness of a conclusion based upon comparison of a single 1947 report on anaesthetised normal subjects (Himwich *et al.* 1947) with one 1987 report on 7 vegetative patients (Levy *et al.* 1987) using vastly different measurement techniques will be addressed in Chapter 6. The second question raised by the claim of equivalence of unawareness in PVS and under barbiturate general anaesthesia assumes that awareness is not possible under anaesthesia. The information available on this point will be considered in Chapter 7.

The three topics on which the accuracy of the M.S.T.F. statement is to be assessed here are the prevalence of PVS, the reliability of prognostication about it and the incapacity of patients to suffer thirst. "Prevalence" refers to the frequency of occurrence in the population at any time of patients with a particular condition in contrast to "incidence" which denotes the frequency with which new cases of that condition appear in the course of a year. To attempt some conversion between these two measurements, it is necessary to have an estimate of the average duration for which any patient newly entering a PVS remains in this condition. The M.S.T.F. estimated this period as averaging between 2 and 5 years. The significance of prevalence of PVS in any community is that it provides an indication about the financial cost of the ongoing provision of care to people in a PVS, a subject to be examined in Chapter 14. The higher the prevalence estimate becomes, the greater will be the projected financial burden imposed by decisions to continue to care and the more compelling the economic arguments to develop and implement general policies to withhold care. However, at this point the issue which I wish to address is not that of the *actual* prevalence of PVS in the United States but that of the *soundness* of the M.S.T.F. approach to estimating this figure. As one of the few quantifiable aspects of PVS, prevalence lends itself to this assessment.

Having acknowledged that the prevalence of the PVS was not known, the statement estimated that "in the United States there are 10,000 to 25,000 adults and 4,000 to 10,000 children in a persistent vegetative state" (M.S.T.F. 1994a: 1503). A notable feature of estimates of PVS prevalence, mentioned above, is that, once formulated and published, they are likely to become the basis for propositions about the financial cost to the community of providing medical resources to the affected patients. The M.S.T.F. estimates of the number of patients in a PVS in the United States have been cited frequently since 1994 in this context. The Task Force did not itself collect new data but relied on collation and interpretation of data that had previously been published by others. Of the 108 literature references provided in the first of the two parts of the statement, no fewer than 20 were cited as the basis for the U.S. prevalence estimates. Inspection of these references provides an insight into the processes underlying preparation of the statement. Apart from one French monograph, all of the cited sources relating to PVS prevalence have been examined in preparing the following assessment. Six of the remaining 19 papers contained no data directly or indirectly relevant to estimation of PVS prevalence in any geographical location (Higashi *et al.* 1981; Levy *et al.* 1978; Gillies and Seshia 1980; Bricolo *et al.* 1980; Levy *et al.* 1981; Braakman *et al.* 1988). These papers contained descriptions of series of patients from a number of institutions but did not provide any indication of the populations from which these series had been drawn or of their representative nature.

Six of the remaining 13 citations of PVS prevalence contained original data related to prevalence. The extent to which they support the inferences drawn from them by the M.S.T.F. will be indicated. A 1977 paper of Higashi *et al.* was based on examination of 110 patients hospitalised in 16 prefectures of western Japan. Inclusion in this series was on the basis of criteria which were acknowledged by the authors to be "arbitrary". Rather than claiming to detect lack of awareness, Higashi *et al.* scored on "defect of verbal and behavioural communication", "loss of expression of attention" and "absence, or at least reduction, of emotional expression" (1977). In describing their patients, Higashi *et al.* recorded that 42.7% initially had "eye-following movements". Whether the clinical features of all patients would have fitted the original description of PVS by Jennett and Plum (1972) and met their specified diagnostic requirements remains questionable. To the extent that they did not do so, prevalence estimates of Higashi *et al.* will be excessive. Of the total series, 37 of the patients of Higashi *et al.*, were located in a thorough survey in Yamaguchi prefecture, implying a prevalence of 25 patients per million population. This would imply a U.S. total of around 6,600 PVS patients assuming that incidence, diagnostic requirements and survival were comparable in the two locations.

A paper of Sato *et al.* (1979) also from Japan, reported a prevalence of 22 PVS patients per million population in the Tohoku District (equivalent to a U.S. total of approximately 5,800). An article on the vegetative existence by Minderhoud and Braakman (1985) reported on a survey of Dutch hospitals and nursing homes undertaken in 1983. An 80% response to this survey identified 53 patients diagnosed as in a PVS which, if adjusted to a national total, gave an overall prevalence for the Netherlands of approximately 4 patients per million, from all causes of PVS (U.S. equivalent 1,060). A 1988 French paper reported a prevalence of 10 PVS cases per million population (US equivalent 2,650) (Brule *et al.* 1988).

Two articles published in 1992 complete the body of primary data on which the M.S.T.F. estimates of U.S. totals ranging from 14,000 to 35,000 was based. The first of these articles (Sazbon *et al.* 1992) contained data from Israel on the frequency with which patients entered PVS exclusively as a consequence of trauma, whilst the second reported on a survey of paediatric cases in the United States. Sazbon *et al.* reported their experience in a Tel-Aviv unit which received all patients from Israel who remained unconscious for a month after trauma. The incidence of cases meeting this admission requirement was 4 per million population. As data on the interval until emergence from a vegetative state, or length of survival of these patients in a PVS was not provided, it is not feasible to calculate prevalence of post-traumatic PVS in Israel. Nevertheless, even making allowance for lack of information about survival and for the restriction of the scope of the report to patients in PVS following trauma, the Israeli data would, if extrapolated, be likely to suggest a figure for U.S. prevalence well below the minimum estimate of the M.S.T.F.

Data on the prevalence of PVS in American children was provided in an article by co-chairman of the M.S.T.F., Stephen Ashwal and his colleagues (Ashwal *et al.* 1992). As it was the only reference cited by the M.S.T.F. which presented information on paediatric PVS patients, the Task Force estimate of 4,000-10,000 was, presumably, based exclusively on it. The data in this report was generated by a survey of members of the U.S. Child Neurology Society. Responses from approximately one third of its members indicated a figure of 1663 children in a PVS. Scaling up from these figures would imply a total U.S. paediatric PVS population, around the lower end of the M.S.T.F. range. However, the survey did not identify patients and, consequently, no allowance for double scoring was possible. To the extent that paediatric PVS patients, especially in the early stages of the condition, are likely to have been examined by more than one neurologist in the course of validating the diagnosis, the extrapolated population estimate could well be excessive.

Seven papers referenced as dealing with PVS prevalence in the M.S.T.F. report remain to be examined after excluding the irrelevant 6 and considering the 6 which provided original data. Of this remaining group, 4 did no more than cite secondary data of variable quality from elsewhere. A report from two A.M.A. Councils (American Medical Association Councils 1990) estimated U.S. prevalence from the data of Higashi *et al.* (1977) in Yamaguchi prefecture. In contrast with the inference drawn from the Higashi *et al.* paper in the text above, the A.M.A. report estimated a considerably greater U.S. prevalence of 15,000-25,000. Whilst it was at the upper end of available estimates, the published A.M.A. estimate of PVS prevalence remained substantially below the earlier estimate of more than 100,000 provided by the same organisation in its *Amicus Curiae* brief in the Cruzan case (American Medical Association *Amicus Curiae* 1990). The A.M.A. estimate acquired honorary status as data when cited in three more of the references which were, in their turn, cited again by the M.S.T.F.. Bryan Jennett (1991) cited the A.M.A. estimates, together with the data of Higashi *et al.* (1977) and Minderhoud and Braakman (1985).

Ashwal *et al.* (1994) cited the A.M.A. estimate (American Medical Association Council 1990) together with the data generated by the Child Neurology Society survey (Ashwal *et al.* 1992). The Institute of Medical Ethics Working Party on the Ethics of Prolonging Life and Assisting Death estimate of PVS prevalence in the U.K. (Institute of Medical Ethics 1991), which had been based on a mix of Higashi *et al.* (1977), Minderhoud and Braakman (1985) and the A.M.A. (American Medical Association Council 1990) was itself referenced as a source of information by the M.S.T.F. The moral would appear to be that any story can be enhanced with sufficient retelling.

In contrast with the preceding four sources referenced by the M.S.T.F., the remaining three cited papers relied on even more indirect inspiration. Tresch *et al.* (1991b), writing in the *Archives of Internal Medicine*, cited an estimate of 5,000 to 10,000 persons in a PVS in the U.S., drawing on an article by Cranford (1988) rather provocatively subtitled "Getting the facts straight". Cranford in his turn had reported the most commonly cited estimate as 5,000 to 10,000, based on epidemiological studies from Japan which had shown

> "approximately 2,000 to 3,000 patients in this condition in that country, and an extrapolation of that data to the United States, taking into account both a doubling in population and our more advanced (and more indiscriminately applied) life-support systems" (ibid: 31).

The second paper of this final cluster of M.S.T.F. references stated, without supporting data, that a Royal Dutch Medical Association special committee had calculated that implementation of a policy of terminating the life of patients in *coma* 3 to 6 months after brain injury from an accident, and one month after its onset from non-traumatic brain disease, would require the provision of this service to approximately 100 patients per year in the Netherlands (Hellema 1991), implying prevalence similar to that observed by Minderhoud and Braakman, as summarised above. In an unequivocal proof of the existence of a sense of humour, albeit mildly warped, on the part of the *British Medical Journal's* editorial staff, this report was juxtapositioned with a cartoon captioned: "Sleeping beauty might not last long these days" (ibid).

Finally, to complete this set of distinctly soft data sources, the M.S.T.F. cited a paper of Spudis, *The persistent vegetative state – 1990* as a source of information on PVS prevalence. To quote the relevant section of Spudis' article:

> "If 1.4 million of the nursing home beds in the U.S.A. are categorized as skilled care or intermediate care and one percent of these have PVS, the total would equal approximately 14,000" (1991: 130).

Whilst the arithmetic in the statement is impeccable, the same can hardly be said of its two conditionals.

I submit that the M.S.T.F. conclusions on PVS prevalence were not in accord with any reliable data on the subject. Insofar as these conclusions are relevant to assessment of the *quality* of the M.S.T.F. statement as a whole, they reflect unfavourably on the calibre of the processes entailed in the preparation of the document in its entirety.

Passing from the question of adequacy of the M.S.T.F. prevalence data to that of its estimate of prognostic error in relation to PVS, the quality of this estimate, has been queried by later authors. Childs and Mercer (1996a), in their report of the occurrence of late improvement in consciousness of PVS patients noted the A.M.A. definition of an acceptable risk of prognostic error as being 0.1% and the empirical estimate of this risk by the M.S.T.F. as being 1.6% (M.S.T.F. 1994b). They contrasted this estimate with the actual data collected in the series of patients documented by the Traumatic Coma Data Bank (Levin *et al.* 1991) which indicated a prognostic error of at least 14%. That is, 14% of the patients who had been assessed as being in a "permanent post-traumatic" vegetative state subsequently regained consciousness. The data from the Bank had been published in 1991 and so it was readily available during preparation of the M.S.T.F. report.

As regards the third topic on which this assessment of the M.S.T.F. statement is based, namely the likelihood of occurrence of thirst following withdrawal of hydration and nutrition, examination of the referenced background to that section of the M.S.T.F. statement reveals this to be particularly sparse. The M.S.T.F. statement reads "patients in a persistent vegetative state cannot experience thirst or hunger" and supports this conclusion with a single reference. This paucity of referencing sits oddly alongside the frequency with which the statement has been cited specifically as an authoritative source on this subject, and its endorsement in the *British Medical Journal* as "a comprehensive and valuable review" (Howard and Miller 1995). The solitary M.S.T.F. reference to possible thirst was to a paper by Ahronheim and Gasner (1990) entitled *The sloganism of starvation* which emanated jointly from the New York University School of Medicine and the Department of Legal Services of the Society for the Right to Die. Examination of the Ahronheim and Gasner article indicates that their statement that deprivation of fluid is not painful was based on citation of four earlier reports two of them describing patients who were terminally ill in the sense in which that description is generally applied. Notwithstanding the origin of these citations being that of *dying* patients, their article relates to PVS patients. The validity of this comparison will be discussed in Chapter 12 when physiological aspects of thirst will be considered.

I submit that critical examination of specific claims in the M.S.T.F. statement does not reveal great precision and accuracy in the document. Apart from this, the general approach of the statement has been questioned by a number of authors. For example, in undertaking a "critical analysis" of the M.S.T.F. statement, Howsepian (1996) criticised both its logic and its language. As a general criticism, he contended that:

> "Many of the alleged 'medical facts' that the M.S.T.F. claims to be summarizing really are pieces of quite complex, contentious and conceptually subtle philosophy" (ibid: 5).

Howsepian noted a tendency for the M.S.T.F. wording to shift ground and to substitute terminology in the course of the argument. For example, there is a transition from "without detectable awareness" to "unconscious" whilst "artificial hydration and nutrition" becomes "hydration and nutrition". Howsepian queried the logic of the statement's description of PVS as entailing "complete unawareness of the self and the environment". He commented that, whilst the M.S.T.F. conclusion that the presence of stereotyped behavioural patterns in response to stimulation of patients diagnosed as in a PVS "is consistent with complete unawareness", in the absence of specific evidence to exclude the possibility, it is equally "consistent with complete awareness". He pointed out that, as the report effectively excludes the possibility of any consciousness, by the wording of its definition of PVS, then

> "any condition diagnosed as PVS in which any degree of consciousness is present is a case of misdiagnosis" (ibid: 10).

Howsepian also charged that the statement selectively quoted from the A.N.A. 1989 position paper on PVS

> "in a manner that includes only conclusions which could be interpreted as fostering the view that not treating PVS patients is morally permissible" (ibid: 26).

3.6 OTHER U.S. REPORTS

Other groups to have promulgated statements on PVS, include the American Thoracic Society (1991), the Child Neurology Society (Ashwal *et al.* 1992) and an Aspen Neurobehavioural Conference of head trauma rehabilitation specialists (Giacino *et al.* 1997). The American Thoracic Society Position Paper acknowledged the right of a competent patient to decline treatment, and of a designated surrogate to do so on behalf of an incompetent patient, but specified that life-sustaining medical intervention can be limited without any consent if, in the opinion of the physician, "meaningful survival" is unlikely to be achieved. Detailed guidelines for the physician in assessing "meaningfulness" from the patient's perspective were not supplied. The permanent loss of cognitive and sentient capacity when the residual life "may be generally regarded as having no value for such an unconscious person" was given as an example of lack of meaningful survival. It was recommended that *lack of meaningful survival* is to be defined without reference to the patient's personal values unless the patient, when capable of doing so, had explicitly specified in an advance directive that such an existence would have value for him or her. This default position represents a substantial change from earlier presumptions, which had been pivotal in U.S. court cases, that the patient *would* have wished for survival unless he or she had specifically indicated to the contrary.

The 1992 report from the Child Neurology Society, prepared following a survey of Society members, revealed some striking contrasts in patient management when read alongside the A.N.A. paper which was concerned primarily with adult patients. Thus, 75% of the responding paediatric neurologists "never" withheld fluid and nutrition from children in PVS (Ashwal *et al.* 1992). Additionally, 75% recommended medications to relieve pain and suffering in these patients. These differences in practice could apparently not be attributed to doubts on the part of the respondents about the accuracy of diagnosis of PVS in children as a large majority of them considered that reliable diagnosis was possible.

The Aspen Neurobehavioural Conference report was prepared by a mix of neurologists and rehabilitation specialists, a difference in authorship composition from other reports, such as that of the M.S.T.F. which is reflected in its output (Giacino *et al.* 1997). The Aspen group was less dogmatic than the M.S.T.F. in pronouncing upon the retention of any undetectable neurological attributes by patients diagnosed as in vegetative states. It acknowledged that there was no definitive way in which to formulate a clinical assessment of internal awareness in a patient unable to express manifestations of awareness in response to external environmental stimuli. In considering prognosis and management it observed that:

> "Many patients do not 'persist' in the state and go on to make further neurologic improvement, some to the point of good functional outcomes by such measures as the Glasgow Outcome Scale" (ibid: 81).

A "significant number" of participants in the Aspen group were reluctant to accept the M.S.T.F. projections of permanence and life expectation in vegetative states. This reluctance was said to be engendered by the very limited data on follow up of vegetative state patients in the scientific literature and by the derivation of these projections from "expert opinion" rather than on any more solid basis. The Aspen Group also expressed concern that misuse of the term "PVS" could encourage

> "the inappropriate withdrawal and withholding of care, failure to refer for rehabilitation services, discontinuation of rehabilitation efforts and tendencies toward less aggressive management of comorbid factors" (other concurrent disease states) (ibid: 81).

3.7 U.K. STATEMENTS

The two major U.K. authorities to have issued statements on PVS are the British Medical Association (B.M.A.) and the Royal College of Physicians (R.C.P.). Even before the B.M.A. release of guidelines on treatment decisions for PVS patients in 1994, the preceding B.M.A. discussion paper (1992) had acquired an authority in the case of *Airedale NHS Trust v Bland* more commensurate with that usually accorded definitive guidelines. The guidelines were reissued in a revised form in 1999. Whilst these guidelines recognised that withdrawal of hydration and nutrition differed from withdrawal of other forms of treatment, all procedures with "the potential to postpone the patient's death" irrespective of their intensity, were lumped together as examples of "life prolonging treatment". The description "basic care" was applied to various procedures offering symptom relief and to oral hydration and nutrition. The guidelines acknowledged that withdrawal of hydration and nutrition differed from not providing other forms of treatment and recommended that "additional safeguards be built into decisions". They also advised that oral nutrition using a cup, spoon or syringe constituted basic care and should not be withdrawn. An interesting aspect of the 2001 revision of a B.M.A. guidance for decision-making in relation to withholding and withdrawing treatment (not exclusively in relation to PVS patients) is its explanation that:

> "Whilst the term 'artificial nutrition and hydration' is used in this guidance, it is recognized that neither the nutrition nor the hydration is, in fact artificial although the method for delivering it is" (ibid: 8).

The R.C.P. recommendations, issued in 1996, suggested the substitution for the term "persistent" vegetative state of two others, namely "continuing vegetative state" (when the condition has remained unchanged for more than four weeks) and "permanent vegetative state" (when diagnosis of irreversibility can be established with a high degree of clinical certainty). In an interesting malapropism, the R.C.P. referred to a patient as *entering* a permanent vegetative state after a specified period. A more accurate statement would be, not that a patient *enters* a PVS after a certain interval, but that he or she is reassessed after that time as *being in* PVS. One recommendation in the R.C.P. paper, destined for variable observance in practice, was the requirement that the patient in PVS should not be able to track moving objects with the eyes. Tracking was regarded by the R.C.P. in 1996 as incompatible with the diagnosis of PVS. A revised document, issued by the R.C.P. in 2003 emphasised that the single, cardinal feature required for a diagnosis of vegetative state is the loss of awareness. Eye tracking was categorised as "compatible but atypical".

In the same year as the R.C.P. recommendations were first issued, the outcome of an internationally constituted working group on PVS was published (Andrews 1996; International Working Party 1996). This group met under the aegis of the Royal Hospital for Neuro-disability at Putney, the major U.K. centre for care of patients in PVS and related states. Its summary commenced with the observation of several neurorehabilitation specialists that there were no formal guidelines for the treatment of patients in the vegetative state (contrasting with the abundance of sources of advice on *non-treatment*). The international working party noted that eye tracking by a patient might only be observed in response to a family member but also cautioned that the presence of tracking, in isolation, was not necessarily proof of emergence from a vegetative state.

Since the release of the R.C.P. recommendations relating to diagnosis, the implications of some specific cases of individual patients have suggested a need for running repairs. On one hand courts have sanctioned withdrawal of hydration and nutrition from patients whom expert testimony had indicated did *not* conform to the R.C.P. recommendations (Dyer 1997a; Dyer 1997b). On the other hand, instances of unexpected late emergence of patients diagnosed as PVS, according to accepted guidelines and recommendations, most spectacularly that of a man who had been vegetative for 7 years, have led to acknowledgment by both the B.M.A. (Macdonald 1996a) and the R.C.P. (Dyer 1997a) that their guidelines may require reconsideration, presumably to tighten them.

3.8 RECAPITULATION

Why has such a profusion of statements and guidelines relating to PVS been issued by distinguished medical groups? I interpret the succession of these articles over a period of 12 years, referred to in this Chapter, as a reflection of ongoing uncertainty about PVS and a continuing need to provide reassurance to the medical profession and the community at large. Some of the earlier statements expressed a degree of certainty concerning their accuracy which has not been so evident in later versions. There has often been a tendency for the degree of certainty expressed by expert groups to vary in inverse proportion to the solidity of the available data on the subject. Notwithstanding their derivative nature, some of the major statements have, in the course of time, been accorded the status of primary sources of information.

The primary purpose of this Chapter has been to test the basis for some of the most authoritative and influential statements on PVS. The statement of the U.S. M.S.T.F. on PVS, undoubtedly the most cited publication on the subject, has been examined in some detail as a means of assessing the quality of the research undertaken in the course of its preparation. This examination was undertaken by selecting pronouncements from the statement and assessing their accuracy *in the light of what was known in the medical literature* at the date of release of the statement.

The history of U.K. authoritative statements on PVS has been briefly touched on in this Chapter. The evolution of these statements has been notable for the influence of two series of events, namely instances in which patients diagnosed as PVS regained consciousness and a series of court hearings to approve the withdrawal of hydration and nutrition from other patients.

In my assessment, statements and guidelines have more frequently been developed in order to close down discussion on the issue of the nature of PVS rather than to encourage wider presentation of competing interpretations. There has been a tendency to gloss over specific aspects on which the quality of information is poor and often to move imperceptibly from evidence-based to value-based pronouncements. Whilst the composition of the drafting groups is not directly relevant to assessing their quality and has not been examined in this Chapter, the interested reader who turns to the original sources may detect a moderately incestuous approach both in the composition of different groups and in their citations.

Given the decidedly limited body of information about the abnormalities of fine structure in the nervous system of patients in a PVS, when compared with that available for many other medical conditions, and of the specific manner in which these structural changes are manifest in clinically ascertainable features, it might well be queried whether PVS lends itself to many of the dogmatic statements it has generated.

CHAPTER 4

CONSCIOUSNESS

> "A detailed analysis of the nature of consciousness is not needed, however, when considering the class of patients in whom all possible components of mental life are absent – all thought, feeling, sensation, desire, emotion, and awareness of self or environment" (President's Commission 1983: 171-192).

Notwithstanding the view of the U.S. President's Commission, cited above in relation to "permanently unconscious" patients, the concept of consciousness remains central to any attempt to understand the vegetative state. Yet, despite the extensive literature on *un*consciousness in relation to the vegetative state, discussion of this clinical condition appears to have been notable for the paucity of discussion of the nature of the attribute which affected patients are considered to lack. As a general principle, one might anticipate that any understanding of *un*consciousness would proceed from an understanding of consciousness. As consciousness is anything but a well defined state about the presence and absence of which there is universal agreement, the common omission of discussion of precisely *what* is lacking is puzzling.

> "Three common maxims about consciousness are:
> (1) those who study consciousness agree about only one thing, namely there is no agreement about its definition;
> (2) consciousness has as many theories as theorists; and
> (3) consciousness is what brain scientists become interested in towards the end of their careers" (Cowey 1997: 54).

These observations by Alan Cowey, Professor of Physiological Psychology at the University of Oxford were said to typify general impressions of consciousness up to 1996. Another conventional perception of consciousness from within the neuroscience community was attributed to the neuroscientist Benjamin Libet:

> "It is okay to be interested in consciousness, but get tenure first" (cited by Searle 1998: 193).

However, as Cowey proceeded to point out, the three maxims were rapidly becoming less accurate representations of the subject as knowledge accumulated.

4.1 RELEVANCE OF STUDIES OF CONSCIOUSNESS TO ITS DEFINITIONAL ABSENCE IN PVS

The intention of this Chapter is not to add anything to the mass of speculation already existing on the subject of consciousness. What will be attempted in the first part is to indicate the relevance of the existing, limited comprehension of consciousness to characterising and diagnosing PVS on the basis of *un*consciousness and the implications that more recent information on consciousness may have for understanding PVS and related conditions. It is surprising that little attempt appears to have been made to incorporate observations made on vegetative patients into the understanding of consciousness.

The second part of the Chapter will leave aside the question of what is known, or more accurately what is *not* known, about consciousness in relation to PVS. It will start with the generally acknowledged propositions that the greater part of cerebral cortical activity is not attributable to, or associated with, consciousness and that much cognitive activity occurs whilst the individual is unaware of it. Unconscious receipt and processing of information bulks large in cerebral activity but is implicitly ignored when consciousness is specified as a prerequisite for such activity. Having considered this topic, the Chapter will conclude by examining the nexus which is often postulated between consciousness and personhood.

The specific topics to be considered in the first part of the Chapter are:
- the terminology and its contribution to confusion about consciousness.
- the significance of *vigilance* in making observations on patients. Reduced levels of receptivity associated with impairment of vigilance can effectively interfere with detection of retained cognition.
- the feasibility of identifying *neuroanatomical and neurophysiological correlates* of consciousness and using these to interpret the pathophysiological processes in vegetative states. The extent of understanding of the relationship of specific structural components of the *normal* brain to consciousness remains limited. Nevertheless, the frequency with which the extent of damage to the brain of specified patients has been inferred to preclude any possibility of consciousness requires that this issue be considered.
- the significance of inability to establish *communication* between observer and patient as a factor in diagnosing and subsequently managing vegetative states. In the absence of some form of communication, detection of any level of retained consciousness becomes impossible.

The remainder of the Chapter will deal with:
- the possible applicability of observations about *unconscious receipt and processing* of information by experimental subjects, whose nervous systems are intact or who have well defined neurological lesions, to individuals with brain injuries of the severity associated with PVS. With occasional exceptions, the PVS literature omits any consideration of the likelihood of unconscious mental activity, a subject which is becoming of increased interest in *normal* brain function following a

long period of neglect. The presumption that anything other than *conscious* activity is of no value underpins virtually all discussion of the interests of PVS patients.
- the basis for the trend to *equate consciousness with personhood*. The condition of "personhood" has been invested with a status, even in some medical literature, that is difficult to reconcile with its imprecision.

Compounding the inherent complexity of the subject, speculation about, and investigation of, consciousness has been approached from within a number of quite disparate disciplinary fields, with little interaction apparent between them. This separation seems to have contributed substantially to the unfavourable reputation the subject of consciousness has acquired, among neuroscientists. Consciousness has been considered by philosophers, neuroscientists, experimental psychologists and, more recently, by those concerned with artificial intelligence, not to mention clinicians. Reading of the clinical literature relating to vegetative states leaves the distinct impression that many clinicians have not taken much account of the views of practitioners in the other four disciplines when considering questions about consciousness and unconsciousness that may be relevant to their patients.

Clinical quarantining from the ideas of others about consciousness finds its most overt expression in definitions that automatically link unconsciousness and vegetative states. As noted in Chapter 1, the original definition of a vegetative state referred to there being "no evidence" of a functioning mind but, in practice, this has come to be understood as "the absence" of a functioning mind. As a corollary of this second interpretation of terms, it is commonly accepted that any patient meeting the clinical criteria for diagnosis as "vegetative" *must* therefore be "unconscious". From first principles, I suggest that one could envisage three combinations of a diagnosis of vegetative state and unconsciousness. One group of patients may be diagnosed clinically as being in a vegetative state but be subsequently found to have remained conscious. Such patients will be specifically considered in Chapter 8 in relation to the subject of "misdiagnosis". Classification as "misdiagnosis" indicates that there was an error in that case but does not raise questions about the validity of the *concept* of a vegetative state (only about the capacity of the clinician to diagnose it). A second group of patients could be those diagnosed on clinical grounds as being in a vegetative state while remaining conscious but in whom this capacity *remained* unrecognised. The third group of patients could be diagnosed as in a vegetative state and also be unconscious. Whilst the second and third groups would differ conceptually, they would be clinically indistinguishable with their relative frequency remaining unknown. A proprietorial position towards the recognition of consciousness has been adopted by some groups, as for example, in the assertion, referred to in the preceding Chapter, that only neurologists have the capacity to pronounce on the subject of consciousness. The proposition that non-neurologists could not determine whether a PVS patient can consciously perceive pain and suffering (American Academy of Neurology 1989) might surprise some of those in other disciplines (and other medical specialties) with an active interest in consciousness. It would certainly amuse them.

4.2 TERMINOLOGY

Definition of consciousness appears to have remained very much a matter of personal taste. Sommerhoff and MacDorman (1994), when considering the reasons for scepticism among neuroscientists about consciousness, drew attention to the concluding, dismissive remarks on the subject in the Macmillan Dictionary of Psychology:

> "Consciousness is a fascinating but elusive phenomenon: it is impossible to specify what it is, what it does, and why it evolved. Nothing worth reading has been written on it" (Sutherland 1989).

They also observed that some major reference books on the cognitive sciences failed to include the term "consciousness" in their index. Cowey has suggested that lack of an agreed definition of consciousness has resulted both from differing choice of words by different writers and from the likelihood that the term itself has been used to describe several states "that will eventually prove to be different and sometimes not even closely related" (1997: 54). An example of the use of words without generally accepted meanings was provided in an article which referred to a distinction, drawn by physicians between the "level" and the "content" of consciousness. By "level", was intended "the degree of arousal" whilst "content" meant the ability "to interact meaningfully with his (i.e. the patient's) environment" (Cranford and Smith 1979). It was explained that:

> "Patients in a persistent vegetative state ordinarily will have a normal level of consciousness but the content of consciousness is severely impaired" (ibid: 204).

Alluding to the variable and quite imprecise use of terms specifically in relation to patients in PVS, Spudis cited the popularisation of

> "such non-clinical words as cognition, self-awareness, introspection, human(hood) person(hood), self(hood) and sapience" (1991: 133).

Giacino (1997), writing for a clinical neurological readership, commented that attempts to establish a consensual definition of consciousness had been confounded by lack of a common vocabulary. He contrasted the synonymous use of the terms "consciousness" and "awareness" in the standard neurological reference text on unconsciousness with an approach from the perspective of experimental psychology. The latter took "consciousness" to be the general capacity for subjective experience while "awareness" represented a specific manifestation of that capacity which was directed and acted to define subjective experience.

Formal definitions of consciousness have ranged from the dismissive to those composed of extended lists of the required attributes. McQuillen, in referring to the "will-o'-the-wisp" nature of the concept, recalled the opinion of the nineteenth century English neurologist Hughlings Jackson:

> "There is no such entity as consciousness; we are from moment to moment differently conscious" (1991: 374).

More recently, clinicians writing in the context of PVS have sometimes opted to define *un*consciousness rather than consciousness. The U.S. President's Commission (1983) followed Jennett and Plum in defining unconsciousness as the inability "to experience the environment". Inclusion of self-awareness, in addition to awareness of the environment, by the Multi-Society Task Force on PVS (M.S.T.F.) (1994a) in *its* concept of consciousness raises the question of the extent to which non-human species are to be regarded as conscious, an issue which will be taken up below.

Some quite trenchant criticisms of both Commission and M.S.T.F. definitions of unconsciousness have been delivered by Howsepian who exemplified "lucid dreams" as an instance in which consciousness was present in the absence of experience of the environment and described the arguments that the M.S.T.F. used in establishing that all PVS patients were unconscious as "conceptually misshapen" and its conception of (un)consciousness as "conceptually incoherent" (1996). In particular, he criticised as untenable the M.S.T.F. requirement for self-awareness as a component of consciousness stressing that detachment from self, without the loss of consciousness, may be achieved during deep meditation. As regards patients with end stage dementia, identified by the M.S.T.F. as in a vegetative state (and so definitionally unconscious), Howsepian (1996) raised the case of the severely demented patient, lacking self-awareness, who nevertheless may still have "qualitatively rich experiences". Another telling dismissal of attempts to equate consciousness with self-consciousness has been provided by the philosopher John Searle who emphasised that most conscious states, such as feeling a pain, do not involve self-consciousness. An exception, noted by Searle, could be the individual who becomes conscious of self as an inveterate worrier (1998: 6).

The American Medical Association (A.M.A.) definition of consciousness, published in 1990 divided it into an arousal mechanism and a separate network controlling learning, memory, self-awareness and adaptive behaviour (American Medical Association Councils 1990). Giacino's (1997) description encompassed wakefulness, the capacity to detect and encode stimuli and the capacity to formulate goal-directed behaviour. Taking account of Howsepian's earlier objections to the M.S.T.F. definition, he noted that consciousness could imply awareness *either* of self *or* of the environment. Sommerhoff and MacDorman have drawn attention to the different constructions likely to be placed on the term "consciousness" by those researching in neuroscience compared with "common usage" (which will usually be that of the families of unconscious patients). Whereas researchers are likely to be especially interested in higher functions such as language and social relationships, the concerns of other members of the community are more likely to include

> "modes of awareness that are not denied to creatures lacking language or social relationships" (1994: 151).

This more popular view of consciousness would not necessarily require retention of higher functions by an individual in order that he or she still be regarded as "conscious". Any definitional requirement for *self*-awareness as an attribute of consciousness has potential implications for non-human species perhaps denying it to all apart from chimpanzees. Inclusion of the latter species within this more restrictive view of consciousness follows from the work of Gallup (1970) demonstrating that chimpanzees, but not macaque or Rhesus monkeys, could recognise their mirror images as self.

Irrespective of which definition is adopted, it remains necessary to be clear about the limits to its application. Any worthwhile definition will deal with *what consciousness is*. *How* consciousness is achieved, irrespective of the discipline within which the answer is framed, is a separate question which may be more amenable to answering. Some commentators have made the point that it is preferable that a definition of consciousness *follow from* a better understanding of the processes mediating it rather than being expected to assist in their investigation. A neuroscientist addressed the relationship between brain processes and consciousness as follows:

> "In an awake brain some events give rise to consciousness, but others, probably the vast majority of events going on in the brain, have nothing to do with it. Unconsciousness is not necessarily attended by a loss or depression of all brain activity. Rather, it is caused by a selective loss of some functions" (Flohr 1995: 158).

There appears to be an increasing awareness of the need for approaches from both philosophy and the neurosciences. For example, a neuroscientist writing on consciousness stressed that the question of the extent to which neuroscience has explained consciousness is "ill-posed".

> "All that neuroscience can do is explain the neural correlates of consciousness, leaving the difficult problem of explaining what consciousness is untouched" (Bennett 1997: 164).

A philosopher writing at the same time advocated consideration of consciousness as a normal biological phenomenon and criticised those of his colleagues who sought to eliminate consciousness by reducing it to something else such as a "brain state" that can be described in terms of a computer program (Searle 1998). He also stressed that the objectivity of science is not incompatible with the study of subjective states.

An example of earlier gaps between neuroscientific and philosophical approaches to consciousness, as seen by neuroscientists, was the response of Sommerhoff and MacDorman to the theories of Dennett (1991) in his book *Consciousness explained*. "The strict methodology, coherent framework and conceptual accuracy" of the neurosciences was contrasted with the approaches of those who

> "allow themselves greater latitude in the choice of their concepts, accepting both metaphors and undefined concepts whose meaning and tacit premises are often far from clear" (Sommerhoff and MacDorman 1994: 153).

Dennett's *explanation* (the italics of Sommerhoff and MacDorman) was described as dependent on abstract metaphors.

In a class apart from the differences attributable to varied disciplinary backgrounds are differences between philosophers themselves. Whilst not always adding much to the understanding of consciousness, they can often be relied upon to provide entertainment for others. For example, in an interchange of views, John Searle wrote of the work of Daniel Dennett referred to above in the following terms: "I regard Dennett's denial of the existence of consciousness not as a new discovery or even as a serious possibility but rather as a form of intellectual pathology" (1998: 143). To which Dennett replied: "No one should be surprized to learn that the feeling is mutual" (Searle 1998: 143).

4.3 VIGILANCE: ATTENTION: HABITUATION

The level of vigilance of persons who are in, or near to, a vegetative state could be impaired, independently of interference with cognition and the circumstances in which such patients are nursed may contribute to this impairment. The possibility of impairment of vigilance says nothing directly about whether an individual retains cognitive capacity. What it *does* say is that the *detection* of any retained cognitive capacity may well become more difficult than has generally been conceded when vigilance mechanisms have been damaged.

The *detection* of consciousness, or of a retained capacity for cognition, in an individual incapable of communicating in a conventional manner depends upon the ability of an observer to detect other forms of response. A prerequisite for the occurrence of some detectable response is an intact afferent (inward directed) mechanism with the capacity to receive a stimulus from a sense organ and transmit this centrally within the nervous system. The central mechanism, if it is functioning, may interpret the transmitted stimulus and formulate a response. If the efferent (outward directed) limb, is to produce a response that can be detected by an observer, it will need to possess not just peripheral motor capacity but also, as stressed by Howsepian (1996) in his critique of the M.S.T.F., the ability to *harness* that motor capacity. Failure in any one of this sequence of components will result in the absence of any "read out" for an observer to detect in response to a stimulus. The question of whether any stimulus can automatically be assumed to have become accessible to mechanisms mediating cognition will depend upon vigilant status. Failure of a patient to produce any detectable response when examined is often deemed automatically to equate with lack of consciousness at the time of testing if not with the ongoing absence of any capacity for cognition. However, all stimuli presented to *non-brain-injured* individuals do not necessarily enter consciousness and this may apply equally to brain-injured persons. Hearing is not synonymous with listening.

The *Oxford Companion to the Mind* notes under its entry on "attention" that the nervous system is subjected to far more stimulation than can be used and that a person remains consciously aware of only a limited amount of that stimulation. It notes that, although much sensory information may be filtered out and not enter consciousness, emotionally important words and phrases may be perceived even when included in a message that is filtered out (Moray 1987: 59-61).

The terminology that has been used in describing studies of vigilance or attention has been as profuse and variable as that characterising the subject of consciousness itself. The term "vigilance" has been used with quite different meanings by neurosurgeons and psychologists. Among the earliest and most comprehensive studies of vigilance were those undertaken by H.N. Mackworth (1968) with radar operators during World War II. In this situation, vigilance was defined as a readiness to detect and respond to certain specified small changes in the environment, occurring at irregular time intervals. The investigation was based on observation of motor responses to signals occurring at random intervals against a continuing background of non-signal events. Continuous attention by the subject was required for signal detection. This is the sense in which "vigilance" will be used in considering its relevance for evaluating the conscious status of patients for whom a diagnosis of PVS is to be made.

A thoroughly documented observation relating to vigilance in normal conscious subjects which should be considered in any discussion of the diagnosis of vegetative states is the failure of *fully conscious* normal subjects to remain aware of stimuli presented when vigilance is diminished. In Mackworth's original experiments, background "noise" included both irrelevant extrinsic stimuli and activity generated within the nervous system rather than being a response to an external input. His studies, and similar research undertaken by others, led to the conclusion that:

> "The only pre-requisite for obtaining a decrement in physiological arousal (ie. vigilance) is that the experimental situation be prolonged and monotonous" (Parasuraman 1983: 38).

The relevance of this conclusion of Parasuraman for individuals with severe brain injury is that background activities in a hospital ward may constitute just such a situation of prolonged, monotonous sensory input.

The legitimacy of taking account of observations made in *normal* individuals during experimental psychology studies of vigilance (as defined by Mackworth) when attempting to explain observations derived from patients diagnosed as in, or close to, a vegetative state may be challenged on the basis that comparable experimental studies have not been repeated in these patients. Nor could this readily be done. However, I believe that the legitimacy of *ignoring* the possible relevance of those studies with normal subjects for patients diagnosed as vegetative is open to much more forceful challenge. The fundamental objection to any extrapolation from subjects without brain injury to those with very severe injury is the definitional one that vegetative patients are deemed to have no residual capacity for cognition (as Cranford (1984) has eloquently expressed himself, "the IQ is 0"). However, to the extent that vigilance and consciousness are regarded as sufficiently discrete attributes to be differentially affected by injury, the possibility of impaired vigilance should be considered before assuming total lack of cognition.

As with consciousness, a specific neuroanatomical location for vigilance functions has not been demonstrated. However, vigilance may be severely impaired in the absence of a comparable level of interference with other neurological functions. Parasuraman (1983) concluded that good vigilance performance was dependent upon the efficient integration of the functional capacities of a number of areas. Consistent with this conclusion, patients who had been submitted to complete surgical section of the corpus callosum, the midline structure connecting the two cerebral hemispheres, sustained considerable impairment of the ability to detect signals (Dimond 1979). Likewise, an impairment of vigilance has also been reported in persons with subcortical epilepsy. The author of the latter report concluded that:

> "Impaired vigilance is an essential feature in the behavioural derangement of the brain-injured subject" (Bruhn 1970: 453).

This 1970 report from a Danish neurology clinic, whilst applying the term vigilance similarly to Mackworth, defined a high level of vigilance as "alertness" (Bruhn 1970). The author used the term "attention" to describe a highly selective orientation of the individual's sensory apparatus. He distinguished the three preceding terms (ie. vigilance, alertness and attention) from "arousal" which was applied to a diffuse excitatory state of the central nervous system. However, "vigilance" has been used by some authors to refer to quite a different entity. Bricolo *et al.* attached the term "vigilance" to re-opening of the eyes of a comatose patient and quite explicitly separated it from the type of attention implied above. Perhaps influenced by the earlier French term "coma vigil" to describe patients some of whom would later be classed as vegetative, Bricolo *et al.* (1980) in a review of a large series of unconscious neurosurgical patients, used "vigilance" only to describe retention of the capacity for eye opening without any implications of awareness, presumably in the same sense in which Jennett referred to vegetative state patients as awake but not aware (Cornwell 1996). They interpreted "PVS as "vigilance" without conscious activity and referred to the

> "dramatic dissociation of vigilance from consciousness expressed in the vegetative state" (Bricolo *et al.* 1980).

Parasuraman (1983) specifically addressed the differentiation of vigilance (using the term in Mackworth's sense) from arousal and emphasised that an individual's capacity for the two states could vary independently. Patients in whom a decline in vigilance could nevertheless be accompanied by a high level of arousal were described as being awake but not vigilant. Giacino (1997), in discussing the inconsistent use of terminology, used vigilance as a term to describe the capacity to sustain over time the orienting reaction evoked by unexpected stimuli. Rehabilitation specialists with particular interests in the treatment of severe brain injury have usually applied "vigilance" in the sense used by psychologists emphasising the frequent dissociation between patients' vigilance or attention and their state of arousal. Wood (1991) emphasised that vigilance (and hence the opportunity for an observer to access any consciousness retained by a patient) may decline without any change in the level of arousal. He also pointed out that the selection of the most appropriate target stimuli for an individual patient may permit detection of vigilance despite the retention of only a low level of arousal (for example, a sleeping person may respond to his or her quietly spoken name but not to other words). This recalls the frequent advice from experienced neurorehabilitation practitioners that stimuli with high personal salience, whether verbal or otherwise, should be provided when diagnosing or assessing patients suspected of being in a vegetative state.

There are several reasons why individuals with brain injuries of sufficient severity to render them candidates for the diagnosis of a vegetative state could be expected to have markedly decreased levels of vigilance. The most important contribution to reduced vigilance is likely to be that of the brain injury itself. Among other factors are the prolonged monotony of the environment, sensory deprivation, the intrusion of a relative excess of irrelevant "background" stimulation, the effect of soporific drugs that decrease vigilance and the relative infrequency with which stimuli that have a high degree of personal relevance are included in conventional neurological assessments. There are additional reasons why the actual level of *retained* vigilance in a patient with brain injury may be overlooked. Of possible reasons for the failure of an observer *to detect* retained vigilance in a person with a severely injured brain, the most important reason is likely to be that impairment of vigilance may result in an inordinately delayed response. As a result of this delay, the response, when it comes, may be regarded as temporally irrelevant to the question. The occurrence of responses, delayed to such an extent that they appear unrelated to the question, is a common feature of patients in minimally responsive states. Equally characteristic is a propensity to tire rapidly, especially during an unsympathetic examination, with the result that responses may become inappropriate or completely lacking. This tendency may be exacerbated by factors such as constipation, elevation of body temperature and unsatisfactory sleep on the preceding night. von Cramon (1978), writing about the experiences of comatose patients has stressed that identical stimuli may evoke more or less differentiated behavioural responses depending upon the level of vigilance. Freeman (1993) has inferred that complete loss of control of a patient's personal environment, and its violation by apparatus such as endotracheal tubes may evoke a "fight or flight" stress response. In the absence of capacity either to fight or flee, the patient resorts to an inward flight and shuts down when examined.

One factor contributing to decrease in the vigilance of normal subjects, which has also been examined in patients with severe brain damage, is habituation, a state in which a subject becomes accustomed to a situation that persists. Habituation has been categorised as one of the most fundamental properties of animal behaviour (Sharpless and Jasper 1958). Investigation of the effect on cortical evoked potentials (the electrical manifestation of receipt of a sensory stimulus by the cerebral cortex) of the habituation of cats to auditory stimuli did not reveal any change in potentials as habituation of arousal occurred. This was interpreted as indicating that the sensory pathways to cortical projection areas were not involved in habituation (ibid). In contrast with that conclusion, study of the habituation of human subjects to visual stimuli revealed a concurrent decline in the amplitude of cortical evoked potentials (Haider *et al.* 1964), an observation which would suggest that the cortex *was involved* in habituation. This might raise the question of whether the cortex is also *required* for habituation to occur.

Mackworth (1968) described the onset of habituation in normal subjects during performance of vigilance tasks. As has been the case with vigilance, there has been little investigation of whether habituation occurs in patients with severe brain injuries. One such study of habituation in unconscious neurosurgical patients suggested that it not only occurred but also that its rate of onset appeared to be independent of the depth of unconsciousness (Gulbrandsen and Kristiansen 1972). Disconcertingly, dishabituation (interruption of habituation) was said to have been achieved in this study by "loud shouting or shaking" of the unconscious patients. Another disconcerting feature of this 1972 paper from Oslo (and an indication that negative attitudes towards unconscious patients are not a recent development) was its repeated reference to the group of patients under study as "the material". Any interpretation of reports of habituation of vigilance in unconscious patients will remain dependent upon the neural mechanism which is ultimately established as the basis for habituation. Should habituation require cortical activity, the case for persistence of such activity in some vegetative patients would be strengthened. At a practical level, Wood, has cautioned that attempts to produce arousal using intensive overstimulation, could lead to the possibility of an increase in susceptibility to habituation with unconsciousness:

> "If, therefore, a non-brain-damaged person's ability to discriminate and respond to frequent and repetitious forms of stimuli is impaired, what hope is there for a vegetative or coma patient?" (1991: 406).

An indication of the likely complexity of testing for the retention of vigilance by a person with severe brain injury, and of the additional complexity in interpretation of that testing has been provided in McMillan's account of his experience with a 24 year old English woman who had been diagnosed as vegetative by 3 out of 5 specialists. After examining this patient on some 16 occasions, each for 20 minutes, he demonstrated that her responses to questions, which she communicated to him by means of a buzzer, were statistically consistent (Fraser 1979). Whilst a number of brain functions have been investigated in patients regarded as being vegetative or near vegetative, there has been very little formal testing of vigilance in comatose or PVS patients. In one report of such testing, Schuri and von Cramon compared the electrodermal responses of a group of patients in coma of different depths to hearing their own name forwards and backwards. Increased responses which occurred only after hearing the correctly pronounced name were observed in individuals who were otherwise unresponsive to all but strong non-specific stimuli (Schuri and von Cramon 1981).

4.4 NEUROANATOMICAL AND NEUROPHYSIOLOGICAL ASPECTS OF CONSCIOUSNESS

Both anatomical and physiological grounds have been cited in statements from neurological bodies to preclude retention of consciousness in patients diagnosed as vegetative (American Academy of Neurology 1989; American Neurological Association 1993). The paper most frequently cited to advance this proposition examined cerebral cortical metabolic activity by positron emission tomography

(PET) and concluded that metabolism was so depressed as to preclude the possibility of any mental activity:

> "Such metabolic hypoactivity has precedent only in deep anesthesia and supports clinical evidence that cerebral cognitive function is lost in the vegetative state, leaving only a body that can no longer think or experience pain" (Levy *et al.* 1987: 673).

Neuropathological findings obtained from autopsy examination of patients who had been diagnosed as in a PVS, and subsequently used as a basis for interpreting the lesions underlying this condition, have already been summarised in Chapter 2. Four reports on the subject published in 1994 suggest, when considered together, that the regions of the brain mediating consciousness are much more dispersed than has traditionally been taught. Kinney and Samuels (1994) from the Harvard Departments of Pathology and Neurology, in reviewing the pathology of PVS, proposed that

> "neuropathologic studies of patients with PVS are crucial for helping to define the anatomic regions essential for human awareness and arousal" (ibid: 549.

One assumption implicit in this conclusion is that the clinical diagnosis of PVS provides a sufficiently reliable and reproducible marker of loss of consciousness to permit a valid correlation of the anatomical lesions in individual patients with their specific functional deficits. A second, unstated assumption is that the technology available to the neuropathologist has the discriminative precision required to identify those components of damage directly responsible for loss of consciousness and to distinguish them from any accompanying pathological changes which have not had this effect.

As discussed in Chapter 2, the autopsy report on Karen Ann Quinlan and the correspondence that it elicited challenged prevailing views that loss of consciousness in vegetative patients reflected cortical damage. The disproportionately severe damage to her thalamus compared with the cerebral cortex was interpreted as indicating a critical role for the thalamus in cognition and awareness, but not in arousal (Kinney *et al.* 1994). As noted in Chapter 2, correspondence in response to publication of the Quinlan autopsy findings included a report of severe thalamic damage with cortical sparing at autopsy in another patient after 4 years in PVS (Jellinger 1994). Another correspondent responding to the M.S.T.F. statement which had been published in the same issue of the *New England Journal of Medicine*, drew attention to the contrast between its assertion that the cerebral cortex is the locus of conscious awareness and the incrimination of the thalamus in this function by the Quinlan autopsy (McQuillen 1994). A fourth report, also published in 1994, concluded on the basis of tracing neural connections in cebus monkeys that the basal ganglia and cerebellum were involved in higher cognitive function. In this report Middleton and Strick (1994) postulated the existence of closed loops between an area in the prefrontal cortex involved with spatial memory and the basal ganglia and cerebellum.

Any attempt to apply a structure : function analysis to the problem of consciousness assumes that it may be considered equivalent to, and analysed in the same manner as, any other physiological function. The philosopher John Searle maintains that the processes underlying consciousness should be regarded as physiological functions in the same way as those which underlie the secretion of bile (Searle 1998: 6). Whilst this is a useful way of emphasising that consciousness *should* be susceptible to explanation in terms of anatomy and physiology, it does not guarantee that defined correlates of consciousness which are as reliable as those applicable to bile secretion not only exist but can be identified. Until this is achieved, it will not be possible to guarantee that damage to specific regions, or combinations of regions, of the brain excludes consciousness. The most frequently cited neurophysiological PET data bearing on the capacity of PVS patients for consciousness will be discussed in Chapter 6. Whilst PET, or any technique for quantifying the activity of brain cells, can measure the level of metabolic activity of those cells, it cannot thereby be assumed to be documenting activity responsible for maintaining consciousness in the absence of independent confirmation that this is so. Flohr (1995) has proposed that:

> "Consciousness is bound to a specific subset of processes that can be characterized physiologically. In an awake brain some events give rise to consciousness, but others, probably the vast majority of events going on in the brain, have nothing to do with it. Unconsciousness is not necessarily attended by a loss of some functions" (ibid: 158).

Whereas it is possible to measure the brain's metabolic activity with precision and to express it in quantitative terms, it is not feasible neatly to apportion some percentage of it to maintaining consciousness or even to the capacity for doing so.

Recognition of consciousness by an observer remains dependent upon the subject's retention of a capacity to communicate with that observer. It inevitably follows that independent validation that decrease in any measurable physiological brain function below a specified level reliably indicates loss of the capacity for consciousness is not practicable unless the observer can distinguish lack of *ability* to communicate from lack of *anything* to communicate. Nevertheless, it is frequently claimed, despite the absence of reliable means of making this distinction or of distinguishing the "vast majority" of brain events referred to by Flohr from those specific to consciousness, that technologies such as PET can measure capacity for consciousness.

Whilst the question of whether measurement of neurophysiological parameters can be used to exclude consciousness in a person diagnosed as in a vegetative state is of clinical importance, a second question, namely that of the precise relationship to consciousness itself of *any* measured attribute which is believed to correlate with consciousness, is of wider interest. A correlate, empirically observed to be an invariable accompaniment of the phenomenon of interest helps to exclude the occurrence of that phenomenon, but a correlate that is on the direct causal pathway to the phenomenon is invariably more informative. Some possible correlates of consciousness clearly are not associated with its production. For example, some studies of intracranial pressure fluctuation in clinically unconscious patients have strongly suggested this parameter correlates well with retention of some awareness. Thus, comatose patients have been reported to develop an increase in intracranial pressure when conversations were *about* them but not when they were merely *over* them (Snyder 1983). Similarly, changes in pulse rate may indicate a patient's awareness. Freeman (2002) has frequently observed that the increase in pulse rate occasioned by medical examination of children, diagnosed as comatose, and not exhibiting other signs of awareness, is reduced when a parent makes his or her presence known. Electrodermal changes that occur exclusively in response to personally relevant stimuli presented to apparently unconscious patients correlate with otherwise undetected awareness but are clearly consequences rather than causes of it (Haider *et al.* 1964).

The second question, namely the exact relationship of whatever event is measured to consciousness, may be taken further back. Are electrical manifestations of brain activity that are consistently observed to be associated with consciousness, and that do not appear to be consequences of it, merely representative of processes underlying and essential to consciousness or are they actually the electrical representation of consciousness itself? Clearly, if the latter situation were to obtain, it might become possible at some time to identify the persistence of consciousness that was otherwise undetectable (subject to the caveat referred to above in discussion of PET, namely that confirmation of the level of consciousness by some independent means would be required to validate the test).

Some of the mechanisms which have been suggested to form the basis for consciousness might lend themselves to the development of clinical tests to detect it. For example, one proposal which has been advanced to explain the control of consciousness of incoming stimuli has been termed the "searchlight hypothesis". This proposal, as developed by Crick (1984), includes a mechanism (which he suggested was located in the thalamus) which exists to search all sensory inputs, to correlate the data from them and then to direct attention to features uncovered by the search. Crick suggested that the searchlight achieved temporary conjunctions of neurones by rapidly modifiable synapses (the interfaces between neurones) to produce transient cell assemblies. One electrical correlate of attention which, it has been suggested, is responsible for linking or "binding" discrete cortical networks is fast gamma rhythms, often referred to as "40 Hz" rhythms. It has been hypothesised that, although these rhythms are correlates of consciousness of information, they do not represent consciousness itself (Jefferys *et al.* 1996).

Whilst systematic studies of 40 Hz rhythms in vegetative patients do not appear to have been reported, there have been reports that these rhythms appear in subjects experiencing rapid eye movement (REM) sleep in a form similar to those recorded from awake individuals (Llinàs and Ribary 1993). Interpretation of putative electrical correlates of consciousness may be further complicated if, as suggested by Llinàs (1988), there is a dialogue between internal states generated by intrinsic electrical activity and incoming sensory information from the external world. Intrinsic electrical activity of this type could represent the physiological substrate for an "inner awareness" or "private" mental activity not dependent upon receipt of stimuli from, or communication with, the external world. However, the testing of this hypothesis and the identification of electric correlates that might indicate the occurrence of inner awareness would not appear to be readily achievable.

4.5 COMMUNICATION

Communication between a subject and an observer requires an active input from *both* and, in the absence of either input, it may be concluded not only that the subject is unable to communicate but also that he or she has no mental activity to communicate. Unlike the measurement of pulse rate or blood pressure which can be completely observer-independent, the detection of a minimal level of consciousness in a subject is likely to be dependent upon the experience, patience and especially the identity of the person seeking to establish communication. Other factors such as the time of day, the intensity of other potentially distracting activity in the ward, any preceding nursing procedures involving the patient and the nature of any sedating medication may also adversely influence the assessment of consciousness.

Observer bias may lead to failure to detect retained consciousness, for example if the observer is dismissive of ancillary devices designed and used in specialised neurorehabilitation centres to monitor weak motor activity. For instance, the response of Ronald Cranford (1996) to a system for communicating with patients at the Royal Hospital for Neuro-disability springs to mind:

> "Videotapes of the buzzer in operation would help to demonstrate to others the usefulness and reproducibility of the system. Until such validation occurs, I must view the buzzer system with some scepticism" (ibid: 5).

It is of some interest that validation is required for tests of consciousness but not for tests of the *un*consciousness which is central to diagnosis of a vegetative state. A false positive diagnosis of consciousness is possible if patient responses are unreasonably over-interpreted by the observer. However, the use of specialised communication devices designed to detect slight pressure changes produced by patient movements, especially if combined with an examination procedure capable of demonstrating statistical significance in a response pattern, may permit observer subjectivity to be minimised (Fraser 1997).

The identity of the observer and the nature of the questions that are presented and, in particular, the personal relevance of each of these to the patient are likely to be critical. This point has often been obscured when the innate advantage that a member of the patient's family is likely to have in communication has been conflated with the risk that the family member may self-delude into seeing what he or she *wants* to see. The rehabilitation literature on management of patients suspected of being vegetative has increasingly emphasised the bridging role that a patient's family can play in establishing communication. This role may be reinforced if a patient retains a capacity for communicating when the selected topic recalls pre-disability experience, but is unable to engage with new and unfamiliar topics. Freeman (1991) has drawn attention to the shedding of tears by a patient, when told by family members that they are about to leave the room, as one of the first indications of awareness. A very common feature after brain injury, even when this is much less severe than that associated with a vegetative diagnosis, is shortening of attention span. Attention is not an all-or-nothing property and it may wane rapidly in a patient with severe brain injury or be diminished as a result of residual drug effects. An unfamiliar and apparently threatening environment may suppress the response of a severely impaired individual, even if attention remains.

4.6 UNCONSCIOUS MENTAL ACTIVITY

> "It has become generally accepted that a large, perhaps even a major part of our mental activities can take place without our being consciously aware of them" (Libet 1965: 77).

Whilst there have been a variety of observations of *conscious* individuals, with and without neurological abnormalities, which indicate that stimuli received, but not consciously perceived, can affect behaviour, enter memory and be responsible for learning, the possible implications of the retention of processes such as these by PVS patients have rarely been explored. The significance of subconscious, or unconscious, activity in *normal* brain function has been adequately acknowledged by psychologists but, because of the impracticability of verifying its occurrence in real time, it has been even less susceptible to anatomical location or neurophysiological correlation than has consciousness itself. Most commentators writing about vegetative states have readily acknowledged that the extent of any inner mental activity in a person incapable of communication cannot be assessed by an observer. Nevertheless, most have also readily conceded that individuals diagnosed as vegetative are unconscious *by definition*, so precluding any further discussion of the possibility of any form of residual mental activity. This section will consider some features of unconscious processing of information in the normal brain and by patients with brain lesions.

Should the retention of any mental state, other than consciousness as defined by the M.S.T.F., be significant in deciding upon patient management? The emphasis placed on the retention of capacity of patients to communicate in some way with an observer attempting to detect consciousness has diverted attention away from any consideration of "inner awareness" as a worthwhile variant form of mental activity. Whilst very limited attention has been given to any possibility of retained inner awareness in individuals diagnosed as vegetative, substantial significance has been accorded by psychologists to unconscious mental states, inaccessible to an observer, in *normal* subjects. Although the significance of unconscious mental activity in the function of the brain in a *normal* person cannot be defined with precision, this has not generally been regarded as grounds for dismissing it as of no consequence in human mental processes. The likely importance of unconscious mental processes in developing ideas and in fuelling insights has been described by Libet (1965).

> "Many instances have been documented in which highly creative and elaborate 'thinking' by scientists, poets, etc. has developed unconsciously, although interplay with conscious experiences is commonly involved" (ibid: 81).

Libet speculated that all instances of intuitively generated ideas or artistic expressions could be originally based on unconscious processes that had preceded their entry into consciousness. In the absence of sufficient data about the structural or functional basis for unconscious activity in individuals with an *intact* brain, it becomes both impracticable and unreasonable automatically to exclude as significant the persistence of such activity in at least some of those persons diagnosed as comatose or vegetative.

Whilst the occurrence of unconscious mental activity cannot be directly observed even in normal subjects, there is ample evidence for the occurrence of unconscious perception in both normal people and those with specifically localised brain injury. It would also appear, that unconscious perceptions can enter into inner awareness or unconscious mental states. Unconscious perception by a normal subject can occur if the stimulus that is presented remains too weak or if the subject's attention has not been focussed upon it at the time of presentation (ibid). Sensory stimuli too weak to be consciously appreciated can, nevertheless, generate cortical evoked potentials in normal subjects (Libet *et al.* 1967). No distinction was observed in these potentials during the transition from stimuli which failed to enter consciousness to other, stronger ones which did so. Dixon and Henley (1991) reporting on the subject of unconscious perception proposed that stimuli of which an individual remained unaware might nevertheless exert a considerable influence on his or her subsequent behaviour or emotions. Discussing possible implications of data from psychological research for clinical practice, Dixon and Henley contrasted the immense information-processing capacity of the brain (when assessed in terms of numbers of neurones and their interconnections) with the extremely limited extent of conscious channel capacity. They stressed that:

> "The mechanisms whereby the brain receives, processes and transmits information are by no means identical to those that provide for conscious perceptual experiences" (ibid: 243).

A 1997 review of the unconscious mind from the perspective of clinical neurology exemplified some of the contradictions inherent in the neat definitional approach to PVS adopted by many neurologists and authoritative working parties. Acknowledging at the outset that consciousness escapes a satisfying definition, Orrin Devinsky (1997) proceeded to explore some of the features of unconscious mental activity. Discussing the intact nervous system he noted that "boundaries between conscious and unconscious knowledge and behaviors can be discrete or continuous" (ibid: 323). At one point, Devinsky observed that preconscious stimuli such as subliminal percepts and implicit memories can influence thought and behaviour whilst remaining below the threshhold of conscious awareness. Nevertheless, on the following page, the issue of unconscious activity in the brain of the PVS person received only scant attention it being noted that "consciousness is profoundly impaired", an assessment sourced to Jennett and Plum (1972).

An article in a 1992 issue of *American Psychologist*, entitled *Unconscious cognition reclaimed*, reviewed the chequered history of that subject. The author Anthony Greenwald recalled that, following Freud's provision of a theoretical background, the subject of unconsciousness had disappeared from the vocabulary of many psychologists by the 1950s. This was a response to the continuing lack of any evidence to support psychoanalytic theories of unconscious influences on perception (Greenwald 1992). Greenwald then proceeded to emphasise that "recently developed research methods have at last made unconscious cognition a routine subject of laboratory investigation". He concluded that unconscious cognition had become solidly established in empirical research, although the capacity for its analysis appeared to remain considerably below that applicable in the case of attended stimulus cognition.

Blindsight is probably the most dramatic example of unconscious perception by individuals with brain injury. Its significance for better understanding PVS is not that patients with injuries producing blindsight necessarily resemble much more severely affected patients in vegetative states. Rather, localised lesions which permit affected people to retain good capacity to communicate their experiences, can provide an insight into aspects of mental function not testable in severely disabled people who are unable to communicate. A report by Poppel *et al.* (1973) appears to have been the first description of the phenomenon subsequently termed blindsight. They described the visual capabilities of four patients who had sustained injuries to their visual cortex. After defining the area of the visual field in which each patient failed to report any vision, Poppel *et al.*, nevertheless observed responses by the subjects to stimuli presented within this affected area. Another report in the following year described a patient of Weiskrantz *et al.* (1974) who was blind in part of his visual field as a result of damage to his visual cortex. Although this patient had no awareness of "seeing" in his blind field, it was shown that he had knowledge of the identity of visual stimuli presented to this field.

The relevance of the phenomenon of blindsight to inferences about possible retention of unrecognised capacities by unconscious patients is that reception of visual stimuli, in the absence of awareness of them at the time, should not be discounted out of hand in individuals who appear to be unconscious. It may be recalled that most of the patients in Andrews' series of misdiagnosed PVS cases were considered to be cortically blind (Andrews *et al.* 1996). Weiskrantz's patient claimed that he saw nothing and attributed his success in identifying stimuli that had been presented in his blind field, and of which he remained unaware, to "just guessing" (Weiskrantz *et al.* 1974). The mechanism underlying blindsight remains unexplained. Magnetic resonance imaging and PET examination of the damaged visual cortex in a patient with blindsight have both failed to detect any activity in response to visual stimuli, implying that the phenomenon could not be attributed to retention of some cortical function (Stoerig and Cowey 1997). In their review of the subject, Stoerig and Cowey emphasised that patients with cortical lesions could be trained to acquire blindsight. However, they pointed out that the time of patients with such disabilities was usually too valuable to devote to training (or to participation in research), whereas in the case of monkeys bilaterally deprived of a visual cortex, "who have little choice", extensive teaching can enhance blindsight performance. As if to emphasise their point, Stoerig and Cowey commended the doggedness of the researcher responsible for training the monkey Helen for 8 years.

A point which may be relevant to the recognition of blindsight in unconscious patients is its clear differentiation from "residual vision", a state in which consciousness of presented stimuli remains intact (Stoerig and Cowey 1997). Whilst blindsight has attracted most attention and been more thoroughly investigated, it is not unrealistic to suspect that stimulation of other sensory organs may also impact on higher regions of the brain without simultaneously entering consciousness. For instance a group of Stanford neuroscientists has described "blind smell", a phenomenon in which activation of thalamus and cortex was observed by means of magnetic resonance imaging during presentation of an air-borne chemical at a concentration too low for the subjects to detect (Sobel *et al.* 1999).

Whereas blindsight exemplifies the retention, by people with brain injuries, of a capacity to receive stimuli of which they are not aware, the phenomenon of sensory hemineglect illustrates another possibility, namely that of loss of attention in the absence of any motor or sensory impairment. Sensory hemineglect has been observed following severe injury to the parietal cortex in some patients who then behave as though one half of their surroundings does not exist. That this neglect does not reflect interference with the capacity to *receive* external sensory stimuli was graphically demonstrated by a patient with sensory hemineglect who, when afflicted with delirium tremens, described the complete restriction of hallucinations to that side of the body on which attention was retained. Mesulam (1981), when reporting this case, specified the neglect syndrome in the following terms:

> "The deficit is not one of seeing, hearing, feeling or moving but one of looking, listening, tracking and exploring" (ibid: 318).

The possible relevance of sensory hemineglect to the vegetative state lies in the demonstration which it provides that the capacity to attend to, or be aware of, a stimulus that is received by the brain in an otherwise normal manner can be lost. As Mesulam has pointed out, effective execution of attention requires interaction between three attributes, namely intense concentration, inhibition of distractibility and the ability to focus the centre of awareness.

There are some circumstances in which inferences may be drawn about retention of a capacity for mental activity, despite diagnosis of a vegetative state. One potentially instructive situation is that of individuals who, having been diagnosed as in a vegetative state, have regained capacity to communicate and have also retained a recollection of earlier events. Before a person who has been diagnosed as vegetative, but who subsequently regains consciousness, can describe his or her experiences during the earlier period, at least three things are required. First, the affected individual must have something to tell others about. There is a prerequisite for some *experience* whilst in the vegetative state. Second, the person must have a capacity to *recollect* features of that experience. Third, neither of the preceding capacities can be discovered by an external observer unless the patient also has regained the capacity to *communicate* with others by some means. Any inner mental activity that occurred whilst the patient was vegetative will remain undetected, unsuspected and probably denied by others in the absence of memory and communication. If a person's recollection of events whilst vegetative is found to correspond with independently verifiable detail of his or her external environment during that period, this strongly suggests that any mental activity during that period was accessible to sensory input. If it does not correspond, it will be difficult, if not impossible, to locate the timing of the remembered experience accurately. It could antedate or correspond with the vegetative interval or be attributable to the recovery period.

Whilst the general acknowledgment by a British Medical Association spokesperson, Dr Nathanson (Fletcher 1996), that patients in coma were frequently aware of events around them was unexceptionable, the actual accounts of experiences recalled by identified people bring home this point more forcefully. Such accounts have been published both in newspapers and medical journals. One of the best publicised illustrations of the retention of awareness without capacity to communicate this to others was provided by Mark Newton who was regarded as unconscious for 6 months after a diving accident. Having regained a capacity to communicate after admission to the Royal Hospital for Neuro-disability, he indicated that, although aware of activities around him whilst comatose, he was unaware that others could not hear him.

> "I used to talk to people and just assume they could hear me. It never occurred to me that we were not having a two-way conversation. People used to look at me sitting with my Walkman on and patronisingly say 'Ah he's listening to his tape'. I'd be shouting, 'No I'm not. It's finished. Will someone please turn it over'" (Cohen 1996).

His account of the period during which he was regarded as vegetative provides some revealing insights: "I was not in pain. I was perfectly comfortable". The extent to which Mark Newton is representative of patients who are regarded as unconscious over a prolonged period is unknown, and almost certainly unknowable.

Mark Newton's story implies that the proposition to be disproved should not be that of whether *all* persons diagnosed as in PVS could retain consciousness but that of whether *any* can. There is no reason why capacity to *experience* events whilst unconscious should be accompanied by a capacity to recall these events, but experience of which there is no recall could be just as realistic, when it occurs, as other experience that can be subsequently recalled. Similarly the occurrence of unrecognised bilateral sensory neglect in a patient regarded as vegetative would make it extremely difficult to determine whether consciousness remained undetected. Both blindsight and sensory hemineglect have been recognised and well characterised in individuals with localised brain damage and retention of capacity to communicate. Exclusion of attention defects like them in individuals lacking capacity to communicate may be impossible.

It would be difficult to sustain an argument that the recalled experiences of those who had been in a coma or a vegetative state, and who later regained the capacity and the opportunity to communicate, were not relevant to consideration of the cases of others who remained uncommunicative. The primary distinction between coma and vegetative states, namely the occurrence of periods of eye opening in the latter, appears to be quite empirical. Most accounts of patients' recollections of periods spent in post-traumatic coma have emphasised their emotional overtones. In Schnaper's (1975) Baltimore study of individuals who had been in post-traumatic coma, approximately two-thirds of the patients reported, after recovery, that they were amnesic in relation to the period of coma whilst the remainder recalled fantasies or dreams, usually in threatening circumstances. On the basis of these findings, Schnaper nevertheless advocated the presentation only of positive messages to patients who were diagnosed as being unconscious. Tosch's study of patients who had been in post-traumatic coma, produced similar results with approximately half of the patients having some recollection of their period in coma (Tosch 1988). A striking feature of both studies was the marked difference in response to stimuli that had emotional content for the individual patient compared with the response to neutral stimuli. This recalls the common experience of the families of people with severe brain injury. Like Schnaper, Tosch also concluded that the possibility of retention of some awareness by comatose patients required that any discussion of a patient's condition in his or her presence should be couched in positive terms. The implication from these studies that at least some unconscious patients retain an awareness of their environment and/or a capacity for mental activity is consistent with reports of learning by comatose patients (Shiel *et al.* 1993).

Once the possibility is acknowledged that mental functions other than those associated with a detectable conscious state may be retained in an unknown number of those individuals diagnosed as being in a vegetative state, the question becomes that of assessing the *value* to be attached to retention of those functions. In doing so, it is appropriate to anticipate the contrast (to be discussed in Chapter 10) between the assessments of the life quality of people with disabilities that are formulated by non-disabled individuals and by those actually affected by disability. The former are invariably strikingly negative and pessimistic compared with the latter. The contention that (detectable) consciousness is a prerequisite for personhood (which has underpinned the case for excluding PVS patients from this state) is premised on the belief that other forms of (unconscious) mental activity are of no value to the subject (Cranford and Smith 1987). It assumes that there exists a black and white conscious/unconscious separation rather than a gradation of conscious states. This ignores the original proposition of Jennett and Plum (1972) that a "continuum" was likely to exist between a vegetative state and consciousness. To require that only detectable consciousness can exempt a person diagnosed as vegetative from down-grading to the status of some entity less than a person is implicitly to assert that unconscious mental activity in such a person is without significance.

4.7 PERSONHOOD AND PVS

> "The vegetative state has especially kindled the interest of those neuroscientists concerned with the generation of thoughts and with the minimal requirements needed for an individual to qualify as a human being" (Spudis 1991: 133).

> "In fact, we do not know very much about persons in comparison with what we know about kidneys" (Cassel 1996: 147).

Anyone who finds the question of recognition of consciousness in another individual too simple could profitably spend some time considering the recognition of personhood. As Spudis remarked in his review of PVS cited above, one effect of description of the condition has been to popularise non-clinical words such as human(hood) and person(hood). The question of the personhood status of individuals diagnosed as in PVS has been accorded such a level of exposure in the literature on this condition that it has become impossible to ignore in discussion of the attitudes of others to affected patients. Cassel's 1996 paper, also quoted above, commented on the results of a survey of physicians' beliefs about PVS patients. The extent of illogicality and inconsistency manifest in the responses (described with admirable professional politeness as "clinical incoherence" in the title of Cassel's commentary) led him to write of the confusion among neurologists about what is believed to be fundamental to being a person. As he observed, thinking about the nature of persons is not taught in medical schools and whatever capability for doing so any physician possesses will have been "gained through experience in everyday life" (ibid). It follows, although Cassel has not explicitly made this point, that a physician is not necessarily better qualified than any other member of society to assess personhood. In practice, physicians with personality limitations may be less competent than others in their community without such impediments to do so.

"Personhood" is simply defined in the *Oxford English Dictionary* as the quality or condition of being an individual person. A clear definition of the meaning attached to the term "personhood" by authors using it in relation to patients diagnosed as in vegetative states has often been lacking. When used by an ethicist, "personhood" would generally refer to the possession of full moral standing by a member of the human species. Whilst this meaning has provided the basis for an enormous philosophical output, the term "personhood" is itself of relatively recent (1959) introduction. In medical, as distinct from ethical, writing on the vegetative state, the term appears to have been restricted to individuals manifesting certain specified attributes, most importantly consciousness and cognitive capacity. Withdrawal of personhood from patients diagnosed as in a vegetative state seems usually to have been based on the second interpretation, in particular an imputed irreversible loss of consciousness. However, that withdrawal has inevitably led to diminution of these patients' moral standing, especially when management decisions are to be made.

Some commentaries on the PVS have considered that the loss of *self*-consciousness, with persistence of other forms of conscious capacity, is sufficient to forfeit personhood. This position was approached by the U.S. President's Commission (1983a) and it has also been proposed in considering patients with advanced forms of Alzheimer's disease in whom there appears to have been some dissociation between consciousness and self-consciousness. I find the proposition that loss of self-consciousness can be a marker of loss of personhood implausible because varying degrees of loss can occur as a result of damage to the nervous system as well as in individuals with intact nervous systems. In the first category, apart from patients with Alzheimer's disease, are those with neurological lesions which lead to failure to acknowledge large parts of the body as "self" and others such as Mark Newton who failed to associate conversations about himself with that self but thought that they related to another individual. Suspension of self-consciousness, accompanying an intact nervous system, occurs during deep meditation and also in the "out of body" experiences described by some individuals who have been resuscitated after cardiac arrest. The latter accounts are notable for the person's capacity to watch the resuscitation from the perspective of an "independent" observer.

When personhood is allocated primarily on the basis of clinical features, a patient in a vegetative state might be described as a "non-person", albeit one with full moral standing. However, if retention of the "higher functions" of the brain is considered to be an essential condition if an individual is to retain personhood, a patient in a vegetative state could be considered as a "non-person" lacking full moral standing. Irrespective of the basis for classification, both groups of "non-persons" would be considered to be living. Irrespective of the definition of "personhood adopted and the arbitrary components in conferring it on an individual the complementary state of "non-personhood" has been energetically promoted by some commentators as a discrete category suspended between life and death, and accompanied by a corresponding scaling down of the rights of those deemed to fall within it.

The nexus between consciousness and personhood has steadily evolved over two decades. The concept of a state which, while it failed to meet the criteria for brain death, was nevertheless regarded as falling short of perceived requirements for personhood (although this word was not used initially) was expounded by Cranford and Smith (1979). If capacity for consciousness and social interaction were the essential features of human beings, Cranford and Smith specified "neocortical death" as a state in which these capacities were lost, equating it with a variant of PVS in which the EEG was isoelectric. Subsequent investigation has revealed that most PVS patients do not have an isoelectric EEG, and also that the cortical damage which was a definitional feature of the new term was not a consistent characteristic of PVS. A 1987 article, again co-authored by Ronald Cranford, but accompanied by a different Smith, advanced its argument in its title, *Consciousness: the most critical moral (constitutional) standard for human personhood* (Cranford and Smith 1987). It asserted that debate about human personhood had replaced that about definition of death slotting in the category of non-personhood between conventional death (including brain death) and being alive (and conscious). Two potential impediments to acceptance of the new classification were acknowledged but then eliminated. The first was the reliability of the diagnosis of permanent unconsciousness, in relation to which it was asserted:

> "It is possible for neurological specialists …. to determine with an extraordinarily high degree of certainty that there has been a permanent loss of consciousness" (ibid: 237).

The second potential barrier, namely the need to allay any concern that permanently unconscious patients may experience pain or suffering, was also readily disposed of:

> "Direct clinical experience with these patients demonstrates that there is no behavioural indication of any awareness of pain or suffering" (ibid: 240).

By 1998, Korein, who had been one of the earliest to write on brain death in clinical terms, could refer to "an objective biological foundation" for a schema in which the "human organism" existed in ascending phases designated as the "human being" and the "person" (Korein 1998). Referring to individuals who have been diagnosed as being in PVS, he explained that:

> "It should be stated that prior to their illness these patients were in the person phase and are now in the human being phase" (ibid: 42).

A contribution to *A Companion to bioethics*, published in 1998 pursued the question of loss of personhood in an individual who does not meet any of the criteria for death.

> "If one were identical with one's organism, then of course its death and one's own death would be one and the same event (or process). But if one is distinct from one's organism, then one's own ceasing to exist and the death of one's organism are different" (McMahan 1998: 255).

The situation envisaged as corresponding to that of an individual in PVS in this description was "that one might die or cease to exist while one's organism would continue to exist".

Whilst PVS has been advanced as the archetypal condition which exemplifies the separate nature of "personhood" and "life", a similar issue has been raised in relation to patients in the most advanced stage of Alzheimer's disease. Nevertheless, some commentators such as the ethicist Daniel Callahan (1995) have been at pains to isolate PVS from Alzheimer's disease, excluding the former from any arguments advanced in support of retained capacities in those affected by the latter. Other authors have classified the most advanced stage of Alzheimer's disease as equivalent to PVS. Many of the arguments that have been advanced in relation to personhood and PVS have also been presented in discussion of personhood and Alzheimer's disease and the responses to them have relevance to PVS. The association between personhood and cognitive ability implicit in the non-personhood concept has been vigorously criticised by Kitwood and Bredin (1992) in discussing care of the demented. They dissented from the increasing preoccupation with presumed "cortical" processes in personhood.

> "The two have been bound up too closely in western psychological theory, especially of late; its 'hypercognitivism' is something of a disadvantage for a humane understanding of dementia, and needs to be resisted" (ibid: 278).

They emphasised the distinction between capacity for cognition and personhood, noting that some of those who have reached zero in cognitive terms "still appear to be faring well as persons" (ibid: 280). Rather than deferring to specialists to define personhood, it would be worth recalling the distinction drawn between the perspectives of neuroscientists and patients' families by Sommerhoff and Dorman (1994). They pointed to the different meanings likely to be read into the term "consciousness" and suggested that families of patients were more concerned than neuroscientists with attributes other than those requiring the higher cognitive functions. Many families may be more prepared to accept as a person their member who has been diagnosed as in a PVS than are some of the commentators I have cited. Kitwood and Bredin stressed that personhood should be envisaged in social rather than individual terms and criticised the focusing of attention overwhelmingly on the demented subjects as the problem while the professional staff caring for them are "not problematized at all" (ibid: 272). Whilst much of their discussion is directed to patients who, although demented, retain capacity for interaction with others, the points that they raise would extend without any cut-off to those cases of dementia who have been claimed to fall within a vegetative classification.

Even though the concept of "personhood" has been criticised as non-clinical (Spudis 1991) and not falling clearly within the comprehension of many clinicians (Cassell 1996), claims have been made to underpin it with a scientific basis, albeit a patently simplistic one. For example, the 1998 bioethics volume referred to above, deftly simplified any problem with an anatomical basis for personhood by assigning it to "the higher brain and in particular the cerebral cortex" (McMahan 1998: 251). Proposals to define personhood objectively may be interpreted as one component of a "coping strategy" to assist medical and nursing personnel dealing with patients lacking signs of cognition (Kitwood and Bredin 1992). As the available evidence increasingly implicates brain structures beyond the cerebral cortex as contributing to consciousness, attempts to isolate "personhood", as a property defined by consciousness and cognitive capacity, to a specific location in the brain run counter to this scientific trend. The question of whether unconscious, or subconscious, activity could provide a basis for ongoing personhood has been ignored. Cassel (1982) has pointed out that a person has a past and without a past is incomplete. Whether some individuals, diagnosed as having entered PVS, either as the end stage of Alzheimer's dementia or following a more acute episode, may retain an "inner life" sustained, not by contemporary inputs, but by recollection of things past remains unknown. Writing about the experience of being demented, "a phenomenon which may appear to some to be a contradiction in terms", Foley (1992) has suggested that the absence of emotional "display" is too often assumed to indicate "that no emotion is being experienced".

One potential difficulty, which would be raised by a "*cerebral death*" definition but could be avoided by substituting "*non-personhood*", is that of explaining how death could be a species-dependent issue. Schema that seek to classify a state of "cognitive death" (Cranford and Smith 1987) on the basis of conscious status must run foul of species distinctions. Thus, if "self-awareness" is held to be an essential component of consciousness as authorities such as the M.S.T.F. on PVS have held, then only humans and chimpanzees can ever be conscious. These are the only two species that appear to be able to recognise self as such when confronted with a mirror. If a member of the species *homo sapiens* who can breathe unaided and who can be maintained in good physical health by the simple expedient of feeding (i.e.

two of the characteristics of many persons diagnosed as in a PVS) is to be certified as neocortically dead, it may be awkward to explain why a dog in a biologically identical state is not also automatically considered to be dead. However with the introduction of a novel category of personhood which is forfeited by a human individual in PVS, the nexus with other species, apart from self-aware chimpanzees, can be severed. The notion of a withdrawable state of "doghood" does not appear yet to have entered the philosophical literature.

Entrenching personhood as a state could have legal implications extending beyond the relatively harmless and irrelevant arena of academic debate. Tom Stacy, writing in the *Cornell Law Review*, may have foreshadowed future developments in pointing out that existing medical and legal definitions of death have moved away from "using purely biological terms" (Stacy 1992). He extended the proposition that brain dead patients no longer retain a right to life to include the PVS patient. Having argued that

> "a capacity for consciousness constitutes a necessary condition of *any* (his emphasis) plausible conception of life" (ibid: 501),

he concluded that

> "a being irretrievably bereft of consciousness has no claim whatsoever to the right to life associated with personhood" (ibid: 501).

Cranford and Smith (1987) have spelt out some of the practical implications of stripping the PVS patient of personhood:

> "Society may also wish to reduce the criminal sanctions if a defendant causes the death of someone already in a persistent vegetative state" (ibid: 244).

On the other hand, they suggested an increase in the penalty for an offender who causes another person to become permanently unconscious.

4.8 RECAPITULATION

Consciousness is what is lacking in, and the lack of which defines, PVS. The question of the nature of consciousness has been attacked using the methodologies of a number of diverse disciplines, seemingly without much interaction between them. It is universally acknowledged that the consciousness of one individual is not accessible to an external observer and that, in consequence, that observer can do no more than draw inferences about the individual under study. Having made this *de rigueur* point at an early stage, most commentaries on patients in a PVS then proceed to ignore it. It is paradoxical that clinical certainty about recognition of loss of consciousness can coexist with an overwhelming uncertainty about *what* has been lost.

The burgeoning of interest in PVS in the last two decades might have been predicted to lead to critical questioning of what contribution to understanding of consciousness an improved understanding of PVS might make. This does not seem to have occurred. On the other hand, there appears to me to be some information about conscious states in normal subjects, and others with brain injury much less severe than that which accompanies PVS, which may be at least partially applicable to PVS patients. One essential prerequisite if an individual is to manifest signs of consciousness is that he or she must be *attentive* to external happenings. A substantial body of research exists on the subject of vigilance and its impairment and it is highly likely that, to the extent that capacity for vigilance has been lost following brain injury, the *recognition* of any retained consciousness by an observer will become increasingly difficult.

Well established correlations between normal anatomical structure and corresponding physiological functions will often enable one to infer what clinical signs will be produced by any specified pathological change in a body organ, and vice versa. Such a structure : function correlation is not available for consciousness. I do not believe that any reliable equation exists, backed by sound data, to enable the conclusion to be drawn that loss of a specified proportion of specified neuroanatomical structures is *incompatible* with any possibility of consciousness. Yet this conclusion has been persistently drawn.

There is ample evidence indicating that *unconscious* receipt and processing of information constitutes a major (probably *the* major) part of mental activity. The extent to which this type of activity could continue in any individual after severe brain injury is unknown and almost invariably unconsidered. Quite apart from any impact that the possibility of retention of unconscious mental activity by any patient in a PVS might have on attitudes towards such patients, this possibility should certainly influence management practices, especially as these relate to conversations about those patients in their presence. Also, as with vigilance, the *recognition* of retained consciousness in another is dependent on the establishment of effective communication between observer and patient. As the word suggests, *co*mmunication requires the active participation of two individuals. Diverging assessments by medical practitioners of whether a specific patient, suspected of being in a PVS is, or is not, conscious are not infrequent.

Finally, PVS has been considered by some to be inconsistent with personhood. This argument as I read it, runs that subject ‘A’ is permanently unconscious; consciousness is the be all and end all of brain activity, therefore ‘A’ is no longer a person; only a neurological clinician can undertake this exercise. The extent to which one buys this argument may depend on the level of cognitive competence one regards as essential for a diagnosis of consciousness. The assessment of a neuroscientist and a patient’s family on this may differ.

CHAPTER 5

SENTIENCE

The term "sentience", which has occupied a central position both in the evolution of the PVS concept and in shaping attitudes towards affected patients, has had different meanings attached to it by different authors. This Chapter will deal with some of the propositions that have been advanced on the issue of sentience in vegetative states and will also consider sources of additional information. The meaning attached to "sentience" will be the ability or capacity to feel or perceive external stimuli that are presented to sensory organs. The issue of capacity for feeling or perception of thirst, an example of sensory information generated entirely *within* the body, will be considered in Chapter 12.

Sentience and consciousness usually coexist, but that coexistence is not synonymous with their being two descriptions of the same phenomenon. Both terms occur frequently in discussion of vegetative states and are often regarded as interchangeable. For instance, Stacy (1992), in opting to use the term "consciousness" to denote the ability to experience sensation, deemed the inability of an unconscious individual to experience sensation to be "true by definition". I believe that the discrete nature of the two terms is best evidenced by the clinical potential for their independent impairment. Thus, depending upon the attributes one regards as essential for consciousness, an individual who is sentient but lacks cognitive capacity may not be regarded as conscious. Alternatively, patients with the most severe manifestations of Guillain Barré syndrome may remain fully conscious although deprived of sensory input from their body. Less drastically, a patient may lose sentient capacity in any single modality, or combination of modalities, without any question of loss of consciousness. Discussion of the management of patients diagnosed as in a PVS commonly attaches different significance to the loss of sentience and of consciousness. Insentience implies that the possibility of patient distress need not be a concern: permanent unconsiousness is often understood to connote loss of personhood.

Reference to loss of sentience usually occurs in the context of pain sensation with relatively infrequent reference to other sensory modalities, an oversight which is at odds with the potential for enlistment of any retained modality in further attempts to detect patient awareness and also in designing positive strategies to enhance any residual capacity for communication. Freeman (1993) has emphasised the counterproductive consequence of any testing for a suspected PVS patient's capacity to perceive unpleasant stimuli, namely that he or she is likely to "shutdown". In contrast with this advice, the approach of Gulbrandsen and Kristiansen (1972) to achieving dishabituation of unconscious patients with loud shouting and shaking (Chapter 4) could not be regarded as consistent with good management.

The issue of pain sensation has dominated much of the discussion of the sentient capacity of individuals in PVS because of its obvious implications for patient management. Incapacity to experience pain has often been expressed in emphatic terms:

> "By the very nature of PVS, patients are not capable of suffering since they are totally unaware of their environment or themselves" (Cranford 1984: 40).

The "definitional" approach to guaranteeing that no PVS patient can experience pain has been used to preserve the integrity of the PVS concept. Any patient who *does* feel pain is, by definition, considered not to be in a PVS, so any question of whether a patient in a PVS could ever feel pain is rendered moot. Some neurologists have pointed out the potential for inaccuracy in the "definitional" approach to excluding sentience on the part of PVS patients. For example, Zeman in a 1997 review article on PVS in the *Lancet* used the heading *Lingering doubt*. He proceeded to ask:

> "Can we be absolutely certain that patients in a vegetative state cannot experience anything?......The oft-repeated answer that these patients are insentient by definition begs the question. We cannot be absolutely certain about the experience of another individual" (Zeman 1997: 798).

A report from the Aspen Workgroup on vegetative and minimally cognitive states in the same year noted that:

> "Patients in PVS are *thought* to be incapable of experiencing pain and suffering" (my emphasis) (Giacino *et al.* 1997: 87).

As with the question of the possibility that an individual can be conscious but in a PVS, the issue of whether a PVS patient can retain a capacity to experience pain will depend upon one's definition of a vegetative state. (Whether a patient is diagnosed as in a vegetative state or in a *persistent* vegetative state should not affect the question of whether pain can be felt *at any specified time*. It may affect that of whether pain is likely to be felt at some future time). If one adopts a definition that precludes pain sensation in a vegetative state, then any patient who retains pain sensation can *not* be in this state, even if this is an enduring diagnosis. Again, as with consciousness, retention of pain sensation in another individual can only be inferred on the basis of an observable response to a noxious stimulus. Lack of response may be attributable to impairment of motor capacity or of its coordination. An observed response is likely to be identical irrespective of whether it is associated with pain or is a reflex without this accompaniment. The individual with an intact nervous system is likely both to display a reflex and feel pain after exposure to a noxious stimulus. His hand, exposed to a flame, will be reflexly withdrawn before the full extent of the pain is experienced. Any patient diagnosed as in a vegetative state by a clinician who considers that this condition excludes capacity to experience pain, is likely to be managed accordingly.

Notwithstanding the preoccupation with pain sensation in the literature, the importance of each of the other sensory modalities for any consideration of PVS should not be overlooked because of the potential they may offer to others for establishing communication with the patient. For example, while the value of vision as a means of receiving external stimuli that could elicit responses is self evident, many of Andrews' series of individuals who had been misdiagnosed as in a PVS had lost their sight (Andrews *et al.* 1996). Communication was dependent on retention of capacity for hearing. Although hearing appears much less likely to be lost as a result of the neuropathological lesions usually associated with PVS, it could be affected in some patients who nevertheless retained function in other sensory modalities. Additionally, people with pre-existing hearing deficiencies are as likely as others with intact hearing to be affected by the trauma and vascular accidents that can lead to risk of misdiagnosis of PVS especially if communication is impaired by the pre-existing condition. The likelihood that a capacity for hearing, and perhaps for listening, may be retained by an undefined number of comatose patients and others who appear to satisfy the specified criteria for PVS, as exemplified in the case of Mark Newton, referred to in Chapter 4 (Cohen 1996), has led a number of authors to stress the importance of care when holding conversations in the patient's presence (La Puma *et al.* 1988). Whilst other sensory modalities, such as those of taste and smell, are not usually tested in determining whether a patient has become completely insentient, both of these have been exploited in attempts to provide sensory stimulation to vegetative patients. Irrespective of which sensory modality is tested, a patient's capacity to respond and so to indicate that some capacity for sentience has been retained, remains dependent on ability to initiate action.

An extreme consequence of inferred insentience, could be that the definition of death was changed so as to include permanent loss of sentience thereby enabling PVS patients to qualify. This proposal is as old as is PVS itself. One writer on the subject observed that there were some strategic advantages in this approach in that it could "settle the definition of death" on grounds that were "independent of moral and legal considerations" (the basis for the latter assertion eludes me) but which responded to the question "Is the patient still among us?" He foresaw some complications to implementing his proposal in that it could be taken for "definitional gerrymandering" and to counter this he anticipated that the "argument for classifying vegetative patients as dead must be made convincing independently of the uses to which it would be put" (Wikler 1988: 44). He suggested that although the *body* of the PVS patient was still alive, the *patient* was not and introduced the analogy of the guillotined individual whose body was no longer the person to support this. Passing over its dualistic implications, the analogy was previously introduced to support the concept of brain death. That the brain of the patient in a PVS indisputably retains considerable neurological activity, whereas that in the isolated guillotined head stacked in the basket does not, and that the patient's brain and body remain integrated in their functioning is a fundamental flaw in the analogy.

5.1 STATEMENTS ON SENTIENCE FROM AUTHORITATIVE SOURCES

> "No conscious experience of pain and suffering is possible without the integrated functioning of the brainstem and cerebral cortex. Pain and suffering are attributes of consciousness, and PVS patients like Brophy do not experience them" (Cranford 1988: 31).

Such a statement from the *Amicus Curiae* brief submitted by the American Academy of Neurology (A.A.N.) in the case *Brophy v New England Sinai Hospital Inc.* hardly admits of any response. The emphasis placed on the A.A.N. statement by Cranford, in citing it, was adequately conveyed by his article's subtitle, *Getting the facts straight.*

Seven years after the Brophy case, when the American Neurological Association (A.N.A.) released *its* definitive statement on PVS intended for exposure to a much wider (and potentially more critical and more medically aware) audience than that likely to fill a Massachusetts courtroom, it ran rather differently:

> "The question as to whether patients in a vegetative state feel pain and undergo suffering may not be resolved scientifically to everyone's complete satisfaction …. postmortem examinations support the belief that they lack awareness of self and surroundings" (American Neurological Association Committee 1993: 387).

As with similar, autopsy-based arguments for the impossibility of any residual awareness, this argument is quite circular. It infers that a specified neurological capacity can be known to have been lost because a sufficient proportion of particular structures within the brain can be demonstrated at autopsy to have been damaged. However, in the case of the sentience of a PVS patient, there is no way of independently determining that this capacity has been lost and so of correlating the extent of loss with the extent of damage, or even with its location. The argument relies on nominating, on an arbitrary basis, both the location and the extent of structural damage required to preclude function and then inferring that sentience *must* have been lost in individual cases on the basis of observation of structural damage of the selected severity and distribution.

The dogmatism of the A.A.N. *Amicus Curiae* brief in the Brophy case was matched by that of a 1990 statement published in its Journal by the American Medical Association (A.M.A.):

> "Pain cannot be experienced by brains that no longer retain neural apparatus for suffering" (American Medical Association Councils 1990: 428).

There are two assumptions implicit in this statement. The first is that the precise nature and extent of those structures in the brain which must be inactivated to eliminate the possibility of pain have been characterised. This requires more than specification of those structures *normally* responsible for pain sensation. Knowledge of alternative structures and pathways which have the potential to take over this function is also required to preclude pain sensation. The difference between knowing which pathways normally transmit sensation and which others can substitute for them is illustrated whenever theoretically adequate neurosurgical procedures such as cordotomy, intended to relieve the pain of malignant conditions, are unsuccessful because of the preservation of alternative pathways. The second assumption implicit in the A.M.A statement is that all patients who are diagnosed as being in a PVS have similarly extensive underlying neuroanatomical lesions which will suffice to inactivate all possible pain mechanisms. One is assumed to be dealing with a pathologically homogeneous condition. Whilst both assumptions remain questionable, the A.M.A. statement has, nonetheless, been regularly cited, for example, by the U.K. Institute of Medical Ethics Working Party on PVS:

> "We agree with the American view that there is no remaining neurological mechanism to make pain or suffering possible" (Institute of Medical Ethics 1991: 97).

Information on the views of neurologists has been provided in a review of PVS by Spudis (1991) published in the *Journal of the Neurological Sciences*, which gave an account of a June 1990 survey of members of the A.N.A. Of several hundred respondents, 44% indicated that they were uncertain about whether PVS patients perceived pain. Presumably, this indicated uncertainty about *what* was actually entailed in PVS rather than uncertainty about whether a well understood condition was being inaccurately diagnosed. A national survey of 250 members of the A.A.N. and 250 from the American Medical Directors Association by Payne *et al.* (1996) sought information about beliefs in relation to PVS patients. Sixty eight percent of the members of the A.A.N. responded. In contrast with the opinions in the A.A.N. statement, 25% of respondents believed that PVS patients could experience feelings of pain. In reporting this outcome, Payne *et al.* noted, that there was a similar prevalence of views on the subject among A.A.N. and non-A.A.N. respondents.

Similar differences between the official A.A.N. and A.M.A. positions and the assessments of a substantial proportion of practitioners have been disclosed in other surveys. For example, a survey conducted for the U.S. Child Neurology Society and released in 1992 indicated that 20% of respondents believed that infants and children in a PVS experienced pain and suffering. Twenty-eight percent of the respondents "always" gave medication for pain whilst a further 14% "frequently" did so and another 33% administered medication "sometimes" (Ashwal *et al.* 1992). A personal description, from a very experienced observer, of responses of PVS patients to potentially painful stimuli was provided by Andrews:

> "Very few patients in the persistent vegetative state are so severely brain damaged that they demonstrate no response, and most respond to pain either by withdrawing or grimacing" (Andrews 1993b: 1601).

Andrews' assessment emphasises that PVS patients do not conform to the stereotype that much of the literature seems to imply, but comprise a clinically heterogeneous group. It also implies that he did not regard complete loss of sentient capacity as an essential requirement for diagnosis of PVS.

Questioning of "authoritative" statements on sentience issued by distinguished groups has tended to evoke rather dogmatic rejoinders. For example, responding in the correspondence pages of the *New England Journal of Medicine* to criticism of the M.S.T.F. report's dismissal of the possibility of pain experience by PVS patients, two members of the M.S.T.F. asserted that:

> "An even smaller minority (of neurologic specialists) continue to maintain that patients in a vegetative state can experience pain or suffering" (Ashwal and Cranford 1994: 1381).

Such an uncompromising claim sits rather uneasily with recent trends towards "evidence based" medicine, not to mention the conflicting assessments of substantial numbers of US neurologists summarised above. In deciding upon the weight to be accorded to surveys of the opinions of different groups, it is necessary to take account of the subject of the survey. Any claim relating to a specific scientific question is either correct or incorrect, irrespective of the opinions of individual scientists on the issue. Those *opinions* carry weight to the extent that they have been based on evidence. In contrast, surveys of the opinions held by neuroscientists about issues that can not be simply resolved on the basis of evidence - for example decisions about the rightness or wrongness of an action – are unlikely to be of more value than the opinions of any other member of the community. Issues of right or wrong can not legitimately be resolved by gauging community opinion.

5.2 ASSESSING SENTIENT STATUS - INDIVIDUAL PATIENTS' EXPERIENCE

. As indicated above, the conclusions drawn by canvassing a large group of the "rank and file" may be substantially different from the opinions expressed on its behalf by the leading, and perhaps more advocatory, members of a profession. Having considered medical opinions based on PVS patients in the preceding section, it is appropriate to compare these with information available about individual patients. Apart from accounts of the sentient capability (or incapability) of PVS patients in general, there have been a limited number of descriptions of individuals. These cannot produce statistically reinforced data, but they certainly provide information about more qualitative aspects. Descriptions tendered in courts have provided some insights. For instance, a 1994 English Court of Appeal case in which the Frenchay NHS Trust defended an appeal against the decision of a lower court that it was not necessary to replace a feeding tube in 'S', a young man in a PVS, brought out some points relevant to sentience. The Master of the Rolls, Sir Thomas Bingham, in delivering the reasons for his decision noted that the nurses caring for S were "gravely distressed" by his condition because they were convinced that, at times, he appeared to suffer (*Frenchay NHS Healthcare Trust v S* 1994). It was noted, additionally, that a neurology professor who had examined S referred to him as appearing to suffer pain. Sir Thomas also observed that S was being maintained "on high doses of sedative drugs" and that a consultant from the Royal Hospital for Neuro-disability who examined him had thought that he would be more comfortable if those dosages were reduced.

Detailed accounts of their experience given by individuals who have been in PVS but have then emerged rarely gain access to the medical literature but have appeared intermittently in the lay press. As emphasised in the preceding Chapter, any account of experience that occurred whilst the individual was diagnosed as unconscious requires, not only that the person actually had some *experience* during that period, but also that he or she is able subsequently to *recollect* that experience. The case of Mark Newton, discussed there and, in particular, his apparently greater access to external input than to his own situation might imply a relatively greater impairment of *self*-awareness than of awareness of his environment (Cohen 1996). Irrespective of the approach adopted, any conclusion about the likelihood that an individual diagnosed as in a PVS could be aware of external stimuli must be based on indirect inferences and be subject to caveats about its interpretation. Ultimately, it may come down to the question of where the onus of proof should lie – with those claiming complete loss of sentience by any patient diagnosed as in a PVS or with those maintaining that some capacity may remain. Descriptions apparently based on information which was acquired whilst unconscious are likely to be dismissed as confabulation if the patient's description is sufficiently at variance with the facts as observed by others.

Recalled experiences of patients who have been clinically unconscious, albeit not in a vegetative state, call into question the assertion that no mental activity was occurring. Accounts of the emotional sequela experienced by patients who have been unconscious for periods of weeks in an emergency medical unit following trauma could provide a guide to the possible experience of some PVS patients notwithstanding the differences in duration of unconsciousness. Such accounts could reflect undetected awareness or "internal" mental activity uninfluenced by external events. Schnaper (1975) provided an account of the recollections of such patients and, without formulating a decision on whether these were internally generated or reflected external events of which patients had some awareness whilst unconscious, emphasised the importance of providing only positive stimuli, in the form of conversation or activities, to unconscious patients. Tresch *et al.* (1991a) sought opinions from PVS patients' families on the subject of patient awareness. Seventy-three percent of families thought that the patient was aware of the presence of family members. Sixty-seven percent believed that the patient could experience pain and 55% said that patients were aware of conversations which took place in their presence. Whilst recognising that sentience cannot be experienced by proxy, it could be argued that the probability that an observer's opinion on the subject of a patient's sentience is accurate will increase as the familiarity of the observer with that patient, and the time spent with the patient, increases. This suggests that the observations of nursing staff and family members could be more valuable than those of medical specialists who may have had relatively limited contact with the patient. The alternative contention is that non-specialist observers do not have the requisite skills to discern what may be happening with the patient and, especially in the case of family members, will be too subjective in their interpretations and may automatically assume that reflex withdrawal from a noxious stimulus always indicates that pain is being experienced. The assessments of specialised medical and paramedical personnel who have spent prolonged periods with unconscious patients after the acute stage may be especially valuable.

The issue of whether comatose patients can hear conversations was addressed in an unusual manner in a 1978 paper which reported on continuous measurement of intracranial pressure in unconscious patients in a neurosurgical ward. There was a "frequent and neatly consistent association" between conversations "about the patient" (compared with "neutral" conversations) and increase in the patient's intra-cranial pressure (Mitchell and Mauss 1978). This association was regularly observed both in alert patients and in others described as comatose. The observations did not lead the authors to question the reliability of diagnosis as comatose. Increased intracranial pressure was also observed in response to potentially painful procedures. The authors concluded that their observations lent credence to the assumption that unconscious patients could process external stimuli long after observable responses were absent.

5.3 ASSESSING SENTIENT STATUS - NEUROANATOMICAL REQUIREMENTS

A possible approach to assessing the sentient capacity of individual PVS patients could be to compare the structural features of their damaged brains with existing knowledge of the normal neuroanatomical requirements for sentience. This approach has been adopted in statements by the A.M.A. and the M.S.T.F. If brain functioning underlying sentience was as well understood as is lung function in gaseous transfer *and* if it were possible to measure the extent to which the structures required for sentient function had been damaged in each individual, as can readily be done for pulmonary function by measuring blood gases, this study would have merit. However, as with the application of a similar approach to consciousness, it is not as helpful for assessing capacity for sentience as might be anticipated. There are several reasons for this. The minimum anatomical requirements for sentience are contested, the location and extent of damage to the brain varies from one PVS patient to another and the capacity to measure those features in the live patient (as distinct from at autopsy) remains incomplete. As noted above, there may be substantial differences between those structures which *normally* mediate pain appreciation and those which *can assume this function* after interruption of the former.

Claims for loss of sentient capacity in all PVS patients based on cortical inactivation depend upon the accuracy of three propositions. The first proposition is that intact function of the cerebral cortex is essential for pain sensation. The second is that it is possible to generalise about the neuropathological features of patients in a PVS. The third is that detailed accurate information about the neuropathological features of any patient can be reliably divined from investigation during life.

Removal of accurately delineated parts of the brain affords a means of differentiating between what is normally involved in sentience and what is essential for it. In addressing the first of the three propositions, observations of patients with well defined brain lesions have implied that cerebral cortical function probably is *not essential* for pain sensation. Extensive study of patients with head wounds, which entailed destruction of different parts of the cortex, did not reveal loss of pain sensation in the corresponding parts of the body (Head and Holmes 1911). Electrical stimulation of many cortical regions in conscious patients undergoing neurosurgery under local anaesthesia (in the 1930s, in experimentation conducted during the course of treatment) consistently failed to elicit reports of painful sensation (Penfield and Boldrey 1937). Pain sensation has persisted on the contralateral side of the body following surgical removal of a cerebral hemisphere (Walker 1942). Proof of the proposition that an intact cortex is necessary for pain sensation will require evidence to disprove the conclusions drawn from these earlier studies. More recently, surgical excision of the cingulate gyrus or cingulum, part of the brain believed to be specifically involved in mediating pain sensation, has been undertaken as a therapeutic measure to relieve intractable pain. The cingulum is part of the limbic system and lies on the inner surface of each hemisphere facing the other hemisphere. Its surgical removal (cingulumotomy) was introduced on the basis that the cingulum is thought to be responsible for bringing pain to the attention of the individual. The cingulum has recently also been incriminated in pain sensation by positron emission tomography (PET) studies. PET activity was detected in the cingulum at the time when normal volunteers reported pain as a result of immersion of a hand in hot water. The activity exceeded the basal record in response to application of heat to the hand at a non-painful level (Jones *et al.* 1991). Cingulumotomy can relieve pain but this relief is often only temporary (Santo *et al.* 1990), presumably reflecting the assumption of this function by other parts of the brain and illustrating the distinction between structures which normally undertake a function and those which *can* do so under abnormal conditions.

The issue of *subcortical* appreciation of pain has been contested. Bernat's review of PVS noted the likely retention of intact pain pathways ascending to the thalamus in patients and also that the possibility of integrating pain experience at the thalamic level had been raised by some neurologists. However, he concluded that:

> "Because it is generally accepted that cerebral cortical integration by thalamocortical connections is a pre-requisite to the conscious appreciation of sensory stimuli, it appears highly unlikely that PVS patients can feel pain" (Bernat 1992b: 180).

A contrary interpretation from another U.S. neurology professor was that:

> "Analysis of the neuroscience of pain leads to the conclusion that pathways sufficient, for the perception and modulation of pain need not arise nor descend to levels generally thought necessary for consciousness" (McQuillen 1991: 383).

This neurologist, Michael McQuillen, also stressed the close correlation, in normal subjects, between the autonomic (sweating and increase in pulse rate) and motor withdrawal responses to noxious stimuli and subjective pain sensation, and inferred that a similar correlation might exist in PVS patients. If elicitation of an involuntary response such as an increased pulse rate is to be accepted as connoting pain in a normal, but not in a PVS, subject, it should be necessary to document a sound basis (independent of the facile reply that the response is associated with pain in the former, but "only a reflex" in the latter) to *explain how* the structures or circuits essential for pain are known to be inoperative in the PVS patient. This would require accurate and comprehensive information on the identity of all structures capable of transmitting pain sensation and on the identity of those structures which had been inactivated in the individual patient.

The anencephalic infant is frequently said to be analogous to the PVS patient in lacking cortical function and is therefore recruited as an additional basis for dismissing the possibility of pain sensation in PVS patients. However, these claims, by groups such as the M.S.T.F., have infrequently been sourced to direct reports from those responsible for the care of anencephalic neonates. In contrast, reports from neonatal specialists, based on their own observation, have attested that anencephalic infants appear to feel pain in a similar manner to intact newborns (Van Assche 1990). Neither normal nor anencephalic neonates are available for interview to recount their respective pain experience. Furthermore, the very limited extent to which normal subjects can recollect neonatal pain experience, at an older age, restricts the extent to which they verify or deny it. Nevertheless, few writers retain the temerity to assert, as once was the case (de Lima *et al.* 1996), that normal neonates are unlikely to feel pain.

Evidence from comparative anatomy and physiology based on non-human species increasingly questions the necessity for a functioning neocortex in order for an animal to experience some painful sensation. Evolution of the forebrain has not entailed its progressive differentiation in successively higher classes of vertebrates. Rather, each class has undergone specialisation of different structures (Sarnat and Netsky 1981) in contrast with other parts of the nervous system in which the progressive refinement of a specific component can be traced through a succession of species. The telencephalon (forebrain) of teleost fish differs considerably from its mammalian equivalent and it is unlikely that any part of the teleost forebrain is a comparable equivalent of the human neocortex. Despite this, the evidence suggests that teleosts such as goldfish can feel pain. Application of a mild electric current to goldfish produces signs of agitation and distress which cease when morphine is added to the water (Jansen and Greene 1970). This morphine analgesia can be reversed in goldfish by naloxone, an agent established as an opiate antagonist in the human nervous system (Ehrensing and Michell 1982). It has also been demonstrated that the capacity of goldfish to learn avoidance of an electric shock is dependent on retention of an intact telencephalon (Overmier and Papini 1986). Taken together, these observations imply that structures with very little resemblance to the human cerebral cortex suffice to mediate experience of some form of pain in other species.

The second and third propositions, identified above as underpinning assertions that PVS patients can not experience pain are that neuropathological features are comparable with each other throughout any series of patients diagnosed as in PVS and that the location and severity of lesions can be accurately measured in living patients. However, as emphasised in Chapter 2 there is considerable variability between the neuropathological features of individual PVS patients, most dramatically illustrated by the failure of the prototype PVS patient, Karen Ann Quinlan, to conform with the preceding generic description of cortical damage. The soundness of the third proposition, namely that the individual's sentient capacity can be deduced from observation of brain lesions, will be discussed in Chapter 6. Claims have been made that techniques such as PET may enable more accurate prediction of patients' functional limitations by measuring metabolic rates in the brain. An associated argument which links the sentient status of PVS patients with that of subjects under general anaesthesia on the basis of PET observations will be examined in Chapter 7.

5.4 ASSESSING SENTIENT STATUS - CLINICAL TESTS

A number of attempts have been made to develop objectively measurable, semi-quantitative assessment tests for sentient capacity in PVS patients. In one test, evoked potentials were measured over the cerebral cortex of PVS patients following the application of a potentially painful electrical stimulus to the body. A fundamental limitation to interpretation of such measurements is the impossibility of determining whether the electrical potential detected over the cortex following a painful peripheral stimulus represents the neuropathological process *responsible* for the actual pain sensation or is only an epiphenomenon that is generated by that stimulus simultaneously with, but *independently of,* the sensation itself. With that qualification, the report of Katayama *et al.* (1991) that cerebral evoked potentials in response to a painful stimulus were increased in PVS patients who had been submitted to deep brain stimulation using implanted electrodes is interesting. Each patient in two groups, one of which had received deep brain stimulation whilst the other served as controls, was subsequently submitted to a painful electrical stimulus applied to a finger and sufficiently strong to produce its reflex withdrawal. Katayama *et al.* suggested, on the basis of the increase in evoked potentials in the group with implanted electrodes, that some of the depression of evoked potentials in response to the application of painful stimuli to PVS patients may be produced by dysfunctional brain activity that is potentially reversible (ibid). Whilst they did not attempt to correlate the extent of increase in response produced by deep brain stimulation with the magnitude of brain damage, it could be suspected that the suggested "*dysfunctional*" group might correspond with those PVS patients found to have less extensive neuropathological changes at autopsy. Interpretation of the findings of Katayama *et al.* would be subject to the limitation that the precise relationship of the evoked potentials to any actual *sensation* on the part of the patient remains unclear. The ethical limitation that one should refrain from the risk of inflicting pain on unconsenting subjects in the course of an experimental procedure is also of concern. A similar concern is raised by a more recent report from Laureys *et al.* (2002) in which strong electrical stimulation, sufficient to cause pain in intact subjects, was applied to a series of non-sedated PVS patients in the course of PET measurement of cerebral metabolism. The activation of thalamus and primary somatosensory cortex, but not of associated cortical regions, was reported.

Another approach to attempting to detect retained sentience in patients in whom conventional clinical neurological testing has failed to achieve this has been to apply semi-quantitative assays based on examination of a wider range of sensory modalities than is usually tested. Modalities such as sensation of smell, hearing, temperature change and vibration have generally been tested much less frequently than sight, touch and pain sensation. In one attempt to achieve this broader testing of sentience, two American rehabilitation practitioners have described a "sensory stimulation assessment measure". Whilst assessing PVS patients by means of the same types of response - eye opening, motor responses and vocalisation - as employed in the established Glasgow Outcome Scale (GOS), they applied a wider range of stimulation to five classes of sensory receptor (Rader and Ellis 1994). This was claimed to be considerably more sensitive than the GOS as a measure of individual clinical change. Subsequently (1997), a "sensory modality assessment and rehabilitation tool" has been developed at the Royal Hospital for Neuro-disability at Putney, by elaboration of an approach originally adopted by Freeman (1996). This test entails the attempted systemic stimulation of seven modalities. It is accompanied by classification of any response to a stimulus into five grades ranging from "no response" to "discriminatory response" (Wilson and Gill-Thwaites 2000).

Yet another possible type of approach to testing PVS patients for sentience has been described by Boyle and Greer (1983) but, to date, tested only on a very limited basis. Boyle and Greer applied operant procedures to several patients in a PVS with the intention of expanding the range of assessment processes available. Requests to patients to undertake specified simple behaviours were followed on each occasion by a reinforcement conditioning procedure, namely the playing, for a short period, of music with which the specific patient had been familiar before entering PVS. This contingent music treatment was observed, by an independent observer, to bring behavioural responses under control in one of the three PVS patients tested.

5.5 RESPONSES OF OTHERS TO THE POSSIBILITY OF RETAINED OR REGAINED SENTIENCE ON THE PART OF A PATIENT IN A PVS

There has been a diversity of response to the recognition of possible sentience in individual patients diagnosed as in a PVS. One response, the accentuation of positive management, has been advocated by rehabilitation practitioners. This approach attempts to "build upon" any indications of sentient capacity to establish procedures for communication between patient and carers with the aim of facilitating communication of the patient's wishes and so improving quality of life. As an alternative response, some have argued that the *retention* of sentience itself becomes a stronger argument than its loss for *ending* the patient's life. For example, Robertson (1991) in an article in the *Georgia Law Review* that discussed the making of non-treatment decisions for incompetent patients concluded:

> "Obviously if the patient was aware of her condition, one could make a strong argument in favour of withholding treatment to prevent her suffering" (ibid: 1159 f/n 84).

Robertson's proposal was that the lives of some patients should be ended not because they have *lost* all sentient capacity but because they have *retained* some. Thus, both loss of sentience and retention of some level are argued to lead to an identical conclusion. Support should be withdrawn because the patient no longer retains a capacity for sentience or because he or she does retain some capacity and so will be appalled by the awfulness of his or her condition.

Robertson's discussion of making decisions on behalf of incompetent patients centred on the case of Nancy Cruzan, a young woman diagnosed as in, or near to, a PVS on whose behalf an application was made to a U.S court in 1990 for withdrawal of hydration and nutrition. In an article on the Cruzan case in the *New England Journal of Medicine*, Angell, noted that Cruzan "would not experience the discomforts of dehydration" (Angell 1990: 1227). Angell buttressed this assessment with a remark attributed to Nancy Cruzan's father to the effect that if she was still aware of pain, then the withdrawal of food and water from her might not generate any more pain than she was already experiencing. While not questioning the father's good intentions, the circumstances which would be associated with their implementation recalls a contemporary publication by a Milwaukee doctor in the *A piece of my mind* series in the *Journal of the American Medical Association*. Its theme was that PVS and Alzheimer's disease patients were vulnerable to mercy killing

> "for the same reason as horses: they cannot object. The patient in a chronic vegetative state .... assumes a vulnerability similar to that of horses: their loved ones, with the best of intentions, can put them to sleep to relieve their suffering, whether or not they want to die" (Goodwin 1991).

5.6 THE USE OF ANALGESIC AGENTS IN MANAGING PVS PATIENTS

A contentious topic related to that of retained sentience is the use of analgesics in managing PVS patients. Administration of drugs for pain relief or mood alteration to any patient totally lacking capacity for sentience appears on first inspection, to be internally contradictory. However, this is not an infrequent occurrence. For instance, the U.K. court hearing in the case of the patient 'S', initiated by the Frenchay NHS Trust to obtain legal endorsement to withdraw food and water, revealed that 'S' was receiving high doses of sedative drugs (*Frenchay Healthcare NHS Trust v* S 1994). Another example was a 1992 report in the *Annals of Neurology* which summarised the logistics of discontinuing the provision of food and water to four children, ranging in age from 5 months to 7 years, who were described as being "hopelessly vegetative". Three of the four children received sedatives, hypnotics and analgesics during the period between cessation of support and death (which occurred from 3 to 10 days afterwards) (Alfonso *et al.* 1992). However, in the case of the fourth child, "a 15-month-old boy with multiple congenital malformations, failure to thrive and severe mental retardation" (ibid: 455), medication was not given to prevent posturing from muscular activity during the course of the dying process, because a juvenile court ruling prevented it. The authors reported that court involvement "hindered the physician's duty to comfort the patient", presumably implying that the infant was regarded as capable of experiencing discomfort, notwithstanding his vegetative status. On the subject of analgesic administration to patients in PVS, it is interesting to note the recently renewed discussion of the merits of providing analgesia to "brain dead" subjects during organ removal. Correspondence on the issue in the journal *Anaesthesia* included the comment that not to provide general anaesthesia to a donor to cover organ removal was "to commit an act of possibly barbarous dishonesty". The writers maintained that:

> "Many anaesthetists clearly have been very uneasy about the transplant lobby's rather rash assumption that organ donors do not require anaesthesia. Many anaesthetists do administer an anaesthetic to these patients" (Wace and Kai 2000).

It may be appropriate to conclude this discussion of sentient capacity in PVS patients by recalling the article by Hoffenberg *et al.* which opened Chapter 1:

> "Indeed if patients in PVS are thought to be sentient or capable of experiencing pain, discomfort or distress either before or after a decision has been taken to withdraw food and fluids, a strong case could be made on humane grounds for routine administration of palliative analgesic or psychotropic therapy" (Hoffenberg *et al.* 1997: 1321).

5.7 RECAPITULATION

There are two reasons for including this Chapter notwithstanding the closeness of its subject matter to that of its predecessor. The first reason is to examine the repeated, adamant assertion that any patient diagnosed as in a PVS lacks all capacity for sensation. The second, following from it, is to consider the background to the claim that procedures such as the withholding of food and water, which would distress sentient individuals would not have any adverse sensory consequences for PVS patients. The first point has commonly been "proven" in the literature on a "definitional" basis, namely that complete loss of sentient capacity has been defined as the central non-attribute of PVS patients. If sentience has been retained, the patient is said not to be in a PVS and so no question of PVS and sentience coexisting in the same individual arises. An alternative response would be to maintain that "true" PVS is not associated with retention of any sensation so that any patient, diagnosed as in a vegetative state, who has pain sensation (perhaps unrecognised) is not actually in that state (even if diagnosis remains unchallenged throughout the course of the case). The second point has buttressed the dismissal of any claims that patients might suffer as a result of withholding food and water.

Assessment of the sentient capacity of one individual by another encounters the same obstacles as identified for consciousness in the preceding Chapter, namely that it can not be done on a foolproof basis. It is of considerable interest that unequivocal statements about the total lack of sentient capacity by patients in a PVS emanating from committees and working parties of professional associations have drawn expressions of substantial dissent from many of the members in addition to being at odds with the outcomes of surveys of members.

In order to dismiss responses of an experimental animal to potentially noxious stimuli as *only reflexes*, it would be necessary to satisfy any institutional animal experimentation ethics committee beyond reasonable doubt that this was so. As withdrawal reflexes could be expected invariably to accompany pain sensation elicited by a noxious stimulus, unless muscular activity was impossible, some *independent* demonstration of the impossibility of inflicting pain would be required. Presumably, the standard of proof required if withdrawal from a noxious stimulus by a patient diagnosed as in a vegetative state is to be confidently dismissed as an accompaniment of pain sensation will depend upon assessment of the gravity of a potential mistake.

A prerequisite for believing that *every* pathway in the nervous system capable of processing pain sensation had been permanently inactivated would be an exhaustive understanding of *which* structures in the nervous system could confer a capacity for pain. I do not accept that the evidence exists to exclude retained capacity for suffering by every patient diagnosed as in a PVS. Underlying this position is an acknowledgement of the manner in which alternative sensory pathways not only exist, but may assume the function of other, disabled pathways after injury to the nervous system. The demonstration that any structure is *essential and irreplaceable* for retention of capacity for pain flies in the face of a host of reports of the transfer of this function to other pathways following therapeutic attempts to ablate pain sensation permanently. A crucial question is that of whether cortical function is not only normally involved in, *but is essential for*, pain sensation.

Discussion of sentience, or its absence, in diagnosing PVS has generally tended to equate "sentience" *per se* with "sentience for noxious stimuli". However, if a more positive approach, encompassing rehabilitation measures, is adopted towards PVS, "sentience" assumes a much more comprehensive meaning than susceptibility to pain. The most thoroughly developed protocols for the rehabilitation of patients after prolonged periods of unresponsiveness utilise all sensory modalities on the assumption that the loss of one or more forms of sentience may, nevertheless, be accompanied by the retention of others which can be used to establish communication. Consequently, a comprehensive assessment of an individual's sentient capacity may permit detection of otherwise unrecognised consciousness.

CHAPTER 6

ELECTROPHYSIOLOGICAL AND IMAGING STUDIES OF PATIENTS IN VEGETATIVE STATES

Several technologically sophisticated types of investigation have been undertaken to support clinical inferences about the vegetative state. This has been done both in attempts to understand the nature of the condition itself and in the course of determining the functional capacity of specific affected individuals. One objective of such investigations, at the earliest stages after the initial brain injury, has been the exclusion of remediable lesions which could be causing or aggravating the patient's condition. A second objective has been to formulate a prognosis, either in relation to the likelihood of *entering* a PVS, when the investigation is undertaken whilst the patient is receiving intensive care, or of *emerging* from PVS when this diagnosis has already been made. Investigations have entailed the use of electrical recordings and of imaging. Finally, all of the available technology has been recruited, at one time or another, as a means of attempting to improve understanding of the pathophysiology of vegetative states. Notwithstanding the original description of a PVS as a set of features to be defined clinically, technology has sometimes been introduced as an ancillary measure to assist in its clinical diagnosis and to reinforce that diagnosis in court. The seductive influence of numerals on either side of a decimal point has been reflected in medicine by a trend to replace subjective forms of patient assessment with tests that deliver quantified results and which rely for measurement on technology rather than the human senses.

The first aim of this Chapter is to examine the historical contribution which electrophysiological and imaging procedures have made to the evolution of the present understanding of PVS. The second is to review the current value of the available tests in explaining the condition. Thirdly, some opportunities for future application of technology to interpreting vegetative states, both in individual patients and in general, will be suggested. Use of the different techniques to be discussed has been separated in time over the last 3 decades as they became available. Application of the most recently developed approaches has been confined to a limited number of centres because of the capital expenditure required to support them. For instance, optimal application of positron emission tomography (PET) ideally requires collocation of a cyclotron to prepare the short-lived isotopes that will be administered to the patient. The individual technologies and their value will be considered separately in this Chapter, more or less in the order in which they have come into use.

The techniques to be reviewed fall into three groups. Electrophysiological investigations can provide some indication of the state of overall function of the nervous system. Structural imaging studies, depending upon the resolution of the equipment used, may indicate the location of a lesion with varying degrees of precision. Functional imaging, a more recent development, can enable the level of metabolic activity in a well defined part of the brain to be observed at the same time as the clinical function that it mediates. In the investigation of most organ systems, it is possible to link *normal* function to *normal* structure in sufficient detail, and with sufficient confidence, to enable inferences about abnormal function to be drawn from knowledge of the abnormal structure. The neuropathological heterogeneity that has been described in PVS may, ultimately, be linked to differences in clinical features if patients diagnosed as in a PVS come to be regarded as representing a group of conditions with differing pathology and course rather than the homogenous clinical state often portrayed in standard descriptions. At present, as it remains a clinically defined condition with variable neuropathology, it is not surprising that electrophysiological and imaging techniques have not assumed a central place in diagnosis of PVS.

6.1 THE ELECTROENCEPHALOGRAM (EEG)

At the time that Jennett and Plum first named PVS, the electroencephalogram (EEG) represented the most advanced technique available for examination of brain function. Their 1972 report noted that there was variability in EEG between PVS patients. They also commented upon the lack of information about the significance of later EEG changes (Jennett and Plum 1972). As the functioning of nerve cells is accompanied by a variety of electrical discharges which can be detected by non-invasive means, measurement of the electrical activity originating in the brain of vegetative state patients and its comparison with that characteristic of a normal brain has been envisaged as a means of discovering more about PVS. The EEG is a record of the electrical activity of the brain recorded from electrodes placed on the patient's scalp. Reference has already been made to the expression "neocortical death", and its synonym "cerebral death" as descriptions of patients in whom permanent loss of function of the cerebral cortex had been inferred, a central predicted feature of which was a persistent isoelectric (flat trace) EEG status. The two cases with isoelectric EEG reported by Brierley *et al.* (1971) as examples of neocortical death were found, at autopsy, to have generalised necrosis of the neocortex. The condition of the brain in the five patients categorised by Pollack and Kellaway (1980), as having sustained "cerebrocortical death", all of whom had isoelectric EEGs, was not described in their report. Whilst these patients conformed to the promulgated notion of PVS as "death of the higher brain", they were unrepresentative of most PVS patients who do not have an isoelectric EEG. As Jennett and Plum originally proposed, the lesion in the brain of a PVS patient could be located in the cortex, the subcortical structures of the hemisphere, the brainstem or in any combination of these. Many subsequent non-medical commentators on vegetative states appear not to have appreciated that destruction of the cortex is not necessarily the fundamental pathological feature. Rather, the defining feature, as nominated originally by Jennett and Plum, was *the failure of the observer to detect clinical indications of consciousness, irrespective of the neuroanatomical basis for this*. It is notable that, as early as 1988, Cranford estimated that the frequency with which electrical activity, could *not* be detected in patients in PVS was likely to be less than 5%.

Correlation between clinical features and EEG recordings could, in principle, be attempted in either of two ways. One approach would be to compare EEG patterns in patients who have sustained increasing degrees of impairment of consciousness with those of a normal control group. Alternatively, EEG data from individual patients at different stages of recovery could be compared with their clinical status at those times. In an example of the second approach, Hansotia (1985), reported a prolonged study of the clinical course of 8 patients in PVS and observed EEGs "that showed a range of patterns that were unchanged from the comatose through to the vegetative state" (ibid: 1048). Any EEG changes that were observed in these patients were not well matched by corresponding changes in the patients' clinical condition. The variability of EEG manifestations that has been observed between patients sharing identical clinical features of PVS has led many neurologists to discount both the diagnostic and the prognostic value of this technology.

In differentiating PVS from brain death using the EEG, Hansotia (1985) noted that absence of EEG activity was understood to characterise the latter. However, the impact of this statement was considerably weakened by a report from Grigg *et al.* (1987) that one fifth of their patients who had been clinically diagnosed as brain dead nevertheless retained EEG activity for a further average period of 36 hours. This observation ran counter to the impression which originally prevailed about electrical activity after brain death. For instance, in differentiating between PVS and brain death in their original paper, Jennett and Plum (1972) had noted that "the EEG is always isoelectric" (ibid: 735) in the latter patients whilst Cranford (1988) in contrasting vegetative states and brain death in his article on *Getting the facts straight* referred to "electrocerebral silence as in brain death" (ibid: 30).

More recent evaluations of the usefulness of the EEG in PVS patients have generally failed to rate it more highly than earlier reports of its variability had suggested. Rothstein *et al.* (1991) did not observe any consistent EEG changes in a prospective study of 40 coma patients. They attributed this outcome to the pathological heterogeneity of PVS. Their conclusion was reiterated by Zeman in a 1997 review. He emphasised that the frequent EEG evidence of continuing cortical activity in patients diagnosed as in a PVS indicated that the clinical diagnosis does not imply cortical silence in these individuals (Zeman 1997).

In contrast to the preceding negative conclusions, a minority of reports have attributed diagnostic value to the EEG in patients suspected of being in a PVS. Hawkes and Bryan-Smith (1974) suggested that the EEG could be valuable in diagnosing the presence of the "locked-in" syndrome (LiS), and so excluding PVS (The term LiS is applied to patients who, although remaining conscious, have severely limited capacity to communicate, typically restricted to eyelid movements).

They recorded a reactive alpha or theta EEG rhythm, said to be consistent with consciousness, in all but one of a series of 7 LiS patients. However, their report did not present EEG data from patients diagnosed as "vegetative" rather than "locked-in" to support the value of the test in discriminating between the two conditions. A reliable distinguishing test for LiS and PVS based on electrical activity in the brain would be of value not only in diagnosis of specific patients but, perhaps, in supporting the discrete nature of the two clinical conditions. If the EEG patterns identified by Hawkes and Bryan-Smith as connoting consciousness in LiS patients are accepted as such, and one operates within a definition of PVS that excludes consciousness, then any reports of the persistence of similar EEG manifestations in patients diagnosed as in PVS should raise some interesting questions.

The EEG has been accepted in court as confirmation of a PVS diagnosis, for example, in a case involving Carrie Coons, the first New York resident to have a right-to-die petition approved on her behalf. In April 1989, the New York Supreme Court upheld an earlier ruling allowing the removal of a gastrostomy tube from Mrs Coons on the grounds that she had been diagnosed as in a PVS. Evidence was tendered in court that both her CT scans and EEG supported the clinical diagnosis of PVS (Steinbock 1989). Six days after the appeal court decision, Mrs Coons unexpectedly regained consciousness and expressed strong reservations about removal of the feeding tube. A request for repetition of the CT scan to confirm the original diagnosis was rejected by Mrs Coons' family.

Another recent instance of advocacy for the use of the EEG (together with neuroimaging procedures) in diagnosing PVS came from one of the most prominent PVS commentators, Ronald Cranford (1996), when criticising the report of Andrews *et al.* (1996) on the frequency of PVS misdiagnosis. Cranford believed that it was unfortunate that Andrews *et al.* had not made use of a range of investigation techniques (EEG, CT, MRI, and PET). In particular, he emphasised his belief that such tests would help to distinguish vegetative states from locked-in syndromes. He also drew attention to the assessments of the U.S. M.S.T.F. and the U.K. Royal College of Physicians' working group on PVS that these tests were of some use in diagnosis.

Apart from study of the EEG as a prognostic aid in PVS patients, its relationship to simultaneous clinical features has been examined. Validation of any correspondence, while it might contribute little to formulation of a prognosis for the individual patient, could assist in understanding the diverse nature of PVS. Attempts to correlate EEG results with the clinical status of individual patients have been directed to both the daily cyclical sleep/arousal pattern characteristic of affected individuals and to changes in levels of the patient's (un)consciousness over longer periods. Raps *et al.* (1991) remarked on the previous absence of any studies of the relationship of EEG to cyclic arousal/sleep patterns when reporting the results of 4 year's continuous collection of video/EEG data from one PVS patient. They identified periods of relative EEG synchronisation and desynchronisation, of which the latter correlated well with times of arousal. A more recent study of parallel EEG and video recordings, albeit over a 24 hour period, produced the surprising result that, of 12 patients deemed to be vegetative, 4 failed to display sleep/wake cycles although otherwise indistinguishable from the remainder (Isono *et al*. 2002). This diagnostically confusing feature was likely to have been a consequence of impairment of the motor innervation of the eyelids.

A thorough study of relationships between clinical status, EEG and CT scans in 15 PVS patients was undertaken over a period of time at Établissements Helio-Marins, a French institution specialising in the care of people in vegetative states. The authors of this report, Danze *et al.* (1989) observed a slight progressive improvement in EEG, with some striking, transient EEG changes sometimes superimposed on this pattern. They also noted the occurrence, in some patients, of prolonged periods during which the EEG remained isoelectric. These periods were followed by the resumption of activity. On the basis of their observations, they queried the frequent assumption that loss of observable *function* can be automatically attributed to and equated with *structural* lesions. This point precisely foreshadowed the point raised by Byrne and Nilges (1993) writing 4 years later in relation to brain death, namely whether cessation of function can automatically be interpreted as destruction of the organ responsible for that function.

To summarise the present position in relation to EEG assessment of PVS patients, there appears to be considerable acceptance of the proposition that the EEG contributes little to diagnosis of the condition and nothing to its prognosis. Nevertheless, refinement of EEG technology may ultimately augment the value of the technology in adding to an understanding of the varieties of pathophysiology that can underlie PVS. One development of EEG technology which has recently undergone trials as a means of monitoring awareness in patients with disordered consciousness (O'Connor *et al*. 1998) and in anaesthetised volunteers (Kearse *et al.* 1998) is bispectral analysis. The bispectral index is computed from examination of the coherence among component EEG waves. Its application to patients diagnosed as being vegetative at different stages of their clinical course, together with clinical correlation, might ultimately provide information not available with existing technology. A recent report describing the application of quantitative EEG analysis, a technique requiring statistical measurement of cross-correlation between two EEG signals, as a possible prognostic aid concluded that it was no better as a prognostic tool applicable to comatose patients than visual assessment of the EEG (Kane *et al.* 1998). In a cautionary comment, the authors observed that outcome was likely to be influenced, not only by the severity of the brain injury, but also by intrinsic patient characteristics and social circumstances.

> "It may not be realistic to attempt prediction of complex psychosocial outcome from early assessments, but this limitation does not alienate its need" (ibid: 249).

6.2 SOMATOSENSORY EVOKED POTENTIALS (SEP)

Somatosensory evoked potentials (SEPs) are records of cerebral electrical potentials elicited in response to the application of various forms of sensory stimulation to the patient's body. The eliciting stimulus may be visual, auditory or tactile. The latter, which is the most likely to be used, consists of stimulation of a nerve in the arm, accompanied by placement of electrodes on the head to detect electrical impulses transmitted to the brain. Recognition of impulses transmitted from the arm to the cerebral cortex in a recording requires the use of techniques to average out background electrical activity which is often of considerably greater amplitude than the potential under examination. SEPs have proved to be more informative than the EEG, particularly in relation to estimating prognosis of patients in a PVS. The hypothesis underlying this test is that the transmission of an electrical impulse from the arm to that location in the cerebral cortex underlying the scalp electrode should indicate that the inward (or afferent) pathway to the cortex is intact. This is especially so if transmission occurs at a normal velocity. Judson *et al.* (1990) reported that the absence of SEPs during the first 4 days after head injury was associated with an "unfavourable outcome" as assessed 6 months later using the Glasgow Outcome Scale (their "unfavourable outcome" group was derived by aggregating the 3 worst classes from the Scale, namely severe disability, PVS and death). On the basis of this finding in a series of 100 patients, they recommended early cessation of intensive care for patients with specified SEP abnormalities while recognising that this decision would result in the abandonment of some patients who could otherwise have had a favourable outcome (falling into the 2 better classes of the Scale, namely moderate disability and recovery). The very large series of patients that would have been statistically required in a study designed to reduce this risk to lower levels was acknowledged but considered to be impractical.

Even leaving aside the question of withdrawing support from some patients who would otherwise have had an outcome assessable as "favourable" using the Glasgow Outcome Scale, I believe the breakdown of the series of Judson *et al.* raises serious concerns both on account of the crude nature of the aggregation of patients into the "unfavourable" group and especially because of the insensitivity of the unmodified Outcome Scale itself. Thus, of the 45 whose outcome was classified as "unfavourable", 36 had died, 2 were in a PVS and 7 remained "severely disabled" at 6 months. However, the discrimination between "moderate" and "severe" disability on the Glasgow Outcome Scale rests on the distinction between a person's capacity to live independently, albeit requiring some assistance, and dependency on others for the activities of daily living of a patient who is, nevertheless, cognisant. Acceptance of the proposal of Judson *et al.* for early withdrawal of support from that group of patients who would otherwise have been scored as "severely disabled" after 6 months, if support had continued, requires two assumptions. First, that the potential of any rehabilitation process, applicable to a patient who has regained consciousness after cerebral trauma, has been exhausted by 6 months. Second, that the standard (or quality) of the existence of this group of individuals is not such as to justify expenditure of societal resources. I consider that the experience of skilled neurorehabilitation specialists gives the lie to the first whilst the expressed opinions of severely disabled people (a few of which will be discussed in Chapter 10) call the second into question.

A similar approach to that adopted by Judson *et al.*, namely aggregating death, PVS and severe disability together as unfavourable outcomes, was utilised by Beca *et al.* (1995) in a study correlating SEPs with the consequences of severe traumatic brain injury in children. The practice of aggregating 3 classes of the Glasgow Outcome Scale to produce the "unfavourable" group precluded the identification of the relative frequency of occurrence of each class among children with early absence of an SEP. However the total series of children (not separated on the basis of SEP measurement) with "unfavourable" outcome consisted of 37 who died, 9 diagnosed as in a PVS at 6 months and 13 who were severely disabled (described as "conscious but severely disabled and dependent"). As with the series of Judson *et al.*, the numerically largest subgroup in those with "unfavourable" outcome as assessed at 6 months had died by that time despite receiving the best available treatment whilst, of the survivors, the severely disabled subgroup outnumbered those in a PVS at 6 months.

Whereas the data of Judson *et al.* (1990) was derived from the study of SEPs in patients with traumatic brain injury, Rothstein *et al.* (1991) described the clinical course of 40 patients who had lapsed into coma after cardiac arrest. They found that the continued absence of any record of an SEP over the cerebral cortex following stimulation of the median nerve (in the arm) was the most useful guide in predicting an unfavorable outcome. However, they cautioned that SEPs were only able to provide information about the functional status of part of the cortex. Consequently, the absence of an SEP over that part of the cortex which has been examined may not necessarily indicate a similar absence of the capacity to receive input over the *entire* cortex.

A series of 34 patients in non-traumatic coma were studied by Chen *et al.* (1996) who concluded that SEPs combined with the EEG and clinical examination provided reliable prognostic data. A noticeable difference from the "traumatic" series of Judson *et al.* was the absence of any severely disabled patients from this series (25 deaths, 2 PVS, 7 good recovery). The nature of the patients studied may have explained this difference, no other reason being readily apparent.

Whereas the detection of abnormal SEPs has generally been found to provide a strong indication of an "unfavourable" outcome, the retention by a patient of SEPs that are only mildly abnormal has proved to be less reliable as a predictor of a "favourable" outcome. In an attempt to develop a better test capable of predicting favourable outcomes, Guerit *et al.* (1999) measured potentials following the input of an auditory stimulus. They reported that the presence of these "event related potentials" implied a good prognosis whereas no conclusion could be drawn from their absence. Demonstration of a statistically significant correlation between SEP and the outcome after non-traumatic brain injury (for example, vascular accidents) was reported more recently by Haupt *et al.* (2000) together with a review of a number of earlier studies with similar outcomes. They drew attention to the value of undertaking measurement of brainstem auditory evoked potentials (BAEPs) in addition to SEPs on the basis that the combination of measurement of two independent activities provided a better insight into surviving brain function.

The assessment of clinical outcomes for correlation with SEPs in studies cited above have been based upon the Glasgow Outcome Scale with simplification into only two outcomes, favourable or unfavourable. The Scale provides little information about cognitive outcomes, and so any correlations of these with electrical recordings taken at an early stage are impracticable. A study in which cognitive outcomes were specifically examined, in addition to motor functions, has raised the question of whether SEPs provide any valid prognostic indication of cognitive recovery. Ozbudak-Demir *et al.* (1999) found SEPs to have no predictive power in relation to cognition. They suggested that long-latency SEPs might reflect cortical integration processes better than the sensory input to specific regions of the cortex reflected by short-latency SEPs (that is, responses detected very soon after application of the stimulus).

Munglani *et al.* (1993) reported on tests for correlation between auditory evoked potentials and cognition using normal subjects who had not sustained brain injuries. In view of the limitations to accurate detection and measurement of cognition necessary to validate correlations in patients with impaired consciousness, they adopted a different approach to develop a quantifiable technique which accurately reflected cognition. Munglani *et al.* sought correlations in anaesthetised normal subjects (volunteering anaesthetist colleagues of the experimenters) rather than in patient's with pathological impairment of consciousness and found that, as the subjects inhaled increasing concentrations of the anaesthetic isoflurane, interference with cognition (as assessed by performance in psychological tests) correlated well with decrease in the measured auditory evoked response to standard noise stimuli. While their results do not appear to have influenced assessment of patients in a PVS, a number of subsequent studies of *normal* individuals under general anaesthesia have strengthened the suspicion that auditory evoked potentials may provide information on the possibility of perceptual processing.

A review of the entire literature on prognosis of both traumatic and non-traumatic (anoxic) coma, including the use of EEG and SEPs and employing an "evidence-based" approach, was prepared by Attia and Cook (1998). In the first instance, these authors nominated the need for a reliable "understanding of the natural non-traumatic (anoxic) history of comatose patients and their possibility of recovery" (ibid: 497) Attia and Cook emphasised several general caveats affecting interpretation of studies of coma. The first was the impact of a self-fulfilling prophesy, namely that, in response to a pessimistic outlook, intensive care had been withdrawn or scaled down earlier in particular groups of comatose patients leading to reduced recovery rates. Thus, an unusually high recovery rate in one study corresponded with a protocol that required all patients to receive full life support for at least 3 days. Second, the effect of observer variability in assessing clinical signs could be a potentially confounding factor together with the variable rate of early death from brain injury or unrelated causes. Finally, cumulative mortality from all causes had eroded the statistical power of any prognostic conclusions because of reduction in size of the study group. In assessing more technique-specific impediments to formulating prognoses from electrical monitoring, Attia and Cook (1998) considered the EEG to be inadequate. While favouring usage of SEPs, they advocated deferring prognostication until the third day by which time "approximately half of those patients with no chance of ultimate recovery have died" (ibid: 504). In reviewing patients who were in coma following trauma, Attia and Cook concluded that the EEG and SEPs were more useful than clinical examination.

6.3 IMAGING OF THE BRAIN

Neuroimaging techniques are being refined at a rapid rate and offer the prospect of providing new insights into brain function. Their attraction for investigation of PVS lies in the possibility that they may permit an objective assessment of the state of awareness or consciousness of "vegetative" individuals and supplement clinical judgement. To this end there has been a strong and increasing tendency to assign correlations between a particular level of consciousness and a specified reading on an instrumental recording. For example, writing on coma in the journal *Neuropsychological Rehabilitation*, Jennett (1993a) cited the conclusion from a PET study that the degree of cerebral metabolic hypoactivity recorded in a small group of PVS patients

> "supports the clinical evidence that cerebral cognitive function is lost in the vegetative state, leaving a body that can no longer think or experience pain" (ibid: 101).

There have been declarations that, if a patient scores below a certain level for the test, any consciousness or self-awareness is impossible. However, the assigned minimal test values that are considered to be inconsistent with any possibility of retention of consciousness invariably appear to have been arbitrarily selected. Before any imaging technique can be interpreted accurately to reflect an individual's state of awareness, it would be essential to make allowance for the influence of co-existing neurological deficits. The simplest way in which to allow for the effects of accompanying neurological damage would be to compare results obtained from "vegetative" patients with results from matched "control" patients who, although conscious and aware, manifest all of the *other* neurological deficits of comparable severity to those of the "vegetative" patients.

Of the imaging techniques applicable to PVS patients, computed tomography (CT) has probably been the subject of the greatest number of published reports although its use in neuroimaging is, more recently, being replaced by magnetic resonance imaging (MRI). Measurement of blood flow to specific cerebral regions has had a limited application in both brain death and PVS. Positron emission tomography (PET) has been adopted as a means of measuring the level of metabolism in specific locations in the brain. Although the number of published reports of its application to PVS patients remains relatively small, having increased to only a modest extent since its initial use, it has had a very substantial influence in shaping attitudes towards patients diagnosed as being in a PVS.

6.4 STRUCTURAL IMAGING: COMPUTED TOMOGRAPHY (CT) SCANNING

The usefulness of tomography, a pre-existing technique for obtaining X-ray images of slices through the body, was greatly enhanced in the 1970s by its computerisation. This refinement made it possible to undertake a complete CT examination through the brain in a relatively short time. The results obtainable using CT have often been regarded as having sufficient value in the diagnosis of vegetative states to merit their citation in court cases to decide on the management of specific patients. Reading of the series of decisions in the 1993 landmark U.K. case of *Airedale NHS Trust v Bland* implies that they were substantially influenced by information provided from CT scans of the patient. Lord Goff's perception of the neuropathology of Tony Bland's brain is best conveyed in his own words from a lecture delivered shortly after the judgement reflecting the impact of the CT evidence presented during the hearing:

> "This condition (PVS) can be, and in the case of Anthony was, physically demonstrated, because the space which the cortex of his brain should have occupied was filled with watery fluid" (Goff 1995: 8).

Consistent with this perception from the bench, contemporary media accounts of the case were said to have included the claim, attributed to a medical witness, that Tony Bland's brain was now liquefied (Jarmulowicz 1995). Lord Goff appeared to accept two evidentiary points as factual. He believed both that an objective diagnostic measure for PVS existed (namely CT scans) and also that Tony Bland had tested positive using this diagnostic measure. As a postscript, post mortem examination of his brain revealed atrophy (1007gms) and "extensive and severe anoxic brain damage" distributed irregularly through most regions but *not* the replacement of his cerebral cortex by liquid (ibid).

A well publicised case in which CT findings were accepted by a court as supporting a diagnosis of PVS was that of Carrie Coons who, as mentioned above, regained consciousness shortly afterwards, thereby bringing an abrupt halt to the court's proceedings to withdraw food and water from her (Steinbock 1989). This has not been the sole instance in which CT confirmation of a clinical diagnosis of PVS has come to grief. A 1990 Israeli report comprehensively documented the case of a 60 year old man who recovered and returned to work as a university professor after being in a vegetative state for at least 8 weeks following an episode of cerebral hypoxia. By the time of submission of the report to a journal (4 years post-vegetative state), he had completed two books, written several articles, participated in international speaking engagements and completed a teaching sabbatical at a major U.S. university (Falk 1990). The interest of this Israeli case for imaging technology lies in the extremely well documented results of CT scanning which "revealed generalized cerebral atrophy" that had progressed since his first examination. Another very adequately documented case in which recovery of consciousness (albeit with persisting severe neurological limitations) occurred in an 18 year old woman despite CT evidence of generalised cerebral and cerebellar atrophy was reported by Childs and Mercer (1996a).

An indispensable consideration with *any* quantifiable, objective procedure (be it EEG, CT or PET) if it is to be employed to substantiate a clinical diagnosis of PVS, is that the original validation of the technique has demonstrated a good correlation with the clinical diagnosis. Otherwise any interpretation of the data must remain highly dubious, irrespective of the intrinsic elegance of the technology. However, as the accuracy of clinical diagnosis of PVS has been emphatically called into question in a number of instances, most notably in a 1996 British report which cited a misdiagnosis rate in excess of 40% (Andrews *et al.* 1996), one could justifiably remain circumspect about the feasibility of validating such clinical-technical correlations. The reliability of any correlation will be only as good as the accuracy of determination of conscious status of the patients studied to derive that correlation. Nevertheless, it has repeatedly been the case that clinical observation and CT scan (or other technology) are jointly presented in the same paragraph to bolster the interpretation placed on the other.

6.5 CT INDICATIONS OF BRAIN ATROPHY IN NEUROLOGICALLY INTACT SUBJECTS WITH ANOREXIA NERVOSA

Apart from reports of brain atrophy in CT scans of PVS patients, there exists a very substantial medical literature describing the presence of similar CT changes in other individuals who are fully conscious and who are, for all intents and purposes, as neurologically intact as the researchers reporting on their medical condition. This other group comprises patients who have sustained substantial loss of body weight as a consequence of the condition of anorexia nervosa. The only article that appears to have specifically drawn attention to the possible significance of CT-diagnosed atrophy in anorexia nervosa for interpretation of brain atrophy in PVS has been a paper from Byrne *et al.* (1997). After commenting upon the atrophy of Karen Ann Quinlan's brain, they drew attention to her severe cachexia and questioned whether the mechanism responsible for CT-detected brain atrophy in people with anorexia nervosa could have exacerbated her CT abnormalities. In raising this issue they were questioning the *direction* of causality in the association between brain atrophy and bodily cachexia. To what extent could starvation as a result of inadequate attention to nutrition, as evidenced by the emaciated condition of Quinlan and Bland, *have been responsible for contributing to* atrophy of the brain? Before considering the possible significance of repeated CT indications of brain atrophy in individuals subject to anorexia nervosa, the lack of reference to this detail in any of the guidelines and authoritative statements on PVS reviewed in Chapter 3 should be noted. Perhaps this is an example of the compartmentalisation of medical knowledge.

The best documented evidence of the impact of subnutrition on the brain comes from developmental studies. Reports of the depressive effect of malnutrition on the proliferation of neurones, and on increase in brain mass in malnourished children in Central and South America, had entered the literature by the 1970s (Winick 1974).

Whilst the relevance of subnutritional interference with brain growth to recovery from brain injury was dismissed out of hand when it was believed that any precursors of neurones capable of multiplication were lacking from the postnatal brain, it has been established beyond doubt in the late 1990s that such precursors *are* present and that regeneration of neurones can occur in *adult* brains after injury. Recent reports of the spontaneous division of neurones in the *adult* human brain, together with the identification of stem cells in adult mouse brain (Reynolds and Weiss 1992; Lowenstein and Parent 1999), render it likely that cell multiplication in a damaged brain could be curtailed by inadequate nutrition. Recognition of stem cells in adult brains inevitably raises questions about the relative inattention to the effects of inadequate nutrition during the long term management of patients with brain injuries. This inattention is especially interesting in view of the well documented increased metabolic requirements following brain injury and the retarding effect of inadequate nutrition on neuronal growth. As already noted, the latter was described in a 1974 review of the impact of starvation on growth of the brain published in a volume edited by Fred Plum (Winick 1974). In this review Winick noted that brain weights, and numbers of brain cells, were significantly reduced in infants dying of severe malnutrition in the first two years of life. The rate of brain cell division was most severely reduced in the cerebrum of malnourished children.

Atrophic changes in the brains of patients with severe anorexia nervosa have been repeatedly observed on CT scans since the late 1970s. The summary which follows does not purport to be a comprehensive account of the literature describing CT-detectable atrophy of the brain in neurologically intact, anorectic individuals, but it is presented to indicate the multiplicity, and persistent reappearance, of reports on this subject. The paper of Enzmann and Lane (1977) which may be the earliest report of CT changes in the brain of patients with anorexia nervosa, opened with the observation that this was an uncommon disease unfamiliar to most radiologists. It described abnormal enlargement of the cortical sulci (the small crevices over the cortical surface) in 3 out of 4 anorectic patients compared with an age-matched control group. Two of the affected patients had been dieting for 8 months at the time of examination, whilst the other had been doing so for 5 years. Reference was made to 3 earlier reports on changes in the brain of anorexia nervosa patients demonstrated by means other than CT. Two of these earlier papers described the pathological changes observed at autopsy in the brains of patients suffering from malnutrition and anorexia nervosa while the third was a German report of enlargement of sulci and ventricles demonstrated during life by means of pneumoencephalography in a patient with anorexia nervosa. Of these 3 articles, only one was published in English and that was in a nutrition journal, perhaps as inaccessible to a highly specialised neurological readership as an article in a foreign language. Another report, published in the same year as that of Enzmann and Lane extended the scope of their article with its description of the reversibility of CT-diagnosed cerebral atrophy in a successfully treated 15 year old patient with anorexia nervosa following body weight gain from 30 to 45kg (Heinz *et al.* 1977). Ventricular dilatation was initially present in the CT scan of this patient in addition to widening of the sulci. It was suggested that correction of the metabolic abnormalities had been responsible for reversal of radiologically diagnosed cerebral atrophy. The authors emphasised the prognostic implications of their findings and raised the possibility that similar patients might be mistakenly labelled as having sustained permanent cerebral atrophy.

A CT study of a series of 14 patients with anorexia nervosa was reported in 1980. Seven of these people had cortical atrophy and/or ventricular dilatation (Nussbaum *et al.* 1980). All except 2 of these patients remained neurologically normal on clinical examination. The severity of weight loss correlated with changes in brain scans. Whereas the 7 patients who retained normal CT scans had sustained an average body weight loss of 22.1%, those with cerebral atrophy had lost an average of 35.2% (ranging up to a maximum of 65.5%). Follow up CT examination of 2 patients who subsequently regained body weight revealed improvement of CT scan appearance in only one. Another patient with anorexia nervosa underwent reversal of generalised CT cerebral and cerebellar atrophy over the course of 3 months as weight returned to normal (Sein *et al.* 1981). As an indication of the frequency of reversal of CT-indicated cerebral atrophy following recovery of normal weight, 21 patients in a group of 23 with anorexia nervosa had cerebral atrophy when first examined by CT whilst 7 out of 11 of these patients, re-examined 4 weeks after regaining normal weight had achieved marked reversal of the earlier changes (Kohlmeyer *et al.* 1983). In another series, reversal of cerebral changes seemed to require at least 2 months, irrespective of the occurrence of more rapid body weight gain (Artmann *et al.* 1985).

Whilst earlier observations of cerebral atrophy in anorexia nervosa had been qualitative or at best semi-quantitative, a report from Datlof *et al.* (1986) dealt with *quantitative* measurement of ventricular dilatation and demonstrated statistically significant differences between patients and age-and sex-matched control subjects. As an indication of the extent of atrophy in the brains of the anorectic patients (accompanied by a corresponding enlargement of the ventricles), the CT-assessed areas of the third ventricle in the matched control subjects ranged from 21% to 50% (mean 39%) of the ventricle area in the corresponding anorectic patient. This expansion in the size of the ventricular cavity corresponded to reduction in the area occupied by brain tissue in the CT scan. Each anorectic subject in this study had lost at least 30% of his/her original body weight.

Whereas Datlof *et al.* attributed cerebral changes to malnourishment, a novel proposal came from another study of three groups, namely 50 subjects with anorexia nervosa, 50 with bulimia and 50 age-matched controls. In this study, Kreig *et al.* (1988) observed cerebral atrophic changes in the CT scans of some bulimic patients, albeit of less severity and at a lower frequency than in the anorectic patients. As the bulimic patients were of normal weight, Krieg *et al.* reasoned that their observed cerebral atrophy could not be attributed to bodily emaciation. An alternative explanation was that atrophy might reflect endocrine and metabolic reactions to starvation, irrespective of whether this had led to weight loss as in the anorectic patients or had been imposed by restriction of food intake (with retention of normal body weight) as in the bulimic group who had been placed on diets as part of their treatment.

The repeated detection of cerebral atrophy in CT scans of anorexia nervosa patients should raise at least two questions in relation to PVS. First, it places the onus on anyone proposing that the atrophy which occurs in any PVS patient has *not* been aggravated by inadequate nutrition to prove that proposition. It emphasises the potential importance of improved nutritional status if any benefit is to be obtained from the capacity, recently demonstrated, for regeneration in the adult brain. Secondly, the deference traditionally paid to CT scans in court hearings to determine whether specified individuals were in a PVS should be questioned, given the extreme wasting of Quinlan and Bland. Tony Bland's body weighed 36kg at the time of death some four years after he sustained his injuries. Karen Ann Quinlan's body weight was 27kg.

CT scanning of the brain has not been accorded substantial weight in formal guidelines or statements on the diagnosis of PVS. The M.S.T.F. statement, for instance, noted the lack of established correlations between neuroimaging and development of the vegetative state but remarked that "most patients who do not recover consciousness have abnormal scans" (M.S.T.F. 1994a: 1506). CT scanning has, nevertheless, been presented to support lack of cognitive capacity in PVS individuals. Cranford and Smith's (1987) assessment of the specific value of CT scans is of interest:

> "Until recently, the diagnosis of the vegetative state was entirely clinical: there were no useful laboratory studies available. This has now changed somewhat with the use of CAT and MRI scans. These radiologic studies show massive structural damage to the cerebral hemispheres in the PVS patient and help to confirm the clinical findings" (ibid: 240).

Seven of the 8 reports of CT-detected cerebral atrophy in anorexia nervosa noted above had appeared by the time of this article. Six years later, Bryan Jennett (1993b) reported the (unreferenced) data that, 5 months after brain injury resulting from trauma or interruption of blood supply,

> "10-20% of brain substance has been lost and after 3 years 35%, representing 400gm or more of brain substance has been lost...Evidence of this degeneration can be provided in life by radiological imaging using CT scanning or MRI; these show progressive enlargement of the fluid-filled ventricles and spaces on the surface of the brain" (ibid: 40).

It may be relevant to note that the two preceding quotations were extracted from periodicals dealing respectively with the interfaces of medicine with law and with ethics rather than from publications directed to audiences likely to have more familiarity with technical detail.

6.6 FUNCTIONAL IMAGING: CEREBRAL BLOOD FLOW

As PVS has been characterised on the basis of functional deficits resulting from a variety of structural abnormalities, tests of *function* may be more specific in detecting it than techniques, such as CT scanning, which exclusively detect structural variation. One of the first functional tests applied to examination of patients in a PVS was the estimation of cerebral blood flow. The rate of blood flow through any specific region in the brain has generally been regarded as providing an accurate, albeit an indirect, indication of the current metabolic activity of that part of the brain because of the very rapid increase in blood flow that is observed to follow increased activity of a region.

Cerebral blood flow is assumed to parallel cerebral metabolism with sufficient accuracy that both may be subdivided into two categories. A certain "basal" level of metabolism, and corresponding blood flow, required to maintain the structural integrity of nervous tissue reflects the requirement for a cell to maintain a specific ion balance across its bounding membrane. This basal activity represents the sum of the metabolic activity of both neurones and supporting (glial) cells. Any additional activity, beyond this "maintenance" level will require an increase in both metabolism and blood flow. Measurement of the level of blood flow in the cerebral hemispheres has been undertaken in investigation of brain death and vegetative states, among other conditions.

Correlation between clinical status and cerebral blood flow has been examined in brain dead subjects with suggestions of less than complete correspondence. Thus, whilst blood flow to the cerebral hemispheres has usually been reported to be greatly reduced or undetectable, within the limits of the technique, in individuals diagnosed clinically as being brain dead (Korein *et al.* 1977), the continuation of a detectable level of cerebral circulation has been reported for as long as two days after the attainment of all requirements for a diagnosis of brain death (Fackler and Rogers 1987). The mandatory use of radiological confirmation of cessation of cerebral blood flow has been proposed by a Swedish committee as a confirmatory test for brain death if organs are to be removed from a patient for transplantation, (Swedish Committee on Defining Death 1984). However, this was emphatically rejected by a leading English proponent of brain death lest it give rise to the impression that a greater degree of certainty is required when diagnosing brain death if organ removal for transplantation is envisaged than when further use of the body is not contemplated (Pallis 1985).

Cerebral blood flow in patients diagnosed as in a vegetative state has been measured on a number of occasions. A very substantial reduction in cerebral blood flow might be anticipated in these patients by comparison with normal individuals because of brain atrophy. Blood flow and metabolism should be reduced close to the basal level associated with maintenance of intact, but not functioning, neurones and glial cells in severely damaged regions. Cerebral blood flow in normal individuals has been compared with that of patients in a PVS in attempts to correlate it with both the clinical status and the subsequent progress of the latter group of patients. For instance, a 1989 Japanese study used single photon emission computed tomography (SPECT) after the intravenous infusion of isotopes of either iodine or technetium and compared 5 normal volunteers (radiologists and neurologists) with 5 patients clinically diagnosed as being in a vegetative state, one individual with a locked-in syndrome and 2 comatose patients. Cerebral blood flow in the vegetative state patients, while variable from one to another, fell within the normal limits as established by the control group of volunteer medical specialists (Sato *et al.* 1989). Mean blood flow rate for right and left temporal, parietal and occipital cortices in the 2 vegetative state patients with the highest rates exceeded this rate in all 5 of the volunteer neurologists/radiologists whilst this flow rate in 3 of the 5 patients exceeded that of the volunteer with the lowest reading. The person in a locked-in state had an increased blood flow to the frontal lobe, whilst flow to this region was significantly reduced in the 2 comatose patients, in comparison with the values in normal control subjects.

Not only have cerebral blood flow rates in normal and vegetative patients overlapped, but there has been at least one report of cerebral blood flow *in excess* of normal levels in an individual meeting the clinical criteria for a diagnosis of PVS (Agardh *et al.* 1983). This patient, in whom brain damage had followed a hypoglycaemic episode, also retained a response of increased cerebral blood flow after arousing stimuli. To explain this, Agardh *et al.* (1983) suggested that isolated, preserved cortical tissue devoid of connections with neurones outside the cortex had retained its blood supply. Whilst very few cases of vegetative state result from hypoglycaemia, the concurrence of the clinical features of PVS with retention of normal cerebral blood flow does not fit well within conventional explanations of the basis of PVS. A longitudinal study in individual patients diagnosed as vegetative would be required if variations in cerebral blood flow were to be correlated with clinical features. Nevertheless, if differences observed between comatose patients and others diagnosed as being in a vegetative state (Sato *et al.* 1989), were confirmed with a larger group of patients, this could raise the possibility of significant changes in cerebral function accompanying the transition from coma to vegetative state. Examination of the correlation between clinical status and cerebral blood flow was undertaken in 23 patients treated experimentally with electrical stimulation of the dorsal column of the spinal cord. Eight of these patients, the CT scans of whom had been almost normal previously, showed clinical improvement accompanied by an increase in cerebral blood flow which was not statistically significant (Kanno *et al.* 1989).

Cerebral blood flow has been used as a surrogate for metabolism in studies of the type discussed above. However, attempts to validate this use have produced equivocal results. In a study of 33 normal individuals the two measurements correlated well with each other when the subjects were resting but sensory stimulation resulted in uncoupling with the increase in cerebral blood flow greatly exceeding the local increase in metabolic rate (Fox and Raichle 1986). Failure of blood flow and metabolism to remain correlated in this study of *normal* subjects in response to physiological changes inevitably calls into question the validity of extrapolating from cerebral blood flow to infer the level of metabolic activity of the brain of individuals in a PVS.

6.7 FUNCTIONAL IMAGING: MAGNETIC RESONANCE

Whilst magnetic resonance imaging (MRI) has largely replaced CT scanning as a technique for visualising brain structure, functional MRI (fMRI) is being developed as a technique for examining brain activation patterns. When used for structural imaging, MRI has been reported to have prognostic value in PVS. For example, MRI studies on a series of patients during the second month after traumatic brain injury revealed that lesions in the corpus callosum (the structure linking the two cerebral hemispheres) and brainstem were statistically associated with subsequent failure to emerge from a vegetative state, although the frequency of corpus callosum lesions in patients who recovered (24%) was sufficiently high to preclude use of MRI on its own as a reliable predictor of PVS (Kampfl *et al.* 1998).

Functional MRI has the capacity to permit observation of metabolism in specific regions of the cerebral hemispheres during cognitive activities and, for this reason, has the potential to be used in detecting such activities in patients in vegetative states. In an example of this application Ricci and co-workers from Bologna examined 4 vegetative patients before and after they had regained consciousness (Ricci *et al.* 1997). The relative concentrations of several metabolites in the cerebral cortex differed from normal and ratios changed during return of consciousness, but the nature of these changes varied from patient to patient without any consistent pattern. A relatively recent refinement in which MRI has been used in combination with diffusion tensor imaging may be of special value in identifying damage to tracts passing from the cortex through the white matter (Werring *et al.* 1998).

6.8 FUNCTIONAL IMAGING: POSITRON EMISSION TOMOGRAPHY (PET): THE FIRST STUDY OF PATIENTS IN A PVS

The PET technique has been used to measure the cerebral metabolic rate of glucose by means of detection of the positrons emitted during the decay of a radioactively labelled analogue of glucose in the brain of a patient into whom this analogue has been injected intravenously. Scanning can reveal the extent to which different regions have taken up the glucose analogue and, inferentially, the level of metabolism of glucose by the tissue of that region. As the resolution of the scanning technique improves, it may be possible to measure the level of activity within very small structures in the brain.

The first reported application of PET to patients diagnosed as being in a vegetative state was that of Levy *et al.* (1987). Levy *et al.* sought to develop an objective measure of brain function, which could supplement clinical observation and inferences drawn from pathological examination as to "whether or not all self-awareness was lost during life" (ibid: 673). In recognition of the impact it has had, especially in supporting clinically based inferences about PVS, I will examine it in detail before considering more recent reports on the same subject. Two conclusions drawn from this original article on PET examination of PVS patients require challenge. In the first place, as has been discussed in Chapter 4, the question of whether *self* awareness is retained or lost remains quite separate from that of whether some level of consciousness has been retained: consciousness does not require one to be continually self aware. Secondly, any independent scientific basis to validate a quantitative association between the level of metabolism and the level of consciousness is lacking. How is one to determine whether some objectively measurable phenomenon actually *corresponds* with the biological event responsible for consciousness or merely represents some other linked, but potentially dissociable, process? How is one to establish that reduction in the selected, measurable parameter below some specified level reliably indicates loss of consciousness, as distinct from loss of those *signs* of consciousness that are observable by another person? Even more relevant may be reliable data indicating what level of metabolic reduction ensures that the capacity to *regain* consciousness has been permanently extinguished. It has been hypothesised by Astrup (1982) that a certain level of brain metabolism is required to maintain the viability of neurones that is, as proposed above, to ensure preservation of ion exchange across the cell membrane which is necessary to maintain its integrity while an increase above this level is associated with neuronal activity.

Levy *et al.* examined a total of 7 patients diagnosed as vegetative and 3 others with the locked-in syndrome (LiS). They reported that the mean metabolic rate for glucose had been reduced to less than half of its normal value in the vegetative state patients (2.73 versus 6.82 mg of glucose/100gm of tissue/min. in 18 normal control subjects). In the 3 LiS patients, there was only a 25% reduction in cerebral glucose metabolism (to 5.08mg/100gm/min.). These results were interpreted by Levy *et al.* (1987) as supporting

> "clinical evidence that cerebral cognitive function is lost in the vegetative state, leaving a body that can no longer think or experience pain" (ibid: 673),

a conclusion which has been extensively reiterated in most subsequent reviews and statements, in addition to court cases, on PVS.

The validity of applying the technique for tomographic measurement of cerebral metabolism of glucose used in the PVS study of Levy *et al.* to investigations of *abnormal* cerebral tissue had been questioned, by Phelps *et al.* (1979), the group originally responsible for its development. Phelps *et al.* had speculated that their algorithm might not necessarily be valid if applied to examination of cerebral tissue that was subject to oxygen deprivation. The constant values incorporated in the algorithm ensured its accuracy for measurements of cerebral metabolism within the range of the *normal* subjects examined during its derivation. However Phelps *et al.* cautioned that application of the algorithm, incorporating the same lumped constant which had been appropriate in studying *normal* brain metabolism, might lead to errors if attempts were made to examine subjects whose metabolic rate was well outside the normal range. The specific risk as identified by Phelps *et al.* (1979) was that, in states of low metabolism which could occur if the blood supply to the brain was compromised, the incorporation into this algorithm of a lumped constant value which was suitable for normal subjects could result in underestimation of the metabolic rate for glucose in damaged tissue. Levy *et al.* (1987) did not comment upon this potential source of error and it does not appear to have been discussed subsequently.

Levy *et al.* stressed the important clinical implications of their findings and asserted that they offered

> "little support to therapeutic enthusiasts who claim that the vegetative state is simply a form of sleep that constant stimulation can reverse" (ibid: 679).

It could, however, be contended that the interpretation of these neuroimaging techniques remains at present heavily dependent upon extrapolation from clinical observations of vegetative state patients. The minimal level of cerebral metabolism which Levy *et al.* identified as compatible with consciousness appears to have been of entirely arbitrary derivation and it remains difficult to see how any level could be reliably established. In criticising the conclusions drawn about the conscious status of their patients by Levy *et al.*, Schiedermayer and La Puma (1988) questioned "reflexively deferring these decisions to a technology". The conclusions drawn by Levy *et al.* about level of consciousness based on PET assessment of cerebral metabolism have been criticised also by De Giorgio and Lew (1991) on the grounds that the appropriate control group, if PET was genuinely to differentiate between the presence of awareness and its absence, should have comprised severely disabled survivors of coma following oxygen deprivation who were nevertheless capable of thinking and experiencing pain. Apart from those conclusions that Levy *et al.* drew based entirely on their own data, they drew another inference equating the level of brain function which they observed in patients in a PVS with that occurring in deep barbiturate general anaesthesia. This conclusion was based on comparison of their results with those obtained in a much earlier study and, probably because of its attractive simplicity, has been even more extensively quoted, one suspects by many who have not explored its basis, as evidence for complete loss of awareness on the part of PVS patients.

6.9 THE EQUIVALENCE OF PVS AND ANAESTHESIA?

Levy *et al.* (1987) asserted that a reduction in brain metabolism of the magnitude which they observed in their 7 PVS patients had "precedent only in deep anaesthesia" (ibid: 673). The only data on the level of brain metabolism during human anaesthesia that was cited by Levy *et al.* to support their assertion was a 1947 report of Himwich *et al.* Their failure to consider the massive differences between the technology available to examine brain metabolism at the extremes of this 40 year interval, not to mention the attempt to compare two sets of data collected under such disparate circumstances, together with the frequency with which the similarity has been recited subsequently, demands a detailed examination of their comparison. Notwithstanding its patent deficiencies, both the M.S.T.F. report and a joint report by the Councils on Scientific Affairs and on Ethical and Judicial Affairs of the A.M.A. specifically drew attention to this equivalence (M.S.T.F. 1994a; American Medical Association Councils 1990). The Task Force added the comment, in relation to patients under deep general anaesthesia, that "all would agree (they) are unaware and insensate" (M.S.T.F. 1994a: 1502). Repeated citation of the equivalence of brain metabolism of patients in a PVS and subjects under deep general anaesthesia has extended well beyond authoritative statements from learned associations. For example, James Bernat (1992b), a neurologist writing in the *Journal of Clinical Ethics*, repeated verbatim the claim for similarity between PVS and deep general anaesthesia, and added that the latter represented a state such that, as regards patients in it, all would agree that they "cannot experience pain and suffering".

Two issues have been raised, but not further addressed by the authority that has been accorded to the PVS/deep general anaesthesia analogy. How sound is it to compare results obtained by two very different techniques? How well established is the completely unaware and insensate status of patients under the pentothal anaesthesia on which the "control" study was based? Unless the first question can achieve an affirmative response, namely that the comparison *is* sound, it should not be necessary to consider the second. However, the proposition addressed by the second question has assumed such a life of its own in the PVS literature that I intend to examine it in some detail in Chapter 7. The scientific legitimacy of the comparison advanced by Levy *et al.* will be considered here.

On first inspection, it seems remarkable that the "control group" of anaesthetised patients selected by Levy *et al.* (1987) to establish that their group of 7 patients examined in a PVS were unaware had been investigated using a totally different technique 40 years previously. It is reasonable to infer that the absence of reference to any more recent, comparable study of the effects of general anaesthesia on cerebral metabolism in normal patients as assessed by PET indicates the lack of such a study available for citation at the time of preparation of the report of Levy *et al.* Given this absence, together with the uncertainty prevailing at that time about *what* fully anaesthetised patients might be able to experience, the categorical designation of *any* specified percentage reduction of cerebral metabolic rate in the very small group of patients examined as being "incompatible with any mental activity" seems to be more than a little presumptuous.

As already remarked, the technology utilised to calculate cerebral metabolic rate in the study of Levy *et al.* and in the two other human studies that were cited by those authors, namely those of Himwich *et al.* (1947) and Brodersen and Jorgensen (1974), differed markedly. Whereas Levy *et al.* utilised PET to measure the metabolic rate for glucose in normal (unanaesthetised) and vegetative subjects, Himwich *et al.* calculated the metabolic rate for oxygen in barbiturate-anaesthetised, neurologically normal subjects as the product of cerebral blood flow rate (which was measured using nitrous oxide) and the difference in oxygen concentration between blood entering and leaving the brain. The absence of any reference whatsoever to this divergence in technology, and of its implications for comparison of metabolic rates of anaesthetised and vegetative subjects, by Levy *et al.* is remarkable in view of their caution, that:

> "One must emphasize the importance of comparing results in the study patients directly with those in normal control subjects examined under similar environmental conditions using the same experimental protocol" (ibid: 678).

Brodersen and Jorgensen were incorrectly cited by Levy *et al.* as having conducted a clinical study of cerebral metabolism during anaesthesia. In reality, their study was concerned with patients in coma from a variety of conditions (trauma, cerebrovascular accidents, hypoxia, hypoglycaemia or barbiturate intoxication). They calculated the cerebral metabolic rate of oxygen as the product of cerebral blood flow (measured using xenon) and arteriovenous oxygen difference (an approach similar to that of Himwich *et al.*). It could be noted that the ultimate outcome in the series of patients of Brodersen and Jorgensen (death, vegetative state or recovery) *did not correlate* with individual patient's metabolic levels.

The necessity for Levy *et al.* to cite two studies published 40 and 13 years previously which used substantially different technology, and only one of which actually dealt with the subject for which it was cited, namely cerebral metabolism during anaesthesia, could justifiably raise reservations about the quality of their conclusions. However, more detailed examination of these two papers gives rise to even more concern about the validity of their conclusions. Levy *et al.* stated that the 60% reduction in cerebral metabolic rate for glucose which they observed in their vegetative state patients exceeded the 30-50% decline seen in most experimental and clinical studies of anaesthesia. Himwich *et al.* (1947) had described reductions of cerebral metabolic rate ranging from 35% to 68% in four normal subjects at a stage of anaesthesia adequate for surgery, compared with the rate measured in the same individuals when awake. However, in the course of interpreting this observation, they recalled their own earlier (1941) observations on the extent of depression of cerebral metabolic rate that could occur in hypoglycaemic coma induced by insulin. These results indicated to Himwich *et al.* that the extent of metabolic depression *per se* produced by barbiturate anaesthesia was insufficient to account for the observed extent of loss of consciousness. Thus, those earlier observations had demonstrated that it was necessary for metabolism to be depressed by hypoglycaemia *to* 38% of its original value before consciousness was lost, whereas a similar depth of clinical anaesthesia could be attained, using barbiturate, with depression of metabolism only to 64% (Himwich *et al.* 1941).

6.10 THE INCONSISTENCY BETWEEN LEVEL OF ANAESTHESIA AND DEPRESSION OF CEREBRAL METABOLISM

Repetition of the 1941 observations of Himwich *et al.* on schizophrenic patients who were undergoing treatment with insulin to induce coma as a form of therapy has become impossible, on ethical grounds, since the replacement of full coma insulin as a therapeutic measure by more effective and safer forms of therapy. As noted above, the magnitude of reduction in cerebral metabolism which was required to produce loss of contact with the environment using insulin was much greater than that observed with barbiturates. In the case of patients receiving only insulin, and no anaesthetic agent, loss of consciousness could be attributed *exclusively* to reduction in cerebral metabolic rate. Himwich *et al.* found that cerebral metabolic rate had been reduced to approximately 25% of its initial level in some patients who were comatose as a result of therapy (not cited by Levy *et al.*). Comparison of the effects of hypoglycaemia and anaesthesia on cerebral metabolism and consciousness inevitably led Himwich *et al.* to conclude correctly that barbiturate anaesthesia was mediated by a specific inhibition of nerve function over and above any effect of general metabolic depression. Consequently, it is invalid to infer that *any* specified level of metabolic rate depression resulting from brain damage would necessarily be accompanied by the same depression of consciousness that accompanied barbiturate anaesthesia which happened, incidentally, to be associated with a similar level of metabolic rate depression.

The question of the extent to which loss of consciousness in barbiturate anaesthesia accurately paralleled the reduction observed in cerebral metabolism had been specifically raised by Himwich *et al.* in their 1947 article. In citing Himwich *et al.*, Levy *et al.* chose to ignore this point, tacitly inferring the equivalence of cerebral metabolic level and depth of unconsciousness and leading to the unsupported assumption that a certain level of reduction in metabolism could be taken as certifying the improbability of any residual consciousness. Research in the 50 years following the report of Himwich *et al.* has completely supported their original inference that the general anaesthesia produced by barbiturates results from specific actions on neurones, *not* primarily from any concomitant reduction in cerebral metabolic rate. It is of interest that two of the papers included in the reference list of the paper of Levy *et al.* quite explicitly indicated that loss of consciousness and depression of cerebral metabolism were *separable* phenomena which could vary independently. Carlsson *et al.* (1976) found that diazepam in anaesthetic doses produced only minimal depression of the cerebral metabolic rate of rats. Davis *et al.* (1984) noted that many effective anaesthetics, *but not all*, depress cerebral metabolic rate.

My general aim in this monograph is both to examine the basis to propositions that have historically influenced the development of perceptions of PVS and then to assess the current status of understanding of PVS. The preceding paragraphs have examined the reasoning underlying claims about the use of the PET technique to assess capacity of PVS patients for awareness which were originally included in the 1987 article of Levy *et al.* Before considering later PET studies from other clinics, a 1998 report (Plum *et al.*) from the same clinic as the 1987 Levy *et al.* paper updating the analogy between PVS and general anaesthesia by substituting a 1987 PET study of the latter for the 1947 report of Himwich *et al.* requires attention.

The total literature retrieved by the M.S.T.F. (1994a) directly describing PET measurement of the metabolism of the brain of patients in PVS dealt with approximately 20 patients. Rather surprisingly, a similar estimate was provided in the 1998 article by Plum *et al.* Taken at face value, this would suggest that the subject had been only lightly investigated during the 11 years after the first report. The 1998 paper of Plum *et al.* cited a PET study (Blacklock *et al.* 1987) of cerebral metabolic rate in anaesthetised patients as the control for its observations on patients in a vegetative state. Blacklock *et al.* found a range of reduction in glucose metabolism of from 47% to 67% during barbiturate anaesthesia. This was attributed to reduction of neuronal activity, however the authors also inferred that:

> "Anaesthetic doses of barbiturates may not be required for suppression of brain metabolism" (ibid: 74).

Blacklock *et al.* based this inference on an experimental study by Crane *et al.* (1978) which had shown that the major portion of the reduction in glucose metabolism in the rat brain during induction of anaesthesia could be achieved with as little as 1/5 to 1/10 of the normal anaesthetic dose of barbiturate. That is, the majority of metabolic depression could be accomplished using a dose of a barbiturate anaesthetic which had little impact on consciousness. The best that can be said about the proposition that patients under deep barbiturate anaesthesia and those in PVS share a similar level in reduction of consciousness is that the cited studies have yet to establish this. The very wide range of values for cerebral metabolism obtained when *normal* patients are examined using different scanners, which will be noted below, is an additional factor to be taken into account when assessing the inferences drawn by Plum *et al.* from the data of Blacklock *et al.*

The inconsistency between depth of unconsciousness and accompanying extent of metabolic depression produced by an anaesthetic can be further illustrated by consideration of different anaesthetic agents. A 1998 summary of the state of knowledge of anaesthetic action by Kress and Weigl stressed the diversity in mechanisms of action between different general anaesthetics whilst noting that synaptic transmission between neurones was a likely site of anaesthetic action. In specifically considering the relationship between depression of neuronal activity and decrease in cerebral metabolism during general anaesthesia they drew attention to the divergent patterns of alteration in these two processes produced by different anaesthetic agents. Thus, after completing two PET studies of human cerebral metabolism using propofol (Alkire *et al.* 1995) and isoflurane (Alkire *et al.* 1997) as anaesthetics, Alkire *et al.* (ibid) remarked upon the differing patterns of alteration in cerebral metabolism produced by the two agents, notwithstanding their similar anaesthetic efficacy.

6.11 SUBSEQUENT PET STUDIES OF PATIENTS IN A PVS

Levy *et al.* (1987) sought to equate a certain level of depression of cerebral metabolism with a certain level of impairment of consciousness on the basis of reports of depression of metabolism accompanying anaesthesia. Their argument was completely dependent on the assumption that the degree of impairment would be a direct *consequence* of the degree of reduction of metabolism. But anaesthetic agents do *not*, achieve their effects on consciousness primarily by reducing cerebral metabolism. Hence, to claim that a 50 or 60% reduction in metabolic rate is

> "strong evidence that such bodies can no longer either think or experience pain or suffering" (ibid: 679)

does not follow. The expected ablation of consciousness and sensation in a normal patient with this level of metabolic reduction during barbiturate anaesthesia provides no indication of whether a similar metabolic reduction in the case of a patient in a PVS (even assuming that identical procedures had been utilised to measure metabolic rate in the two situations) would guarantee loss of capacity to experience pain and suffering.

The M.S.T.F. cited papers by Momose *et al.* (1989), Shalit *et al.* (1972) and De Volder *et al.* (1990) in relation to measurement of cerebral metabolism of patients in a PVS. The report of Momose *et al.* described PET measurement of the cerebral glucose metabolism of a single PVS patient before and after electrical stimulation of his spinal cord. The paper by Shalit *et al.* dealt with patients who were comatose rather than vegetative and did not employ PET. Cerebral metabolism was estimated as the product of nitrous oxide measurement of cerebral blood flow and arteriovenous oxygen difference in the blood supply of the brain. Reversal of coma was observed despite severe, acute depression of the cerebral metabolic rate at the time of first examination when the patients were still comatose and it was concluded that:

> "There is no absolute correlation between the cellular metabolic activity of brain tissue, expressed by tissue oxygen consumption, and the functional integrity of brain mechanisms" (Shalit *et al.* 1972: 159).

The De Volder report detailed PET observations made in 12 patients who had previously had cardiac arrests. Of these patients, 7 were examined whilst in a vegetative state (one of whom was subsequently re-examined after regaining consciousness), whilst the remainder were "normally conscious but disclosed focal neurological signs" (that is, abnormalities that could be attributed to lesions in specific parts of the nervous system). All of the patients had been comatose on first admission. De Volder *et al.* (1990) noted a reduction of approximately 50% in mean cerebral glucose metabolism in the vegetative subjects and a reduction of 25% in the other neurologically impaired group who had recovered consciousness. These figures were quoted by the M.S.T.F. (1994a) in its statement but this omitted any mention of the additional detail that there had been an overlap in brain metabolism between vegetative and conscious groups so that the readings for two of the seven vegetative patients exceeded that of the lowest of the conscious patients. One patient had a metabolic rate of 27.6µ mol/100gm/minute whilst vegetative compared with one of 28.7 following the recovery of consciousness. A similar observation in a patient who recovered from a vegetative state sufficiently to resume both walking and speaking was reported by Laureys *et al.* (1999a). Whilst global glucose utilisation levels, assessed by PET, remained essentially the same after recovery of consciousness, modification of the pattern of regional brain metabolism was reported. Observations such as those of De Volder *et al.* and Laureys *et al.* recall the original assessment by Jennett and Plum (1972) that a *continuum* was likely to exist between those patients who *were* in, and others who *were not* in, a PVS. The caveat imposed by Cranford (1996) in criticising the 1996 report of Andrews *et al.* on the high rate of misdiagnosis of PVS, namely that distinction of PVS from severely impaired, but conscious, patients could have been aided by PET, may also be recalled.

In the year following publication of the M.S.T.F. report, the results of PET measurement of cerebral metabolism of glucose in a further series of patients, 5 of whom were comatose and 10 of whom were described as vegetative, were reported by Tommasino *et al.* (1995). The cerebral metabolic rate was reduced to approximately 50% of the normal mean in patients who were in either coma or a vegetative state and to approximately 35% in patients in PVS. Follow up of this series of patients revealed that 3 of them regained consciousness (one having been initially in coma, and the other 2 in a vegetative state after cardiac arrest or trauma). The authors specifically commented upon the lack of correlation between level of cerebral glucose metabolism and ultimate outcome. Thus, one patient who subsequently became conscious had the lowest metabolic rate of the 6 vegetative state patients and had had a lower rate than 3 of the 4 PVS patients (ibid). In view of the confident statements made by Levy *et al.* (1987) about the implications of certain levels of reduction in cerebral metabolic rates for a patient's potential capacity for consciousness, it is of interest to note that the 3 patients who subsequently regained consciousness had shown reductions of 66%, 39% and 30% in cerebral metabolic rate in comparison with the control group (Tommasino *et al.* 1995). Two recent PET studies of cerebral metabolism have identified areas of residual activity in vegetative patients and speculated on their significance. Laureys *et al.* (2000b) reported that, whilst the primary auditory cortex could be activated by click stimuli, auditory association areas were not, suggesting impairment of the integrative processes thought to be required for a normal level of awareness. Schiff et al. (2002) detected preserved brain activity which was interpreted as indicating the retention of intact, but isolated, modules.

When evaluating the propositions of Levy *et al.* (1987) about cerebral metabolic rate and consciousness, it is advisable to take account of some additional aspects of PET measurements of metabolism. The specific aspects to be considered are the range of variation in PET-assessed glucose metabolism between normal subjects, the impact of sedatives on metabolism, the levels of metabolism demonstrated to be consistent with full consciousness in the developing brain and, a more technical consideration, the effect of changes of cerebral mass on the calculation of cerebral metabolism, as assessed by PET.

6.12 INTER-SUBJECT VARIATION IN PET-CALCULATED CEREBRAL METABOLIC RATES

Variation in the level of cerebral glucose metabolism between normal subjects is considerable. This *inter-subject* variability contrasts with the relatively low levels of *intra*-subject variability on re-testing of the same individual. Wang *et al.* (1994) reported that absolute whole-brain glucose metabolic rates in a group of 34 healthy males aged from 20-29 years, ranged from 31.7 to 53.5μ mole/100gm/minute. This could be represented as a "reduction" in excess of 40% of metabolic rate in some normal young males in comparison with others. The range of variation in values for whole brain metabolic rates over a number of different PET centres was much wider than the range observed by the authors within their own clinic. Thus, a review of published values from 26 centres using a number of different types of scanner disclosed a range of from 20 to 68µ mole/100gm/min. as the normal rate. Wang *et al*. concluded that the type of scanner was more likely to account for differences than the age or gender of subjects and timing of the stages of the procedure. Selection of the lumped constant incorporated in the algorithm used for calculation of metabolic rate was recognised as another major source of potential variation. Caution is clearly indicated when comparing the results from different categories of subjects examined in different centres.

As the study of Levy *et al*. (1987) which demonstrated a reduction in excess of 50% of cerebral metabolic rate in PVS subjects compared with normal subjects was examining different individuals, rather than the same individual before and after the onset of PVS, some influence of inter-subject variability cannot be discounted. Levy *et al*. emphasised the importance of comparing any values for cerebral metabolic rate obtained using PET in vegetative patients with values from normal subjects obtained with identical procedures. Whilst their adherence to this precaution should have eliminated variations based on *instrumental* factors, it would not provide protection from *inter-subject* variability.

PET measurements of cerebral metabolism during sleep have served to demonstrate that marked variations occur in different parts of the brain. For example, Maquet *et al*. (1996) observed activation in brain stem, limbic system and cingulate cortex but decreased activity in many other regions during rapid-eye-movement sleep. Whilst an overall decrease in metabolism of the brain as a whole has been reported in non-rapid-eye-movement sleep, this again was not uniform when specific regions were compared with data from the same subjects when awake (Nofzinger *et al*. 2002).

6.13 PET ASSESSMENT OF CHANGES IN CEREBRAL METABOLIC RATE DURING DEVELOPMENT

Cerebral metabolism may vary with the age of the subject. The extent of variation from adult levels that can occur in infants, while still remaining compatible with consciousness, is considerable. In investigating this subject, ethical considerations dictate a limited selection of subjects. As an informed decision consenting to participate in a PET study could not legitimately be provided on behalf of normal children, the available data has been derived from study of children with medical conditions that could potentially have been directly benefited from PET examination (Chugani *et al*. 1987). The values of glucose metabolism assessed at a range of ages from birth to 15 years in these "near normal" children varied substantially both below and above normal adult levels. For example, cortical values ranged from 65-86% of adult rates during the first year of life, whereas global rates (for the entire cerebral hemisphere) of those children examined between 3 and 10 years were equivalent to double the adult level (ibid). The existence of these large variations between apparently normal and near normal individuals should be recalled before deciding to specify a level of PET-assessed brain metabolism at which the retention of consciousness by the subject can confidently be excluded. If a normal level of consciousness can be retained despite a wide variation in metabolic rate, the arbitrary designation of *any* specific level of metabolism as indicative of loss of consciousness will remain highly questionable.

6.14 SEDATIVES AND PET-CALCULATED CEREBRAL METABOLIC RATES

As patients in a vegetative state are frequently receiving sedatives, the possible influence of these on measurements of cerebral metabolism is relevant to most studies of such patients. Two of the vegetative state patients of Levy *et al.* (1987) were receiving phenytoin at the time of examination. Four of the 7 vegetative state patients in the series of De Volder *et al.* (1990) were receiving potentially sedative medication, as were 3 of the 5 conscious but neurologically impaired individuals. Of the patients described by Tommasino *et al.* (1995), 4 out of 6 vegetative state patients were receiving phenobarbital, as were all 5 of the patients in coma. The only infant in a PVS on whom PET study of cerebral metabolism appears to have been reported was receiving phenobarbital at the time of estimation (Larsen *et al.* 1993). Momose *et al.* (1989) did not indicate the medication status of their single patient.

Information about the effect of barbiturates on cerebral metabolism of glucose, as assessed by PET, was published as early as 1986 by Theodore *et al.* from the U.S. National Institutes of Health. Nine patients receiving treatment with phenobarbitone (and, in some instances, other sedative drugs) to control epileptic seizures were examined by PET whilst on therapy. This measurement was repeated following withdrawal of phenobarbital (only one patient could be maintained without any other drug therapy until repetition of PET, so the remaining 8 patients continued to receive other medication) for a mean period of 14 weeks which was required before plasma phenobarbital concentrations dropped to an undetectable level. On re-examination, when this had occurred there was a mean increase of 37% in cerebral glucose metabolism in this group of patients. Expressed alternatively, phenobarbital therapy alone had been responsible for a depression of metabolism to approximately 70% of untreated levels. As a control measure, to quantify the extent to which inherent intra-subject variability could have contributed to such large increases in cerebral metabolism after withdrawal of barbiturates, Theodore *et al.* (1986) undertook repeat PET investigations on a second group of 5 patients whose sedative medication had remained unaltered. The mean intra-subject variation in this second group was very low, being only 7%. Referring to two earlier studies which had failed to demonstrate depression of human cerebral metabolism in response to non-anaesthetic doses of barbiturates, Theodore *et al.* noted that the subjects of those studies had received only a single dose of sedative one hour before measurement of metabolism. As barbiturate blood levels had not been reported in those studies, it was not possible to determine whether these were comparable with the therapeutic concentrations observed in the chronically dosed patients of Theodore *et al.*

Before considering the possible implications of the study of Theodore *et al.* for the 3 larger studies of brain metabolism of patients in vegetative states, namely those of Levy *et al.* (1987), De Volder *et al.* (1990) and Tommasino *et al.* (1995), it is of interest that none of these later reports regarded that study as of sufficient relevance to justify its citation. The only two earlier reports of effects of barbiturates to be cited in these studies had been published almost 4 decades earlier and their estimations were based on a methodology markedly different from PET. Levy *et al.* and Tommasino *et al.* inferred from these that residual barbiturate effects were unlikely to have influenced their observations. However, serum barbiturate levels were not reported in either of these papers nor was any information provided about times elapsed since cessation of barbiturates or any other sedatives.

In the light of the 14 weeks period that Theodore *et al.* had introduced between barbiturate withdrawal and PET examination in order to exclude residual effects of these sedatives, it seems reasonable to infer that they had anticipated that residual depressive effects on cerebral metabolic rates might persist for a prolonged period after withdrawal of sedatives. Apart from the cursory attention paid to the existing evidence of effects of sedatives on cerebral metabolism, an additional point that does not appear to have been considered in any of the reports concerned with cerebral metabolism in vegetative states is that of whether any impact of barbiturates on the heavily damaged brain of such patients would have been adequately mimicked in the relatively normal patients of Theodore *et al.* suffering from epilepsy. Given the well recognised susceptibility of the damaged brain to depressive agents such as alcohol, it would not be unrealistic to anticipate that *any* blood concentration of barbiturate would be more likely to affect metabolism in a damaged, as distinct from a normal, brain.

6.15 INFLUENCE OF BRAIN ATROPHY ON CEREBRAL METABOLISM STUDIES

A final significant technical consideration which should be factored into any consideration of cerebral metabolism in vegetative states relates to the impact on PET data of brain atrophy. Tommasino *et al.* (1995) raised this possibility in discussion of their results, noting that inclusion of metabolically inactive spaces, created by brain atrophy, could result in artefactual lowering of PET measurements of cerebral metabolism. Whilst identifying this potential source of error, they did not attempt to correct their PET metabolic data to compensate for it. Schiff *et al.* (2002) acknowledged that volume distortions due to localised atrophy could have negatively biased estimates of metabolic activity in some regions. The feasibility of incorporating some compensation for brain atrophy into PET-generated data on cerebral metabolism has been examined by Tanna *et al.* (1991). They compared patients with Alzheimer's disease with healthy elderly people. It was found that, when allowance was made for the reduction of brain mass in the Alzheimer patients, their corrected cerebral metabolic rate was increased by an average of 25%. Levy *et al.* (1987) considered the possibility that cerebral atrophy could have produced an artefactual reduction of the measured cerebral metabolic rate in their vegetative patients, but, for technical reasons, the application of a correction for atrophy to their readings was not possible. However, they did not believe that atrophy could have accounted for the extent of reduction of metabolic rate that they had observed but the possibility that an artefact generated by atrophy could have made some lesser contribution to the observed reduction (perhaps abetted by sedative agents) was not canvassed.

6.16 LOCATION OF LESIONS IN VEGETATIVE PATIENTS USING PET

While the use of PET in the reports discussed so far was directed primarily to measuring the overall rate of cortical metabolism in vegetative patients, there have been some recent reports in which the aim was to identify those structures which have been most severely affected. Many of these reports have come from Laureys' group at the University of Liège. As with earlier PET studies, the number of patients examined remains very small and any conclusions based on the results obtained must necessarily be preliminary. In a study of 4 patients in a vegetative state, Laureys *et al.* (1999b) described a common pattern of inactivation of association areas responsible for linking the cortex with other structures. They interpreted their findings as supporting the hypothesis that loss of connectivity was an underlying factor in vegetative states. Subsequently they reported the restoration of connections between thalamic nuclei and some cortical regions in a patient who emerged from a PVS (Laureys *et al.* 2000a). In a further indication of the selective nature of the functional disconnection in vegetative states, Laureys *et al.* (2000b) have demonstrated that some cortical areas remained responsive to external auditory input in 5 patients in a vegetative state. A report from a Cambridge brain imaging centre, described the occurrence of PET-detected activation of part of the cortex in a patient in a PVS following display of familiar faces, but not of control images (Menon *et al.* 1998). This would imply that processing of visual input remained possible in this patient and that some form of response to stimuli, for which the patient would have had memory before entering a PVS, remained possible. PET has also been applied to discriminating between functional inactivation and irreversible structural damage to the brain by means of imaging of those receptors responsible for binding to benzodiazepine drugs on neurones (Rudolf *et al.* 2000). Extension of these approaches may facilitate an improved understanding of the specific nature of structural and functional abnormalities and possibly provide some prognostic indicators.

6.17 RECAPITULATION

Investigative techniques which provide information about a patient's condition beyond that accessible by means of clinical examination alone have played a major part in advancing the diagnosis and treatment of disease. It would be difficult to find a better example of this than the contribution that introduction of CT scanning made to the accurate localisation, and more effective early treatment, of traumatic brain injury. Whilst the full gamut of investigative techniques have been applied to patients who are in, or close to, a vegetative state, they have added little to diagnosis. Nevertheless, results of investigations undertaken on individual patients have been cited and accorded substantial evidentiary value in court hearings in support of the diagnosis of PVS.

The techniques which have been applied to examination of patients in a PVS have entailed either the recording of electrical impulses from the brain or scanning to obtain brain images. Imaging techniques can provide information about either structure or function. The earliest electrical test, the electroencephalogram (EEG) has been generally acknowledged to contribute nothing to the recognition of a PVS, as recordings from affected patients can range from normal to grossly abnormal without any evident correlation with the individual's clinical condition. Another electrical test, namely measurement of somatosensory evoked potentials (SEPs) provides an indication of the integrity of the inward (sensory) pathways from the surface of the body to the region of the cerebral cortex under examination. Recording of the SEP has been used as a prognostic test to predict the likelihood, at an early stage after brain injury, that a patient will subsequently enter a PVS. However, published reports of the application of SEP measurement for this purpose invariably appear not to differentiate between three possible outcomes namely death, vegetative state or a recovery of consciousness that is accompanied by residual disability sufficient to preclude independent living. Consequently, if one considers, as I do, that patients in the latter category can benefit from rehabilitation, SEP measurement, given its lack of discrimination between these outcomes, is not sufficiently informative to justify non-treatment decisions at an early stage.

Structural imaging techniques include the CT scan which has been extensively applied to patients in a PVS and magnetic resonance imaging (MRI) which is likely to replace it. CT scanning has been used to visualise atrophy of the brain of patients in a PVS, in the medium to longer term, and the results of its application have been produced in court to support the diagnosis. I believe that more has been claimed for it in this context than can be validated. There have been numerous reports of atrophic changes in the brain of patients affected by anorexia nervosa who have no history of brain injury but whose food intake has been curtailed. Despite this, reports of CT studies of PVS patients have failed to acknowledge possible aggravation of the atrophy disclosed by scanning as a consequence of the frequently impaired nutritional status of these patients.

Functional imaging techniques may have the capacity to explain much that is presently unknown about brain function as, with increasing resolution, the activity of very localised structures becomes increasingly accessible to observation. Nevertheless, before these techniques could be applied to arbitrate on the conscious status of any patient, it would be necessary to demonstrate that they can reliably differentiate between one patient who is clinically in a PVS and another with brain damage of similar severity who has regained consciousness. Such a discrimination has yet to be accomplished. Quite apart from its technical feasibility, there is likely to be a major conceptual obstacle to achieving it, namely the inherent inability to validate loss of consciousness, or of any other form of mental activity with certainty, by clinical observation. One can only *infer* such loss indirectly on the basis of observation.

Notwithstanding the impediments noted above to the establishment and validation of a technical process whereby one individual can document loss of capacity for consciousness in another, the technique of positron emission tomography (PET) has repeatedly been claimed to have achieved this. Examination of the published data on which this claim has been based suggests to me that this certainly has not been achieved.

CHAPTER 7

AN ANALOGY BETWEEN ANAESTHESIA AND PERSISTENT VEGETATIVE STATE

> "Similar degrees of cerebral metabolic depression have been reported previously only in deep barbiturate anaesthesia" (Levy *et al.* 1987: 679).

The analogy between anaesthesia and vegetative states has been so persuasive that its detailed consideration is justified. If it is reasonable to invoke the analogy to infer what a vegetative patient can *not* do, it is equally reasonable to use it to infer what such a patient *may be able* to do. The original basis for the analogy, namely a comparison between metabolic rates in the brains of barbiturate-anaesthetised patients and others who were in a PVS was examined in Chapter 6. It was argued there that the conclusion that levels of awareness were similar in deeply anaesthetised subjects and PVS patients was seriously flawed on two grounds. In the first place, the two groups of subjects under comparison had been examined using very different technological approaches. In the second, the assumption that cerebral metabolic rate can be used as a reliable index of level of anaesthesia, which was central to the conclusion of comparability between anaesthesia and vegetative status, is incorrect.

In order to interpret contemporary views on similarities of PVS to general anaësthesia it is necessary to trace their origins. Two issues will be addressed in this Chapter. What information about awareness under anaesthesia was available when the M.S.T.F. presented its comparison? What if anything, might be inferred about the condition of PVS patients from the information *currently* available about awareness of normal subjects under anaesthesia? In opting to pursue responses to these questions, I am not retreating from the conclusion in Chapter 6 that the experimental measurements of cerebral metabolic rate in anaesthetised and vegetative patients provide little support for the claimed equivalence of their conscious status but, rather, am recognising that their inadequacy *cannot disprove* the M.S.T.F. proposition. That inadequacy has not dissuaded other commentators on PVS from basing conclusions about patients in that condition on their impressions of the status of anaesthetised subjects: nor need it dissuade me.

7.1 THE ISSUE OF AWARENESS UNDER ANAESTHESIA AT THE TIME OF THE M.S.T.F. STATEMENT

The most efficient way in which to retrieve a perspective on the issue of awareness under anaesthesia at the time when the M.S.T.F. statement was written is to examine a bibliography on this subject to determine what had already been published. A comprehensive review of the subject, prepared by Wang, and published in 1998 has been used for this purpose. This review tabulated research on awareness under anaesthesia into 3 groups on the basis of the nature of the investigation. The first group of papers dealt with investigations in which positive suggestions had been made to patients who were under general anaesthesia for surgery. These suggestions were of a type expected to be beneficial for the patient's post-operative recovery if acted upon. By the time of publication of the M.S.T.F. report, 18 double blind controlled trials of this type had been reported in the medical literature. Wang's summary concluded that two thirds had demonstrated a significant difference between subjects who *had* received positive suggestions while anaesthetised and those who *had not*.

The second group of papers reviewed by Wang described studies in which suggestions were presented to subjects under general anaesthesia that they should spontaneously undertake some specified movement during a post-anaesthetic interview. The majority of the 10 reports on such ideomotor studies published up until 1994 had yielded negative results. The third group of 28 studies examined the efficacy of verbal stimuli administered to anaesthetised subjects in facilitating their subsequent learning. One third of the studies reviewed by Wang gave positive results.

The recurrent acceptance by journals of reports of the investigation of retention of awareness by individuals under general anaesthesia provides a strong indication that this issue certainly remained contentious at the time of publication of the M.S.T.F. statement in 1994. It is equally clear that, if awareness had been retained by a proportion of people under general anaesthesia, the quotation which opened this Chapter would have become untenable. The M.S.T.F. statement dealt with the issue of whether any of the anaesthetised subjects, who were claimed to be equivalent to vegetative patients in their level of (un)awareness could have been aware by ignoring it. There was no hint of uncertainty revealed by the publications on the subject, nor did any of the papers in Wang's bibliography make it on to the list of references cited by the M.S.T.F.

7.2 INFERENCES ABOUT UNCONSCIOUS SUBJECTS FROM STUDY OF ANAESTHESIA

Since attention was first drawn to the issue, acknowledgement of the possibility of retained awareness, both in anaesthetised, but otherwise normal, individuals and in others diagnosed as unconscious as a result of neurological lesions, has been forthcoming from authoritative sources. As regards the first, a 1994 *British Medical Journal* editorial subheading dramatically summarised the possibility of intra-operative awareness, namely *Patients remember more than we think* (Jones 1994). In relation to the second, a British Medical Association (B.M.A.) spokesperson, interviewed following the disclosure, by a man who had recovered after having been unconscious for 6 months, that he knew what was going on around him acknowledged:

> "We know from long experience with coma patients that they can appear to be deeply unconscious yet remember things that have been said to them or done to them afterwards" (Fletcher 1996).

It is not claimed that a common basis exists for awareness under general anaesthesia and in comatose patients. It is suggested that a better understanding of either subject could provide some additional insights into the other.

Whilst not specifically referred to by the B.M.A. spokesperson, there have been some studies of patients' memories of periods of coma. Self-evidently, this information has become available only from patients who subsequently regained consciousness. Insofar as these studies deal with *experiences whilst unconscious*, subsequent recovery with recollection would be required for their retelling, although not for their initial occurrence. The study of Schnaper (1975) referred to in Chapter 4 identified 3 prevailing themes. Those themes were - being held prisoner, wrongdoing to justify imprisonment and death – among the third of patients who were not amnesic following a period of post-traumatic unconsciousness. Schnaper recommended that apparently unconscious patients should be "spoken to, called by name, touched and handled as gently as possible" (ibid: 97).

The possibility that awareness could be retained under anaesthesia was first brought to general attention with the publication of a paper by Levinson (1965). This paper, which is now little more than an historical curiosity, described the simulation of an anaesthetic crisis for 10 patients during dental surgery. This simulation took the form of an alarmed call from the anaesthetist indicating that the oxygen supply to the patient had failed. After recovery from the general anaesthetic, some patients remembered details of the "crisis", whilst most displayed marked anxiety. An attempt to replicate the results of this study in 1995 failed to detect significant differences between patients exposed to a simulated crisis and controls (Chortkoff *et al.* 1995). Nevertheless, these two studies illustrate some of the procedural difficulties inherent in planning and interpreting studies to detect awareness under anaesthesia and, indirectly, in patients unconscious after brain injury.

7.3 RESEARCH PROTOCOLS IN THE STUDY OF AWARENESS UNDER ANAESTHESIA

Andrade (1995) reviewed the subject of learning during anaesthesia and identified the obstacles to this type of research. Despite the very extensive, continuing study of the subject, it was noted that many of the reported studies were opportunistic and deficient in aspects such as standardisation of anaesthetic procedures and post-anaesthetic psychological assessments. In many instances the nature of the procedures applied to individual participants was not concealed and the identity of experimental and control groups of subjects had been apparent to the investigators. Compounding these difficulties, there exist very substantial ethical obstacles in the way of repeating experiments such as Levinson's. Participants in this original study were recruited under false pretences and placed at risk of suffering adverse psychological effects of prolonged duration which might not readily be resolved. Notwithstanding the impediments to this type of study, information obtained with anaesthetised subjects about possible adverse effects of overheard conversations could be highly relevant in managing PVS patients. As will be noted in Chapter 11, some neurologists have advocated talking, in positive terms, to comatose patients (La Puma *et al.* 1988). Intuitively, one might anticipate that adverse stimuli might have an effect on unconscious patients when neutral ones were without effect. However, it is difficult to envisage protocols by means of which this proposition could ethically be tested. Procedures, such as applying painful electrical stimulation and vigorous shaking to unconscious patients, described in earlier Chapters, appear to me to be ethically unacceptable.

7.4 TYPE AND DEPTH OF ANAESTHESIA

The nature of the anaesthetic agent and the depth of anaesthesia might seem, on first principles, intuitively to be relevant factors when explaining the variable results of attempts to demonstrate learning or behavioural modification in subjects under anaesthesia. Could learning during general anaesthesia be adequately explained on the basis that the anaesthesia was inadequate or incomplete in those instances in which learning could later be demonstrated and that patients showing positive results represented instances of undetected residual consciousness? Such anaesthetic inadequacy could be a consequence of the particular anaesthetic agent chosen, or of fluctuations in the level of its administration. It has been suggested that any retained capacity of a subject to receive input might be associated with use of barbiturate anaesthetics but not with that of the more recently available, volatile anaesthetics. However, Wang's (1998) review of awareness under anaesthesia documented instances of retention of awareness using volatile agents and so failed to support this contention.

A study reported by Block *et al.* (1991) specifically addressed the possibility that awareness under anaesthesia correlated with inadequate *use* of the anaesthetic agent. This group of anaesthetists found that learning, as subsequently assessed by behavioural suggestion, word completion and nonsense word tests, did not vary with methods of anaesthesia. Their data contradicted what they characterised as the "widespread, plausible" belief that "light" relative to "deep" anaesthesia would increase the likelihood of retention of any information presented. This belief might have been an accurate interpretation of the situation, provided that learning mechanisms in the brain were progressively impaired as anaesthetic levels increased. However, Block *et al.* concluded, in the light of the lack of any observed correlation between lightening of anaesthesia and successful learning, that:

> "Some information processing functions of the brain evidently continue to function during adequate general anaesthesia" (ibid: 170).

This conclusion has potential implications for patients who are unconscious for reasons other than general anaesthesia.

7.5 POSITIVE SUGGESTION UNDER ANAESTHESIA

As already noted in summarising Wang's (1998) review, several different experimental approaches have been adopted in attempts to present information to the anaesthetised subjects of those studies. Positive suggestion studies have entailed the presentation of positive intra-operative information in an attempt to achieve favourable post-operative outcomes. Most commonly, the information, presented by audiotape, has included messages of encouragement intended to expedite recovery. Assessments of the outcomes in these studies were typically based on one or more quantifiable parameters such as the duration of post-operative stay in hospital and the post-operative requirement for analgesics.

Implicit in the design of positive suggestion studies has been the assumption that, if the subject became aware of the message, he or she would automatically manifest some behavioural modification in response to it. Leaving aside the unarguably indirect nature of such parameters for comparing the influence of intra-operative stimuli in experimental and control groups of patients, major qualifications to interpretation of the results remain. The capacity for *recall* of any information of which a patient becomes aware under anaesthesia is necessarily assumed if a positive result is to be attainable in any studies of awareness in anaesthetised or comatose patients. However, there is no reason why awareness should necessarily be accompanied by recall. Unless some capacity for recall can be demonstrated, whether in a previously anaesthetised or a comatose patient, it is obviously impossible to infer the earlier absence of awareness in these two categories of subject. One assumption on which positive suggestion studies are heavily dependent is that:

> "General anaesthesia is associated with a special cognitive state, in which verbal suggestions have much more powerful effects than when the same suggestions are presented in the normal, conscious, waking state" (Wang 1998: 90).

In other words, instructions presented under general anaesthesia are assumed to have some greater potency than when they are made to awake subjects. Unless this assumption is correct, and there does not appear to be anything to support it, there is no justification for anticipating that there will be a positive outcome to attempts to influence behaviour, *irrespective of whether the subject was or was not aware, while under anaesthesia*.

Apart from attempts to improve post-operative recovery, positive suggestion studies conducted under general anaesthesia have been trialled as a means of modifying post-operative behaviour both in a trivial fashion, for example, in one study suggesting that subjects repeatedly touch their ear during post-anaesthetic interview (Bennett *et al.* 1985) and for more substantial purposes, for example, to achieve cessation of a smoking habit (Hughes *et al.* 1994). A large group of studies have attempted to initiate learning during anaesthesia. Typically, they have entailed the presentation of taped information to one group of subjects, while anaesthetised, followed by attempts to determine, at a subsequent interview, whether that group is more likely than a control group to recall specific information. Recall of experience under anaesthesia could be an example of explicit or implicit memory:

> "Explicit memory involves conscious recollection of some previous episode and is what most of us understand as recall during anaesthesia. Implicit memory, however, refers to any effect on a person's experience, thought or action that is attributable to a past event, even if that person does not remember the event" (Cork *et al.* 1996: 492).

Anaesthesia may affect these two forms of memory differentially.

7.6 EMOTIONAL CONTENT OF STIMULUS

Whilst there have been few studies such as that of Levinson, designed to have an adverse impact upon the participants, this is the type of study most likely to be relevant to PVS patients. As most authoritative neurological specialists and groups proclaim that PVS patients are totally unaware of their environment, the likelihood is that conversations with distinctly negative implications (for example, concerning deprivation of fluids and food) may take place in the presence of the patient. Apprehension about the inadvertent infliction of distress upon patients in a PVS and in coma as a result of prognostically negative conversations in their presence has evoked admonitions *not* to discuss such patients in their presence and to attempt to converse with them (La Puma *et al.* 1988). On the other hand, some physicians have dismissed attempts at talking to unconscious patients by family and medical attendants as self-delusory:

> "But to expect the unfortunate, overwhelmingly damaged brain to receive the message in intelligent form is, we believe, scientifically absurd" (Levy *et al.* 1988: 288).

If this inference of Levy *et al.* is correct, there would be little point in refraining from talking about and over the patient.

It has been suggested, in discussing studies which attempted to test for intra-anaesthetic awareness by providing *neutral* information, that material with a stronger emotional significance, specific for the anaesthetised subject, may have produced a positive outcome. If such information is to be incorporated into studies of awareness under anaesthesia it becomes more difficult to design reproducible protocols which will be equally relevant to all subjects studied. Reports that anaesthetised patients may be able to receive emotionally significant, but not irrelevant, stimuli parallel the experience of many of those caring for people in the process of emerging from a vegetative state. It has often been observed then that awareness by the patient first became apparent to others as a response to stimuli with specific relevance to the patient. Two rehabilitation specialists recognising this, advocated use of stimuli with personal relevance in attempting to communicate with unconscious patients (Watson and Horn 1991). This would be building upon an existing *data base* of the patient. In reporting the outcome of a study in which post-operative memory for lists of neutral words, presented under anaesthesia, could not be demonstrated, Parker *et al.* (1994) referred to the possible importance of measures to enhance the impact of the material presented and described Levinson's original experiment as "perhaps the most extreme form of saliency enhancement". Translating their nice turn of phrase into more basic terms, if one attempts to scare anaesthetised (or unconscious) subjects out of their wits, this may have more impact on post-anaesthetic memory. Heightened ethical sensibilities have tended to curtail such studies in recent years.

7.7 AMNESIA FOLLOWING ANAESTHESIA AND UNCONSCIOUSNESS

The capacity to recall is essential if retention of awareness during any form of unconscious state is to be demonstrated. The analogy between unconscious and anaesthetised subjects serves to draw attention to the discrete nature of experience and its subsequent recollection. Most investigations of awareness by patients under general anaesthesia have been based on interviews conducted after cessation of anaesthesia. A positive result, suggesting that an individual had been aware whilst appearing to be unconscious, would require not only that awareness had been present at the earlier time, but also that the individual was able to *recall* any information that was processed. The most likely impediment to remembering by a normal individual who has experienced general anaesthesia is the anamnestic effect of some of the drugs used as ancillary agents in association with an anaesthetic agent. In the case of a patient diagnosed as in a vegetative state, failure to recall information could reflect pathological impairment of capacity for memory, irrespective of whether awareness had been present *at the time* that the patient was observed to be unconscious.

The impact on PVS patients of sedatives and other agents with amnesic effects should not be ignored. Whilst the "textbook" descriptions of these individuals depict them as static occupants of beds, the administration of sedative and tranquillising drugs to them is not uncommon as a nursing measure. This practice could well appear illogical on first (and subsequent) inspection. If a patient can be classed as completely unaware of anything with the degree of confidence professed in authoritative statements (Chapter 3), the administration of sedatives is absolutely superfluous. Whilst it is not in dispute that some patients diagnosed as vegetative may be disruptive to a ward regime in the absence of the administration of sedative agents, the likely adverse effects of sedation on recovery of any level of awareness (and also of recognition of that recovery by others) should be stressed. If a vegetative patient is totally unaware, as conventionally stated, sedation contributes nothing that is in *his or her* interests. On the other hand, if any reservations remain about whether a patient is completely unaware, then he or she should not be treated as though it were so. Information on medication of PVS patients has tended to be revealed only in those situations in which it is relevant to the subject to be discussed.

Three examples of situations in which information about sedative use is of particular interest are the diagnosis of PVS, scientific investigation of its nature and the terminal management of affected individuals. The contribution of sedatives to misdiagnosis of PVS in a series of demented patients in U.S. nursing homes will be considered in Chapter 8. Secondly, sedatives can have a prolonged effect on cerebral metabolism as already discussed in Chapter 6. Finally, the administration of tranquillisers or sedatives appears to have been practised in PVS patients when food and water is to be withheld (see Chapter 13).

One approach to the problem of detecting awareness under anaesthesia which obviates possible confounding amnesic effects of some agents is to ascertain the extent of the patient's awareness of stimulation *at the time this is applied* instead of relying upon a post-anaesthetic interview. The isolated forearm technique entails the application of a tourniquet to the arm sufficiently firmly to prevent blood inflow. The patient is asked to indicate awareness of others by a designated movement of the isolated forearm. It has been employed in an attempt to assess the current state of awareness in anaesthetised patients (Wang 1998). The reason for isolating the subject's forearm is to prevent its paralysis by muscle relaxant drugs administered to facilitate surgery. Limitations of the technique are the impossibility of maintaining the inflated tourniquet in place indefinitely and the difficulty which may be encountered in distinguishing spontaneous movements of the isolated forelimb from purposive movements in response to a request from the examiner.

Despite these limitations, the technique may provide information about awareness under anaesthesia that is not otherwise available. Wang has drawn attention to instances in which intra-operative episodes of coherent motor responses to request were demonstrated in anaesthetised patients by the isolated forearm technique when there were no clinically apparent signs of awareness. Discrepancy between responses demonstrated by the isolated forearm technique and more conventional evidence of awareness could be interpreted in either of two ways. It could be indicative of inaccuracy inherent in the technique or it could reflect the insensitivity of conventional clinical approaches to assessment of the level of a patient's awareness. Similar interpretations are applicable to the specialised communication strategies which have been developed for use with unconscious patients.

In discussing the isolated forearm technique, Wang (1998) remarked in his review that:

> "There is now good evidence that, not only is there typically large variation in levels of consciousness in the patient during surgery under a general anaesthetic, but that anaesthetists are remarkably poor at detecting such variation" (ibid: 91).

Perhaps a similar caveat is applicable to some misdiagnosed cases of vegetative state. One British anaesthetist who has made extensive use of the isolated forearm technique reported that 72% of women undergoing major gynaecological surgery using one particular anaesthetic regime responded to a request to indicate awareness

(Russell 1993). However, conventional observation failed to distinguish these patients from non-responders. Few of the responding patients could recall being aware when questioned post-operatively leading the anaesthetist to infer that inability to remember did not guarantee unconsciousness *during* surgery. He recommended that the particular anaesthetic regime not be generally applied.

Extrapolating again from the anaesthetised patient to the vegetative patient, as proposed in the M.S.T.F. analogy, the isolated forearm technique or a similar procedure would not be applicable to the latter group of patients. Whilst patients in a vegetative state would not generally have paralysis of motor neurone end plates similar to that in patients under the influence of muscle relaxants, they are likely to lack the neurological co-ordination required to *harness* motor neurones and so to indicate responsiveness (Howsepian 1996). Lacking capacity to indicate a response at the time of questioning, and potentially also lacking capacity for recall, the analogy with general anaesthesia, if pursued, could allow for the possibility of some vegetative patients retaining undetectable awareness.

In an editorial article that touched on an issue central to perceptions of patients in a vegetative state, Griffiths and Jones (1990) contrasted alternative concepts of anaesthesia. In one account, general anaesthesia is envisaged as a threshold event with loss of consciousness, pain perception and capacity to recall occurring in an all-or-nothing manner at one time. The alternative position is to consider anaesthesia as a continuous spectrum. According to this position, there would be three broad levels of awareness, namely conscious awareness with explicit recall, conscious awareness with no explicit recall and subconscious awareness with implicit, but no explicit, recall. The possible existence of a stage of no awareness remained unclear (Jelicic *et al.* 1992).

Similar alternative descriptions of patients in vegetative states could be envisaged. The concept that anaesthetic agents might effect a dissociation between explicit and implicit memory has received experimental support in a 1996 report from Cork *et al.* (1996). They studied a group of patients who received propofol sedation during surgery under local anaesthesia. When the patients' ability to recall words presented under the influence of propofol was tested, a few exhibited free recall, indicative of explicit memory. The remainder gave no sign of explicit memory but all evinced significant priming in free association tests, indicating that implicit memory had been established.

A final point which might be extracted from the analogy between general anaesthesia and vegetative states is that it appears increasingly unlikely that a single state could adequately explain the former. The heterogeneity, in terms of physiological changes and retained capacities, that characterises general anaesthesia would appear to be equally applicable to the spectrum of conditions conveniently grouped as the vegetative state.

7.8 RECAPITULATION

This Chapter has been concerned with the evidence for and against retention of awareness in subjects under general anaesthesia, not about retained awareness in patients in a PVS. The reason for its inclusion is that PVS patients have frequently been compared with deeply anaesthetised subjects and said to be as unaware as they are. The original observations on which this comparison was based were considered in the preceding Chapter and it was suggested there that the scientific validity of the analogy was highly dubious. However, the analogy has thrived since its presentation in the M.S.T.F. statement and is a persistent feature of description of PVS.

The point was made in this Chapter that the complete unawareness of patients under deep barbiturate anaesthesia was *not* a universally accepted fact when the M.S.T.F. statement was prepared (nor has it since become one). The issue of retained awareness under general anaesthesia has generated a large body of research with divergent results. However, the M.S.T.F. statement, and subsequent recitations of it, have invariably omitted any reference to the uncertainty surrounding this subject. Certainly, credible evidence has been obtained for the continuation of information processing functions in some deeply anaesthetised normal subjects.

Studies of awareness in deeply anaesthetised individuals have suggested that stimuli with strong personal relevance for the subject have a greater likelihood of being received as also have topics related to knowledge possessed by the subject before anaesthesia. These findings parallel the practice, in some facilities caring for patients unconscious after brain injury, of presenting positive messages related to the patient's previous interests and of refraining from holding pessimistic conversations about the patient in his or her presence.

It is possible to eliminate the amnesic effects of medication associated with anaesthesia, and the necessity for a subject to *recall* experiences under anaesthesia in order to establish that they occurred by using a research technique that can detect awareness *at the time of stimulation*. This technique is not applicable to patients unconscious after brain injury, however it is of interest that it has been used to demonstrate that awareness under deep anaesthesia *occurs* in a larger proportion of subjects than those who are able subsequently to *remember* it.

CHAPTER 8

DIAGNOSIS AND MISDIAGNOSIS OF VEGETATIVE STATES

> "If one can say this at all in medicine, the accuracy of the diagnosis of PVS is 100%" (Ivan 1990: 994).

This quotation from a Canadian neurologist addressing transplantation specialists implied a degree of certainty in diagnosis of PVS not held at that time (1990) by all neurologists. The imprecision inherent in diagnosis of PVS was identified, in the same symposium, as a fundamental feature differentiating it from brain death (Wikler 1990). The claim of 100% accuracy in diagnosis of PVS became increasingly ludicrous with the publication of reports of misdiagnosis of PVS from the early 1990s.

Diagnostic criteria may be developed both for determining whether a specific patient meets the requirements for diagnosis of a specific condition and also to assist with the general characterisation of that condition and so achieve its effective delineation from other conditions that could potentially overlap with it. The outcome of a diagnostic decision in each individual case may have major implications for management of that patient and some of the practical difficulties reported in relation to the diagnosis of PVS in specific patients and groups of patients will be examined later in this chapter. When diagnosis is required to define the margins of a condition, it can become part of the process of validating the existence of that condition.

The Multi-Society Task Force (M.S.T.F.) addressed the issue of the relationship between a diagnosis of PVS and unconsciousness in the following terms:

> "By definition, patients in a persistent vegetative state are unaware of themselves or their environment..... There is, however, a biologic limitation to the certainty of this definition, since we can only infer the presence or absence of conscious experience in another person. A false positive diagnosis of a persistent vegetative state could occur if it was concluded that a person lacked awareness when, in fact, he or she was aware" (M.S.T.F. 1994a: 1501).

The criteria to be applied in diagnosing PVS have became central issues in cases referred to the higher courts, especially in the U.K. and U.S. The immediate issue in every case has been the status of the individual patient under consideration. When management decisions regarding withdrawal of hydration and nutrition from a specified individual are to be directed by a court decision of an "*on/off*" type, it is inevitable that both the existence of PVS as a discrete condition and its delineation from other conditions should come under scrutiny. Given the probabilistic nature of the diagnostic process as it relates to vegetative states and the balancing of probabilities entailed in legal reasoning, it is inevitable that objectivity in this decision-making process is dependent on the objectivity of the data on which the decisions are based.

The importance, for PVS, of diagnostic criteria becomes evident when it is recognised that the existence of PVS as a discrete entity has been questioned. The entity has been described as a "collection of symptoms" by a Californian professor of nursing (Hall 1994), and a "behavioural syndrome" by a neurological rehabilitation specialist (Berrol 1986a). It has been perceived as "a catch-all to describe someone who looks as though they are never going to recover from a coma" in a London newspaper (Editorial *The Daily Telegraph* 1997) and a concept "mainly of social and legal interest" rather than a genuine diagnostic category by a correspondent to *The Lancet* (Colover 1997). Responding to the latter criticism, the author of the review of PVS which had evoked it observed that other conditions such as epilepsy and depression, which have been accorded medical recognition may nevertheless be diagnostically imprecise (Zeman 1997). Furthermore, it was pointed out that the fact that journalists, lawyers and the public at large had taken an interest in PVS does not invalidate its credentials as a diagnosis.

Questions about the adequacy of accepted diagnostic criteria for recognising PVS and, much more fundamentally, about *what* those criteria are actually diagnosing have arisen most clearly in court proceedings in which the diagnostic testimony of medical specialists about a patient has been at variance with published guidelines. The evolution of U.K. court decisions in relation to where the "cut-off" point lies, for withdrawal of food and water, will be discussed in Chapter 15. However, a brief account of the medical evidence on diagnosis of PVS as provided in one case during that evolution will be included in this Chapter to illustrate the way in which diagnostic practice can gradually diverge from guidelines on diagnosis.

8.1 THE PLACE OF GUIDELINES

> 'Ms Baxendale QC: Some of the witnesses we have had have described these guidelines as a framework, within which to work..... Does that fit in with how you saw the guidelines?
>
> Lady Thatcher: They are exactly what they say, guidelines, they are not the law. They are guidelines.
>
> Ms Baxendale QC: Did they have to be followed?
>
> Lady Thatcher: Of course they have to be followed, but they are not strict law. That is why they are guidelines and not law and, of course, they have to be applied according to the relevant circumstances.

> Ms Baxendale QC: They are expected to be followed?
>
> Lady Thatcher: Of course they have to be followed. They need to be followed for what they are, guidelines (Hurwitz 1998: x).

In citing this dialogue from the Scott Inquiry into the Arms for Iraq Affair in the introduction to his monograph on *Clinical guidelines and the law*, Brian Hurwitz identified it as highlighting the complex issue of the extent of the authority of U.K. guidelines. This issue was prominent in consideration of the case of Miss D in the Family Division of the U.K. High Court.

Miss D had been diagnosed as being in a vegetative state 6 months after spontaneously losing consciousness. Twelve months after diagnosis, her gastrostomy tube was accidentally dislodged and, 3 days after this mishap, the Trust responsible for her hospital care applied to the Court for a declaration that it would be lawful to discontinue feeding her. In the course of the hearing, it was indicated that she failed in three respects to meet the 1996 Vegetative State Guidelines of the Royal College of Physicians (R.C.P.). Specifically, she could track moving objects with her eyes, she evinced a "menace" reaction (blinking in response to threat) and she responded with nystagmus (to and fro movements of the eyes) after the introduction of cold water into her ear (Grubb 1997b). According to the R.C.P. Guidelines in place at the time, all of these responses should be absent before a patient can be diagnosed as being in a vegetative state. However, expert medical evidence before the Court established to its satisfaction that, notwithstanding failure to meet the Guidelines, Miss D was totally unaware of her surroundings, had no meaningful life whatsoever and was in a permanent vegetative state. The barrister appearing for the Official Solicitor on behalf of Miss D proposed that it was necessary for the Court to decide whether patients in a near-PVS should be treated in the same way as those actually in PVS (Anon. *The Daily Express* 1997). In the words of the neurologist James Bernat (1992), writing 5 years previously on the boundaries of the PVS, the Court effectively decided that, she was "as good as in a PVS". A commentary in the *Medical Law Review* neatly captured the spirit of the court proceedings when it remarked:

> "It is clear – and *Re D* affirms this – that the diagnosis of PVS is very much an art and not a science, requiring clinical experience and persistence in observation to avoid mistakes" (Grubb 1997b: 226).

The concept of evidence-based medicine has yet to impinge on the diagnosis of PVS.

The court decision to approve discontinuation of feeding Miss D prompted the commentator for the *Medical Law Review* to ask, "Where does this leave the Royal College of Physicians guidelines?" (ibid). His response was basically to recognise the authority of these Guidelines *in general* but to conclude that the actual medical evidence in any case would be determinative. It is interesting to recall that the same Guidelines (and other, similar formulations) have been subject to periodic questioning, not for being too restrictive but for not being sufficiently strict, whenever reports have been published of individuals who have regained consciousness *despite* having met the Guidelines (Chapter 9).

A reaffirmation of the original Guidelines appeared in a 1999 article providing practical guidance on diagnosis of PVS and co-authored by a rehabilitation specialist and the Official Solicitor to the Supreme Court. This proposed that, whilst visual tracking of large objects could occur in PVS patients, its presence "should always prompt careful evaluation of the state" (Wade and Johnston 1999). However, in discussing a menace reaction, the same article noted: "There should be no response such as eye closure to direct visual threat". Whilst the tenor of the comments cited to this point could suggest that the diagnosis of PVS, and perhaps by implication its discrete nature, remain to be unequivocally established, other comments allow no equivocation on either issue. A 1996 *Lancet* article, co-authored by a member of the Voluntary Euthanasia Society of Scotland, argued for the introduction of specific legislation on PVS (in which the 'P' denoted "permanent") (Mason and Mulligan 1996). It considered the persistent – or permanent – vegetative state to be "the most obvious candidate for isolation" (from other situations in which euthanasia might be proposed). However, the implication that recognition of the condition and its distinction from other, related conditions could be made with great confidence has increasingly been called into question by reports of misdiagnosis.

A distinction exists between the relevance of diagnostic criteria for individual patients and for the general concept of the PVS. Bernat (1992b) has analysed the impact of individual cases, such as that of Nancy Jobes on perceptions of the nature of PVS itself. He compared the reports provided to a U.S. court by four expert neurologists, each a widely respected expert in the evaluation of patients with altered consciousness. Two of the experts concluded that Nancy Jobes was in a PVS, the third considered that, although severely brain damaged, she was not in a PVS, while the fourth concluded, without qualification, that she was not. The two reports diagnosing the patient as in PVS concluded that there was a lack of emotional responses, dismissing fluctuations in the patient's facial expressions on the grounds that they "did not convey a sense of emotional content", arguably not the most objective of criteria. Having acknowledged the common position of the American Medical Association (A.M.A.) and the American Academy of Neurology that "PVS is a clinical diagnosis that can be made at the bedside by a skilled examiner when the essential diagnostic criteria are present", Bernat nevertheless concluded with masterly foresight that "the certainty of diagnosis of PVS may be limited" (ibid: 176).

Bernat's 1992 article, written before reports of misdiagnosis of PVS became more common did not specifically highlight the point that, in order to decide whether an individual patient meets the criteria for diagnosis of any condition such as PVS, it is necessary for there to be some certainty about those criteria. Perhaps the concept of *what* PVS actually represents may undergo adjustment as has occurred in the case of brain death, another entity defined by clinical criteria. As explained by Bernat in an article on *Refinements in the definition and criterion of death*, modifications were required to insulate the concept of brain death from clinical observations which effectively vitiated the dictum that all functions of the organism as a whole must be lost in brain death. The original brain death definition became unworkable following reports that many individuals meeting the clinical diagnostic criteria retained function at least in the posterior pituitary gland, a part of the brain.

The attitudes of neurologists or neurosurgeons have often been markedly different from those of rehabilitation specialists towards many aspects of vegetative states, such as the possible quality of life of affected individuals and the value of a positive approach to management. Two rehabilitation authors, Giacino and Zasler (1995) highlighted controversial issues in relation to *diagnosis*. They stressed that a diagnosis of PVS is essentially made exclusively on the basis of negative features whereas in relation to the essential *conceptual* feature, that is the absence of consciousness and cognitive function, they commented that:

> "There is no way that we are aware of to clinically assess 'internal awareness' in a patient who is otherwise unable to express awareness relative to external environmental stimuli" (ibid: 42).

Giacino & Zasler (1995) also emphasised that subcortical responses such as the increased heart rate and sweating after application of painful stimuli, the appearance of sleep-wake cycles, grasp reflexes and roving eye movements are as typical of patients in a minimally responsive state as they are of those in a vegetative state. None of these responses which were included as features of PVS in their original description by Jennett and Plum, can

> "be considered pathognomonic of the vegetative state as these findings may also be seen in patients who demonstrate neurobehavioural evidence of environmental awareness" (ibid: 42).

Whilst the prime diagnostic features are all negative (that is, they relate to the *absence* of some feature), none of the positive features ascribed to the condition is unique to PVS. As a final commentary on the inappropriateness of some of the conventional neurological forms of assessment when applied in the longer term to the rehabilitation of patients with severe disabilities, Giacino & Zasler noted that the Glasgow Coma and the Disability Rating Scales do not retain "their predictive utility subsequent to the acute period and are relatively insensitive to subtle changes in neurological responsiveness over time" (ibid: 44).

8.2 PROBABILITY AND PREDICTION

As any diagnosis of PVS is an expression of a probability, any constraint in making it will depend upon the extent to which the individual making the diagnosis is prepared to risk being wrong. Attempts to predict outcomes for comatose patients have run into some statistical and logistic limitations. The original report of Jennett and Plum (1972) in which the PVS was first named as such emphasised that diagnosis was, of necessity, based on the patient's behaviour (or lack thereof) and that the term did not presume the presence of a specific pathological lesion. Given the lack of well demarcated attributes exclusive to PVS (as Jennett and Plum acknowledged "a continuum must exist between this vegetative state and some of the others described" (ibid: 737)), it is inevitable that prognostic assessment of any individual patient will have to be based on probability. However, whereas the term *vegetative state* allows for a component of probability in the *diagnosis,* the addition of *persistent* conveys *prognostic* information and consequently tends to constrain the qualification of probability in this aspect of management. Substitution of *permanent* for *persistent* purports to substitute certainty and eliminate probability.

One of the earliest attempts to predict outcomes in vegetative state patients was outlined in a 1985 article from Levy *et al.* in Plum's department at the Cornell Medical Center. This sought to predict outcomes of patients in hypoxic-ischaemic coma by deriving a set of rules to distinguish between patients with good and poor prognoses early in their clinical course. In a study of 210 initially comatose patients, none of 52 characterised at the time of initial examination as lacking pupil responses to light regained "independent daily function" (in ambulation, bathing, dressing, food preparation, eating and toileting). Of 93 patients who could be identified by other unfavourable criteria on the day following onset of coma, only one subsequently regained independent function. On the basis of their observations, Levy *et al.* (1985) derived an algorithm from which a set of rules to predict outcomes was generated.

A different approach to prognostication of an irreversible condition, with markedly different conclusions, has been advocated by Shewmon (1987). His article, subtitled *The inherent impossibility of validating criteria for brain death or 'irreversibility' through clinical studies*, dealt with the use of diagnostic criteria for brain death in young children and for irreversible loss of consciousness at all ages. Shewmon's contention was that, in the absence of any criteria for the diagnosis of PVS that are self-evident *a priori*, no clinical study, irrespective of the number of patients entered in it, could adequately prove that it was possible to make this diagnosis on the basis of other criteria without a non-negligible (and therefore unacceptable) risk of error. That is, the only way to establish that a diagnostic criterion is valid *a posteriori* (as a result of a study of outcomes in patients manifesting it) would be to establish that it had self-evidently been valid *a priori*. In the absence of any criterion applicable to the diagnosis of PVS meeting this *a priori* requirement, Shewmon concluded that the risk of misdiagnosis could not be negligible. Applying Bayesian methodology to a hypothetical study of outcomes in N patients, Shewmon calculated that the risk of making a false positive diagnosis of PVS in the next patient meeting the selected criterion would be approximately 1/(N+23). On the basis of similar calculations, the chance of having at least one false positive diagnosis among the following (N+1) patients who satisfied the criterion would approximate 50% (ibid). If applied to a series of 100 patients, all of whom met the selected diagnostic criteria and none of whom emerged from a vegetative state, these calculations would indicate that there remained a 1% chance that the next patient to whom that criterion was applied would be misdiagnosed as being in PVS.

Theoretical considerations aside, the validity of algorithms such as that of Levy *et al.* for diagnosis of PVS has been directly challenged on the practical grounds both of reports of clinical misdiagnosis and of inadequate statistical technique. As an example of potential hazards for this algorithm that have been introduced by misdiagnoses, Brown (1990) in an article in the *Postgraduate Medical Journal* subtitled *Time for caution*, pointed to

> "disturbing case reports which seem to undermine not only the accuracy of proposed algorithms for predicting outcome but also our understanding of the pathology underlying the PVS" (ibid: 697).

He commented that:

> "It need only take one recovery to invalidate the thesis that all patients in a PVS with poor prognostic features will fail to achieve a reasonable and significant improvement in their lives as persons – and not merely as bodies" (ibid: 698).

In presenting a comprehensive criticism of the rationale underlying diagnosis of PVS, Shewmon and De Giorgio (1989) endorsed an earlier observation by Levy:

> "Specificity (not making the false-positive error of predicting poor outcome in someone who does well) is more important than sensitivity (not predicting poor outcome in everyone who does badly)" (ibid: 824).

Addressing the question of the size of the sample population required if the risk of a false positive diagnosis of PVS is to be reduced to a "negligible" level, they concluded that a subset of 4603 patients "who met the (nominated) criterion, survived at least 3 months and remained in a chronic vegetative state" would be required (ibid: 834). In making this calculation, they applied the Bayesian approach previously adopted by Shewmon to determine the size of a study group that would be required to ensure a risk of no more than 1 false positive diagnosis in 1000 cases.

Patient numbers in any longitudinal study of the vegetative state will be subject to a substantial early attrition from death. Shewmon and De Giorgio, using the data of Levy *et al*., pointed out that, of one group of 70 unconscious patients initially meeting a candidate diagnostic criterion, only 36% were alive at the end of the first week and only 9% after a year. Depending upon the time that is nominated as necessary to establish a diagnosis of PVS, it is inevitable that the subset surviving until this diagnosis can be made will be much smaller than the starting population. It follows that the size of the starting population required in order to establish a negligible risk of misdiagnosis would have to be considerably larger than that indicated above for 3 month survivors. An additional impediment to formulating predictions on the basis of available data, emphasised by Shewmon and De Giorgio, is the frequent failure of surveys of the outcomes for PVS patients to distinguish long term vegetative survivors from non-survivors and severely disabled, but non-vegetative, survivors.

Formulation of a poor prognosis for unconscious patients is likely itself to contribute to a high early death rate. Shewmon and De Giorgio acknowledged an irresolvable conflict between good science and good patient management and observed that, whereas a study to validate early predictors of neurologic outcome after cardiac arrest in cats and dogs would require provision of maximal life-saving measures, such a course could be contrary to a human patient's best interests or previous wishes. Nevertheless, physicians have experienced increasing pressure to provide predictions for unconscious patients at an early stage. Shewmon and De Giorgio remarked on changes in attitudes to vegetative patients and suggested that, prior to the widespread acceptance of the practice of discontinuing tube feeding in PVS patients,

> "the only opportunity to facilitate the nonsurvival of such patients was perceived to be during the relatively brief phase of ventilator-dependency early in the course of coma" (ibid: 837).

The importance of establishing reliable predictors of PVS may have decreased in inverse proportion to the growing acceptance of withdrawal of feeding support from PVS patients. Finally, Shewmon and De Giorgio stressed that the likelihood of development of a chronic vegetative state, expressed as a percentage of the starting population, was low and recalled that in the 1981 study of Levy *et al*. only 6 of 120 patients categorised on admission as having virtually no chance of regaining independent function, survived for more than 2 weeks.

When considering the extent to which the diagnosis of PVS can be confidently made, there can hardly be a more appropriate source than the remarks of Richard Beresford (1997) at the festschrift to mark Fred Plum's retirement. In identifying the boundaries of neurological expertise, Beresford observed that, if making a diagnosis of PVS is the principal contribution that neurologists can make to management of affected patients (if no treatment is available), then the *reliability* of that diagnosis "assumes overwhelming importance". Taking account of the estimate in an article of Childs and Mercer (1996a) that the probability of regaining some awareness after a year in a vegetative state was 14%, Beresford concluded that:

> "The question then emerges as to how certain neurologists can be when they offer their opinions to families, primary providers, ethics committees or courts" (ibid: 392).

His conclusion was that such opinions failed to reach the standard of "beyond a reasonable doubt". The nomination of a standard of "beyond reasonable doubt" by Beresford represents a considerably more specific interpretation of the level of confidence required in diagnosis than that spelt out by the A.M.A. in 1986. This referred only to the irreversibility of a patient's coma being "beyond doubt" without any further qualification (American Medical Association Council 1986).

Disagreement with the nomination of a standard as demanding as that proposed by Beresford is sometimes raised on the basis that misdiagnosis as vegetative of a patient who retains some level of awareness would not necessarily be a bad thing if it enabled hydration and nutrition to be withdrawn so accomplishing the ending of life which the patient may have wanted. However, I believe this attitude of "the diagnosis was wrong, but it turned out well in the end" flies in the face of the principle that a practitioner should strive *first* to diagnose accurately and *only* then to decide on management.

8.3 FREQUENCY OF MISDIAGNOSIS OF PVS

The claim of 100% accuracy of diagnosis cited at the beginning of this Chapter reflected majority opinion at the time it was made. A 1991 review article cited two Councils of the A.M.A. to the effect that "the chance of error in diagnosis would be approximately 0.1%" (Spudis 1991). However, reading of the original A.M.A report fails to reveal any estimate of the risk of *misdiagnosis* (most commonly representing failure to detect evidence of awareness in a patient who retains any awareness). It does, in the course of discussing cognitive *recovery*, estimate that "the odds of recovery are less than 1 in 1000" (American Medical Association Councils 1990). Distinction between an original, earlier misdiagnosis and a later recovery following accurate diagnosis may be quite difficult in some individual cases. However, inability to distinguish between the two discrete concepts in a review article written by a neurologist is disconcerting.

Pressure on clinicians to ensure that a diagnosis of PVS can be made with complete confidence has increased considerably as a result of the acceptance of withdrawal of hydration and nutrition as a popular option in management. In arguing the case for an improved standard of diagnosis, Andrews (1997) specified several prerequisites that need to be met in making that diagnosis. The first of these was that the patient should be "generally healthy", implying that nutritional status be adequate and bowel and bladder optimally managed. The second prerequisite was that each patient should be assessed sitting out of bed "in a well supported seating system" which afforded the person the best opportunity to be alert. Finally, he stressed the importance of repeated assessments undertaken by a skilled team for short intervals over a period of 4 to 6 weeks, as offering the best opportunity of being able to observe any responsiveness.

While this monograph is concerned primarily with patients who enter a vegetative state as a result of an acute episode of trauma, cerebral anoxia or some combination of these, it is relevant to note the frequent misdiagnosis as being in a PVS of people in the end stages of a gradually progressive dementia. The issue of whether "PVS" is an accurate description of their condition will not be considered. Walshe and Leonard (1985), in extending the PVS syndrome to include such cases noted that there was an inconsistency in response of affected patients to some tests (such as elicitation of nystagmus and fixation of eyes on the examiner) which were considered to be diagnostic for vegetative states as originally conceived. They also reported the existence of intermittent vegetative states in which periods of apparent unawareness were interspersed with awareness. Some of their patients (temporarily) satisfied their prime diagnostic criterion of "a seemingly awake patient who has no interactive behavioural function" due to over-treatment with sedatives or an intercurrent illness. A report on the incidence of misdiagnosis of PVS in a group of nursing home residents, many of whom had been regarded as having gradually entered PVS after a period of dementia, was published in 1991. As already cautioned, its conclusions can not necessarily be applied to other patients, many of them much younger, diagnosed as vegetative after an acute episode of trauma, cerebral vascular accident or cardiac arrest. Nevertheless, of 62 residents of Wisconsin nursing homes who had been identified by nursing home personnel as being in PVS, 11 were found, on re-examination, not to meet the PVS criteria (Tresch *et al.* 1991b).

Awareness of the likelihood of misdiagnosis of PVS in patients who have become unconscious acutely has increased since the early 1990s. A 1993 report from Texas, specifically on the accuracy of PVS diagnosis, reviewed 49 severely brain injured patients from the U.S. and Canada who had been referred for neurorehabilitation over a 5 year period with a pre-admission diagnosis of coma or PVS. In introducing this report, Childs *et al.* (1993) noted that whilst many acknowledged the confusion that existed in diagnosing PVS, there was little research on the accuracy of the diagnosis. A post-admission diagnosis had been formulated for these patients within the first 7 days. In the case of 18 individuals (37%), this resulted in a change of diagnosis to indicate that the patient was *not* in a PVS. The high rate of misdiagnosis was attributed to a combination of confusion over terminology and lack of extended observation by the referring physicians. Some physicians have acknowledged that the risk of misdiagnosis was *not* a fact which suddenly emerged in the 1990's. Highlighting the difference in attitudes and perceptions between neurologists/neurosurgeons and rehabilitation specialists, a position paper from the American Congress of Rehabilitation Medicine (1995) pointed out that knowledge of diagnostic inaccuracies related to the PVS was longstanding and that improvement was not occurring. The position paper considered the findings of Childs *et al.* to be, "particularly alarming". Addressing the question of probability of misdiagnosis in a much less formal way than Shewmon, the paper made the point that:

> "Assignation of the term PVS denotes 100% certainty and the existing body of scientific knowledge does not support this level of confidence" (ibid: 206).

Whilst the position paper referred to *persistent* and *permanent* vegetative state, the abbreviation was identified with the former. In seeking to discern the reason underlying misdiagnosis, the paper examined the requirements for an observer to decide whether a putative response from a patient was "meaningful or purposeful". It suggested that frequency and appropriateness of the presumed response were critical in the context of reaching this decision.

Without question, the greatest impact on discussion of misdiagnosis has been that made by a report of Andrews *et al.* (1996) from the Royal Hospital for Neuro-disability. Forty patients referred to the hospital with a diagnosis of vegetative state were studied. Of these, 17 (43%) were assessed as having been misdiagnosed. With a single exception, all of this mistaken diagnosis group had been referred by a neurologist, neurosurgeon or rehabilitation specialist. In order to reduce the likelihood of erroneously classifying patients, who had been accurately diagnosed but were in the process of emerging from a vegetative state, as instances of misdiagnosis, anyone who had been unconscious for less than 6 months was excluded from the study. Of the 17 patients re-classified as misdiagnoses, 7 had been presumed to have been in a vegetative state for longer than a year and 3 of these had been so presumed to be for over 4 years. The condition of the group of 17 incorrectly diagnosed patients of Andrews *et al.* remained one of severe physical disability but almost all were able to communicate, to varying degrees, with others. Fifteen of the group relied on pressing a buzzer as their only functional movement for communication. Andrews *et al.* described one patient on whose behalf a communication mechanism could not be established until joint contractures had been corrected permitting the use of "a slight shoulder shrug". In seeking to explain the previous misdiagnoses, it was found that 11 of the group were either blind or had severe visual impairment. Whilst the subject of hearing was not addressed in the report, it would be reasonable to speculate whether any of the remaining 23 patients in the series, regarded as correctly diagnosed as vegetative, retained awareness that was undetected because it was accompanied by visual *and hearing* impairment.

The report of Andrews *et al.* initiated discussion in the lay press about the value of the existing sets of guidelines for diagnosis of the vegetative state and their relevance to future court applications for withdrawal of hydration and nutrition from patients diagnosed as vegetative. It evoked criticism from Ronald Cranford in the same issue of the *British Medical Journal* as the Andrews *et al.* paper. Cranford queried the representative nature of Andrews' patient sample and the validity of the communication techniques. "I must view the buzzer system with some scepticism" (Cranford 1996). He also questioned whether some of the cases represented emergence from a genuine vegetative state rather than its misdiagnosis and objected that assessment should have been accompanied by use of techniques such as CT scans and PET.

Passing from scepticism about the validity of Andrews' claims of misdiagnosis, Cranford directed his argument to the condition of the misdiagnosed patients. He proposed that the re-diagnosed state of the 17 Andrews *et al.* patients was more horrifying than the vegetative state itself, presumably implying that their continued existence was even more to be deplored.

> "Most people would find this condition (patients who are close to, but not in PVS as defined in guidelines) far more horrifying than the vegetative state itself and some might think it an even stronger reason for stopping treatment than complete unconsciousness" (ibid: 6).

Without questioning Cranford's entitlement to think this way, it appears to me to undercut the rationale previously presented to justify the withdrawal of support from patients diagnosed as in a PVS and to replace it with a very different line of reasoning. The original rationale maintained that complete loss of awareness (or, more accurately, of any indication of it that was detectable by others) signified loss of personhood. It was all over. Hence it was reasonable to withdraw all support. Cranford's variant response was that *incomplete* loss of awareness could be a more cogent reason for withdrawal than the complete loss (of awareness, personhood or whatever) that had inspired the original proposal.

Rejoinders to Cranford's criticism of Andrews' findings were provided from two neurological rehabilitation specialists in a later issue of the *British Medical Journal.*

Wade (1996) noted that the term "PVS" should not be applied to patients who have been unconscious for less than 12 months. Whilst the Andrews *et al.* series had only excluded those diagnosed for less than 6 months, Wade nevertheless considered it to be improbable that the rate of spontaneous recovery from the vegetative state could account for those 9 instances of patients in the study group of 40 who had been previously diagnosed as in PVS for 12 months or longer. In stressing the need for thoroughness and experience on the part of any clinician attempting to diagnose PVS, Wade advocated

> "interviewing at least one nurse who knows the patient well, interviewing at least one relative who has been close to the patient" (ibid: 943).

In another letter to the editor, Childs and Mercer (1996b) re-entered the lists and responded to Cranford's commentary in no uncertain terms:

> "Aside from the implication that physicians who provide rehabilitative care are scientifically suspect, Cranford shows his inexperience in the neurorehabilitation of brain injured patients when he doubts the veracity of the buzzer system".

Delivering another riposte, Childs and Mercer noted Cranford's comment that neurodiagnostic tests (Eg PET, CT etc) have some use in the diagnosis of the vegetative state and contrasted this with the earlier negative assessments of the M.S.T.F. on PVS (of which Cranford had been a member) about the value of such tests in making the diagnosis.

It would appear to be improbable, as noted above by Wade, that the patients of Andrews *et al.* who had been unconscious for periods between 6 and 12 months had emerged from an accurately diagnosed vegetative state rather than being the subject of frank misdiagnosis. Nevertheless, the distinction between late emergence and misdiagnosis may become complex in individual cases. In a review in the *Journal of Head Trauma Rehabilitation*, Berrol (1986a) speculated that some of the cases of late recovery from PVS reported to that time may have attained significant, but overlooked, improvements in the first year of unconsciousness.

Reports of systemic misdiagnosis of vegetative states have not ceased with that of Andrews *et al.* Wilson *et al.* (2002) described a series of 12 patients referred as vegetative, to a specialist hospital in Northern Ireland during 1995-7. Four of these patients, when assessed at admission, were considered to have been misdiagnosed. As with the patients reported by Andrews *et al.*, the possibility of correct original diagnosis followed by emergence existed but this seemed unlikely, especially in the case of two who had been regarded as vegetative for more than a year.

Apart from queries about the validity of reports of frequent misdiagnosis of PVS, the initial response to an increase in general awareness that misdiagnosis of PVS was not an extremely rare event was to call for more reliable guidelines that would reduce or eliminate mistakes. Such a call assumes, of course, that the nature of the condition permits their formulation. A similar response followed reports suggesting that emergence (as distinct from primary misdiagnosis) was not a "one in a million" event. A variant response to misdiagnoses has been to advocate widening of the purview of existing guidelines to ensure that they accord with the condition of some patients who have emerged from, or were never in, PVS. The principle underlying this approach is that some patients are "as good as in PVS" (Bernat 1992b). The U.K. case of Miss D already referred to, illustrates some of the implications of this policy of more generous allocation of the PVS diagnosis. Two published comments on that case from divergent sources queried the notion that near enough (to PVS) was good enough. The editor of the *Bulletin of Medical Ethics* was quoted to the effect that there were "constant attempts to quietly push back the frontiers" (Macdonald 1997b). Writing 4 days later in another London newspaper, a Scottish cardinal queried whether the "right-to-die" outlook was being transformed into a "duty-to-die" attitude (Winning 1997).

8.4 DIAGNOSIS IN COURT

Preceding consideration of the precision possible in diagnosis of PVS noted the argument that lack of precision in the diagnosis of other conditions, such as epilepsy, did not diminish their reality. Where the similarity between diagnosis of PVS and epilepsy ends is in the frequency with which a diagnosis of PVS is tendered in legal proceedings of critical significance for the individual concerned. In the case of Miss D, the clinicians were in agreement with each other about her diagnosis but were in conflict with the R.C.P. Guidelines whereas, in the case of Mr 'S', there was a disagreement between clinicians on the diagnosis. This 1994 case in the English Court of Appeal was concerned with withdrawal of treatment from 'S', a young man diagnosed as in a vegetative state. In upholding the request from an NHS Hospital Trust for withdrawal of hydration and nutrition from 'S', the Master of the Rolls noted that he was required to decide between conflicting evidence on the question of whether 'S' possessed any degree of awareness (*Frenchay Healthcare NHS Trust v S* 1994). Testimony was given by a neuropsychiatrist that 'S' appeared to suffer pain and by a consultant at the Royal Hospital for Neuro-disability that he showed some responses. Reference was made to the conviction of his nurses that he appeared to suffer. In response to this, the Master concluded that the evidence that 'S' was in a PVS was not as emphatic and unanimous as in the Bland case (to be considered in Chapter 15). He nevertheless felt that the Court should not attach great weight to the points of distinction from the Bland case. He concluded that there was no reason to question the conclusion of 'S's' consultant that it was in his best interests for no action to be taken to resume feeding (ibid). Disagreements on the question of whether a particular individual was in a PVS have emerged in expert testimony before other courts and, as in the case of 'S', the diagnosis has been in the hands of the presiding judge. The case of 'S' illustrated the paradox of regarding diagnosis of PVS as an "all or nothing" decision but, at the same time being prepared to accept that one patient might be "more in" or "less in" than others.

An example of one legal approach to the question of PVS misdiagnosis published in the Cornell Law Review estimated the risk as 0.004% on the basis that "approximately 100,000 patients" had entered the PVS during the twenty years preceding 1992 and only four reported cases had "resulted in even partial recovery"

(Stacy 1992). Working on this basis, Tom Stacy proceeded to raise the question of the level of possible error that would be acceptable. To establish the inevitability that any human activity will entail risk of some error he cited a philosopher, Anthony Flew:

> "It is an inescapable feature of the human condition that no one is infallible about anything, and there is no sphere of life in which mistakes do not occur" (ibid: 526).

Stacy's estimate of 0.004% for the frequency of misdiagnosis is so much at variance with published experience that it has to be a strong candidate for acknowledgement as the most eloquent demonstration of human fallibility. A better assessment of the risk of misdiagnosis, again from a legal perspective was provided by Beresford (1997) in considering the "boundaries of neurological expertise". He speculated about whether neurologists could

> "confidently assure decision makers that individuals whose eyes are open and who move and make sounds nevertheless cannot experience pain or pleasure" (ibid: 392).

8.5 THE ULTIMATE MISDIAGNOSIS – LOCKED-IN SYNDROME

The issue of accuracy of diagnosis of PVS, which had attracted considerable public attention in 1996 with the publication of the article by Andrews *et al.* was forcibly brought to the attention of the English public again in 1999. The case of Marian Sallery, who had been clinically diagnosed as in a vegetative state, attracted considerable attention with the disclosure in the media of the findings of neuropathological examination of her autopsy specimens. This revealed that "her higher brain functions had remained intact" – as judged by pathological findings at autopsy (Brennan 1999). *The Sunday Times* reported that discussion between her medical attendants and her family on the issue of withdrawing hydration and nutrition had taken place in her presence. Her parents were said to have believed that Marian was aware of her surroundings and it was recalled that she had responded emotionally to television reports on football matches (apparently one of the most distinctive environmental stimuli available to English patients with severe brain injury). The inference drawn from preservation of her cerebral cortex was that Marian had indeed been aware of events around her, including discussions about her fate. That is, to the extent that diagnosis of medical conditions can be based on neuroanatomical lesions, Marian Sallery had suffered from the locked-in syndrome, and was not in a vegetative state.

When outlining the neuropathological features of PVS in Chapter 2, it was indicated that the term LiS was originally applied exclusively to patients with a specific pathological lesion affecting the pons (part of the brain stem) but completely sparing the cortex. It was inferred that such patients could remain completely aware, assuming that there were no accompanying cerebral hemisphere lesions. However, with the growing awareness that a significant number of patients may have been misdiagnosed as vegetative, despite retention of some level of awareness, and that others may have regained consciousness after being vegetative, it has become recognised that patients who have retained or regained consciousness, with little capacity to communicate, such as the patients of Andrews *et al.* (1996) could legitimately be described as "locked in". With this caveat, the account given in this section deals primarily with patients who have been described as LiS.

The term "*locked-in syndrome*" (LiS) was pioneered in a monograph by Plum and Posner (1966) and was as readily adopted as another of Plum's suggestions, the "PVS" itself, was to be 6 years later. Illustrating the manner in which a succinct title can influence not only the recognition of a medical condition, but also the frequency with which it is described, Bauer *et al.* (1979) remarked that, although there had previously been some quite extensive reports of the condition it "did not become popular among neurologists" until it was named as "locked-in syndrome". Entrenchment of a memorable, descriptive title can assist in formulating the perception of the condition it describes as a discrete entity (as has happened with PVS). For example, the Canadian neurologist, already cited at the start of this Chapter for his views on reliability of diagnosis of PVS, when referring to the distinction of LiS from PVS declared that: "the PET scan is quite specific" (Ivan 1990). Given that the total published literature on PET in the LiS to which he referred was 3 cases at that time one might retain some reservations about the claim.

The simple statement that LiS is readily distinguished from PVS by the retention by affected individuals of the ability to communicate with a variety of signals may be diagnostically misleading and raises questions of classification. As already noted, a patient may be effectively "locked in" without displaying typical features of the LiS. Should the ability to communicate be regarded merely as a convenient means of making a differential diagnosis between LiS and PVS or as a defining attribute of the former with significant implications for the status of the patient and, in consequence, for the manner in which affected patients are regarded and managed by others? As has been the case with PVS itself, the issue arises of the legitimacy of splitting off parts of a continuous spectrum by means of nomenclature. It is not difficult to assume that entities designated by such clear, memorable and descriptive terminology as PVS and LiS *must* also designate discrete conditions. As already noted in Chapter 2, the impression frequently given in the literature that people in PVS have a consistent neuropathological status centred on destruction of the cerebral cortex, has not been supported by autopsy reports. Whilst the literature relating to the pathological features of the LiS is much less extensive than that spawned by PVS, there are nevertheless strong indications that the neuroanatomical features of LiS patients may also be quite variable and this may have diagnostic implications.

As early as 1974, Karp and Hurtig concluded that the locked-in syndrome should not be regarded as synonymous with the type of brain stem lesions that were then, and have generally been, considered to be pathognomonic of it (Karp and Hurtig 1974). A review of LiS by Patterson and Grabois (1986) a decade later suggested that the size and location of the neuropathological lesion could differ significantly between patients with similar motor deficits. The absence of a completely consistent association between neuropathology and neurological function presents a qualification to the retrospective diagnosis of LiS in the case of Marian Sallery mentioned above. On the other hand, if there was good neuropathological evidence of preservation of normal structure in her cerebral cortex, the *onus* of establishing that she had lacked awareness (irrespective of whichever term was chosen when diagnosing her condition) should devolve upon anyone asserting this. Levy *et al.* (1987), when introducing their report of the application of PET to distinguish vegetative from locked-in patients, drew attention to the considerable variation in the extent of cerebral hemisphere damage. They noted that it was "difficult to infer on pathological grounds alone whether or not all self awareness was lost during life" (ibid: 673). In commenting upon the differential clinical diagnosis between PVS and LiS, Levy *et al.* considered that this was straightforward, being based on the ability of locked-in patients to communicate using coded eye movements. However, the occurrence of patients such as that of Andrews *et al.* who could only communicate by shoulder shrug and the existence of a "total" locked-in state (see below) in which eye movements are not possible, although full awareness is retained, would seem to void this argument.

The review of Bauer *et al.* (1979) describing the variable manifestations observed in a series of patients in LiS and attempts to classify them into sub-groups of "incomplete", "classical" or "total" LiS has raised some very substantial issues about both the discrete nature of the condition itself and the reliability of its diagnostic distinction from PVS. Incomplete LiS was defined as a condition in which other movements, additional to vertical eye movements and blinking, remained possible. Classical LiS patients retained only these two capacities. Total LiS, two examples of which were identified in the series of 12 patients, was described as entailing

> "total immobility including all eye movements combined with preserved consciousness" (ibid: 84).

Bauer *et al.* surmised that such people retained a capacity for

> "existing inner monologue and awareness of external and internal stimuli as far as the corresponding pathways for sensory perception are spared by the lesion" (ibid: 84).

Recognition of total LiS in two of the patients of Bauer *et al.* was assisted by the normality and near-normality, respectively, of their EEG recordings. Another patient in this series, whose case Bauer *et al.* found to be "especially instructive", had transiently entered LiS following temporary impairment of blood flow to the brain stem. This person, who had a slightly abnormal EEG during this episode, was reported as remembering

> "all details of the locked-in condition, and related vividly his feelings during his general flaccidity" (ibid: 83).

The *diagnostic* implications for PVS of the "total LiS" state are considerable, but appear not to have been widely appreciated. One review of the case of Anthony Bland noted that the question of whether a person could be "locked-in" and *also* have lost the capacity for eye movement had been raised with an expert witness but not pursued (Borthwick 1996). If a condition of "total LiS" as described by Bauer *et al.* exists, then the response of the expert witness clearly should have been in the affirmative.

The capacity of a patient in the LiS to communicate with others may vary from time to time. Whether such variation could occur independently of changes in conscious state or whether it reflects a temporary deterioration in this is unclear. For example, Giacino (1997) described a patient, diagnosed as locked-in, whose eye movements deteriorated over repeated trials and eventually became unintelligible. As an additional consideration, it should be evident that any capacity of locked-in persons to communicate, whether by eye movements or by any other means, will only become and remain apparent if they retain the capacity to *receive* communication from others. This is likely to have been the principal reason for misdiagnosis in the series of Andrews *et al.* (1996). As reported by Andrews *et al.*, some of their patients who retained awareness but had been misdiagnosed as PVS were blind, probably as a result of cortical damage. Communication with these originally misdiagnosed patients was dependent upon retention of their capacity for hearing. If hearing has been impaired, whether as a result of the events leading to the LiS or as part of pre-existing or unrelated pathology, attempts to communicate with a patient could be thwarted, irrespective of his or her retention of cognition and of the capacity for eye movements. In this situation, the inference would probably be drawn that the individual was completely unconscious. Whilst there is little if any published information specifically on the subject of pathological interference with hearing in LiS patients, damage to afferent (sensory) nerve pathways can extend to the auditory pathways (Patterson and Grabois 1986).

The perceptions of the diagnosing practitioner in relation to the frequency of occurrence of LiS and its typical features are likely to determine the risk that LiS could be mistaken for PVS. For instance, if a condition is *regarded* as being extremely rare (irrespective of whether this actually is the case), there may be reticence in diagnosing an individual case if only because an incorrect diagnosis may constitute an embarrassment for the practitioner. Similarly, if the descriptions of a condition most readily available in the literature are not representative, the likelihood of its recognition may be reduced. Uncertainty appears to prevail in the literature on both of these points. As regards the frequency of occurrence of LiS, Nordgren *et al.* (1971), from the Rochester Medical Center, NY, concluded, on the basis of having encountered 7 patients in 12 months, that LiS was a more common condition than previously acknowledged. On the other hand, Giacino and Zasler (1995), in a comprehensive review of outcomes after severe traumatic brain injury, referred to LiS as "relatively rare". They, nevertheless, also indicated that LiS patients were often misdiagnosed as comatose or vegetative. Patterson and Grabois (1986) commented upon the possibility that the published papers relating to LiS may not represent a true sample of this condition and, in the course of reviewing a large series compiled from the literature, observed that:

> "Case histories which are unusual or show a successful therapeutic approach are submitted for publication while the routine cases are not" (ibid: 762).

Apart from its diagnostic implications, retention or loss of eye movements raises conceptual implications for LiS. Thus, it is difficult to discern any sound neuroanatomically based reason for postulating that preservation of the brain stem structures necessary for retention of the ability to blink should be a basis for *also retaining awareness or cognition* as distinct from providing means for *others to recognise it*. The concept of PVS has been constructed so as to have as its dominant feature the total lack of any awareness by the affected individual. In contrast, the LiS patient is demonstrably aware and, potentially, may be as aware as his or her medical attendant. On the basis of these constructions, the PVS patient is dismissed by some commentators as no longer being a person (and to be treated accordingly) whilst the LiS patient usually attracts sympathy and support (with the qualification to be noted in the following section). Yet the only *observable* differences between the two classes of patient may be that the LiS patient is still capable of blinking. Reduced to its most simplistic form, why should the ability to blink be a prerequisite for personhood?

8.6 IMPLICATIONS OF A DIAGNOSIS OF LOCKED-IN SYNDROME FOR PATIENT MANAGEMENT

Recognition that an individual represents a case of LiS rather than being in a PVS may well influence management decisions. Some published reports on survival rates in the two conditions suggest that LiS patients may receive better treatment. One correspondent to the *New England Journal of Medicine* in the aftermath of publication of the statement of the M.S.T.F. on PVS contrasted the conclusions about survival of PVS patients in that statement with his own experience of much better survival of a cohort of patients who had remained in LiS for more than a year (Haig 1994). It was suggested that there should be little physiological difference between LiS and PVS patients. However, the correspondent suggested that the much lower survival rate of PVS patients could reflect conscious or unconscious neglect by care givers.

In contrast with the proposition that patients diagnosed as in LiS might, as a consequence, receive more treatment, others have argued strongly against this possibility. Braithwaite and Thomasma (1988) advocated the application of an "anti-cruelty policy" which would direct the withdrawal of "life-sustaining treatment" from any patient with a "hopeless injury". "Hopeless injury" was defined so as to include "no observable pleasure or happiness in living aside from immediate and transitory physical satisfaction" (ibid: 711) and patients with the LiS were cited as an example of it. Braithwaite and Thomasma's dismissal of LiS patients would hardly appear to be applicable to the world's best known such individual, Jean-Dominique Bauby, founder of the Association du Locked-In Syndrome and author of an account of living in LiS (Bauby 1997). As described by his publisher, Bauby's "poignant and often wryly humorous" account illustrated his ability to "invent a life for oneself in the most appalling of circumstances". However, the proposition that patients in LiS may be even more appropriate candidates for withdrawal of support than accurately diagnosed PVS patients has been forcefully presented.

8.7 RECAPITULATION

Opinions about the certainty with which PVS can be diagnosed have varied with the identity of the person expressing the opinion. The diagnosis is made on clinical grounds, there being no reliable confirmatory technology, and it has usually been stated that any competent neurologist can make it. Nevertheless, the large group of patients in the 1996 report of Andrews *et al.* who had been mistakenly diagnosed as in a PVS had been examined by specialists. A diagnosis of PVS is likely to have major implications for the future treatment of the affected person. It is likely to be regarded as of high evidentiary status by a court. Nevertheless, it remains a probability rather than a certainty.

To some extent reflecting the probabilistic nature of the diagnosis, sets of diagnostic guidelines have been developed. A characteristic of any description of the diagnostic process to be applied to PVS is that the most distinctive feature of the condition is a negative one, namely loss of capacity for consciousness. On the other hand, none of the positive features is unique to PVS as all may occur in conscious patients with severe brain injury.

Attempts to improve the diagnostic efficiency of PVS could be directed to research at the level of populations of patients or to fastidious compliance with optimal requirements for assessing the individual patient. The most common research approach, namely that of the prospective study of a group of patients sufficiently large to provide good statistical power, does not readily lend itself to PVS because of the inordinately high rate of early attrition of any starting population of patients with very severe brain injury as a result of death. Diagnosis of the individual patient, if it is to be done properly, requires that physical condition first be optimised, that repeated examination be undertaken and that attention be paid to any observations of nursing staff or family members who are familiar with the patient. It also requires that potential confounding factors, such as visual impairment, be excluded.

Reports of misdiagnosis of patients as in a PVS have usually attracted one of three types of response of which the first is denial. Secondly, such reports have prompted calls for improved diagnostic guidelines. Thirdly, it has been concluded that the situation of a misdiagnosed patient who retains awareness must be more horrible than that of others who are genuinely unaware. An offshoot of this response has been to advocate an "anti-cruelty policy" of withdrawal of support from patients diagnosed as being in a "locked-in" rather than a "vegetative state".

CHAPTER 9

EMERGENCE FROM A VEGETATIVE STATE

> "Anecdotal rumors of dramatic recovery are common but are seldom reported in detail" (Dougherty *et al*. 1981: 997).
>
> "Furthermore, the lay literature is replete with dramatic, but unfortunately unsubstantiated and inaccurate reports of dramatic recoveries from coma" (Cranford 1984: 38).

These neurological appraisals from the early 1980s are indicative of a dismissive attitude towards reports that have not appeared in "mainstream" medical journals. Any consideration of the question of emergence from a vegetative state requires recognition at the outset of the potential difference between *emergence* and *recovery*. As the crucial definitional feature of the concept of a vegetative state is that the affected person is completely unaware of his or her environment, it follows that *any* indication of awareness on the part of an individual who was genuinely lacking this previously, represents emergence from the vegetative state. The extent of emergence, and its continuation, may vary between different patients.

Apart from differentiating "emergence" from "recovery", it will also be necessary, to differentiate between primary misdiagnosis and accurate original diagnosis followed by genuine emergence. Whereas emergence from a state diagnosed as "vegetative" or "persistent vegetative" could be consistent with either possibility, emergence from a "permanent" vegetative state *always* indicates misdiagnosis. Additional complexity is sometimes introduced into recognition and acceptance of emergence when the observations pointing to it have been made in the first instance by the patient's family rather than by a physician. In contrast with the relatively defined meaning of "emergence", the term "recovery" may have quite different connotations for different assessors, ranging from very modest improvement, such as the regaining of consciousness by a person who remains totally dependent upon others, to a complete restoration to good health. Undoubtedly, some disputes about the likelihood of "recovery" from vegetative states reflect a failure to distinguish between emergence alone and more extensive recovery.

This Chapter will be concerned exclusively with the issue of emergence, whilst the question of *what level* of recovery could be regarded as worthwhile by a patient, and by others, will be considered in Chapter 10. The question of "dramatic recovery", whatever that may be, referred to in the quotations above is even further from the scope of the present Chapter.

Whilst caution about accepting non-medical accounts of a patient's history, for example those provided by the patient or family, because of their variable evidentiary quality, is a feature of most medical specialties additional factors are likely to be operative in the case of patients diagnosed as being in a vegetative state. One factor that cannot be ignored in evaluating medical responses to such reports is that those individuals who are the subject of claims for delayed emergence from a vegetative state have frequently already been excluded from ongoing neurological and rehabilitation care because they were considered unsuitable for it and unlikely to benefit. Consequently, reports of their improvement may be taken as direct criticisms of their earlier medical assessment and management. Another factor leading to disputation is the frequency with which family members have claimed to have communicated with a patient diagnosed as vegetative when the medical attendants have determined that this could not be possible. In balancing the conclusions of family and physicians it is necessary to acknowledge that the former can be at risk of deluding themselves into seeing what they hope to see. It is also necessary, however, to recognise that the family is likely to have spent much more time in the company of the patient than has the physician and that the family will be much better attuned to those topics of communication that are likely to interest the patient.

Although the distinction between misdiagnosis of a person as being in a vegetative state and later emergence, after being accurately diagnosed as vegetative, may be extremely difficult in retrospect, Andrews *et al.* (1996), were confident that the series of patients whom they described represented misdiagnosis. As already noted, if the term *permanent* vegetative state has been applied, any instance of "emergence" must be, by definition, an instance of misdiagnosis. Whilst emergence was described, in the medical literature as extremely rare, or a non-event until, the mid 1990s, accounts of individual patients and series have since become more frequent. A major practical concern raised by confusion between initial misdiagnosis and subsequent emergence from a vegetative state is the loss of opportunity for early attempts at rehabilitation of misdiagnosed patients. This disadvantage may be compounded if additional impediments to communication, such as contractures, are superimposed before recognition of the patient's status.

The possibility that any patient regarded as being in a PVS could regain consciousness has become of growing concern as the withdrawal of hydration and nutrition from these patients has been increasingly advocated and practised. This heightened concern has been based on the possibility that some patients who subsequently might have regained consciousness, if the provision of care had been continued, have been prevented from doing so by death following the withdrawal of feeding. The countervailing argument is that total certainty that consciousness will not be regained should not be necessary before a decision is made to withdraw feeding, and so end a patient's life. In practice, there has been considerable variation in the degree of certainty that has been required in making this decision.

One argument that has been advanced is that a degree of certainty consistent with that prevailing in community acceptance of other types of mistakes that cost a life is appropriate. In presenting this argument in relation to PVS Stacy (1992) has drawn an enterprising analogy with capital punishment which, when he wrote, had been adopted in 37 U.S. States "despite the inevitability that innocent persons will be executed" (ibid: 523). He buttressed the argument by citing the case previously advanced for the death penalty by van den Haag:

> "I do not doubt that, over a long enough period, miscarriages of justice will occur even in capital cases. Despite precautions, nearly all human activities such as trucking, lighting, or construction cost the lives of some innocent bystanders. We do not give up these activities, because the advantages, moral or material, outweigh the unintended losses. Analogously, for those who think the death penalty just, miscarriages of justice are offset by the moral benefits and usefulness of doing justice" (van den Haag 1986: 1664).

Were this analogy to be probed more extensively, the extent to which one is *obliged* to avoid misadventure in trucking, lighting or construction might be examined. It would also be reasonable to take account of the relative intensity of intervention required to reduce the risk of death by misadventure in the course of trucking and of caring for vegetative patients.

The possibility that instances of vegetative patients regaining consciousness could affect community attitudes to the management of patients in vegetative states has been dismissed on account of their reputed rarity, and perceptions of the poor residual condition of these patients. Some commentators have emphatically claimed that a person who retains, or has regained, some awareness is in a worse predicament than others still considered to be in a vegetative state and is even more deserving of consideration as a candidate for withdrawal of hydration and nutrition. Failure to recognise early signs of emergence in patients diagnosed as vegetative is likely to reduce the intensity of attempts at rehabilitation and of treatment of accompanying medical conditions. Perhaps in compensation for diminution in the force of the argument that patients never emerge from PVS, the limitations of patients who had been vegetative have been increasingly emphasised as cases of emergence have come to light. Fred Plum wrote to a U.S. President's Commission that:

> "Even those few in whom late evidence of cognitive awareness has reappeared had to be classified as having a severe disability both from the standpoint of physical and intellectual residua. I know of no example of such a patient who has returned to what can be considered independent intellectual or motor function" (President's Commission 1983a).

A forcefully expressed opinion on the subject of emergence from PVS and its aftermath was that of Schneiderman *et al.* (1990):

> "The mythologic power of the coma patient who 'wakes up' apparently overrides the rarity of documented confirmation of such miraculous recoveries (which have resulted moreover, in incapacitating mental impairment or total dependence)" (ibid: 952).

Whilst media reports of emergence may fail to emphasise residual disability, and be unduly optimistic, journalistic hyperbole about PVS can be equally pessimistic. Thus, an English journalist, writing in 1997 about patients in vegetative states, asserted that:

> "Their bodies have shown all the signs of life, but when they die autopsies have found their brains shrunk to the size of a walnut" and "there would not have been sufficient brain cells in their skulls for a self to have existed" (Nicolson 1997).

Leaving aside the question of *how many* nerve cells are required for a self, distortion of the general perception of the vegetative state in non-medical writing has not been exclusively related to accounts of miraculous recoveries.

9.1 FREQUENCY OF EMERGENCE FROM PVS

Of many impediments to the collection of accurate data on the frequency with which patients have emerged from PVS, variable application of the term "persistent" at different periods and in different clinics has been among the most important. Variable levels of unresponsiveness of people grouped under the common nomenclature of "PVS" effectively precludes the assembly of a homogenous starting population for prolonged observation. The existence of a "spectrum" of patients, as foreseen by Jennett and Plum (1972) in their introduction of the term "PVS", and evident in the underlying pathological heterogeneity underpin this. Andrews' (1993b), account of the variability among patients in response to potentially painful experience is in accord with this, as is his reference to Anthony Bland as the most unresponsive PVS patient he had seen (*Airedale NHS Trust v Bland* 1993: 828).

Another impediment to data collection is introduced by attrition among any starting group of unconscious patients which is likely to frustrate epidemiological studies aimed at determining the frequency of emergence among those who come subsequently to be diagnosed as in a PVS. A majority of such a starting group is likely either to die or to regain responsiveness, albeit with varying degrees of residual disability. The small number of patients who remain alive but unresponsive over a prolonged period may be dispersed to nursing homes, domiciliary care or other placements further decreasing the likelihood that their long term outcome will be ascertainable. A constraint that is commonly imposed on any attempt to follow patients as a consequence of this dispersal is that indirect approaches such as the administration of questionnaires or telephone interviews to carers which can adversely affect data quality may be required.

Implementation of follow-up processes at widely spaced intervals runs the risk of imposing artificial "cut offs" on a continuous process and this may translate into conclusions that emergence is considerably rarer than is actually the case after specified temporal milestones. For example, a substantial study reported by Heindl and Laub (1996) commenced with 127 paediatric patients who remained in a vegetative state for at least 30 days following traumatic or hypoxic brain injuries. Having achieved a high level of retrieval of patients, they concluded that less than 5% of either group of patients emerged from PVS after 9 months. This percentage, however, was calculated using the starting population as the denominator. If the frequency of subsequent emergence of *those patients remaining alive and unresponsive after 12 months* is recalculated from the data in their report, it was 25% (8 out of 31). This is, presumably, the information which would be of most value to the families and medical attendants of this subpopulation of patients.

The wide range of variation in quality of care reflecting geographic, economic and other distinctly non-medical aspects of individual cases will confound tracing of outcomes. It would be patently nonsensical (unless one believes that outcomes for these patients are absolutely pre-ordained) to lump together those who have been "warehoused" from an early stage with others who have had the opportunity to be managed and continually re-assessed in an institution specialising in the care of patients in states of prolonged unresponsiveness. The locality, or health authority, relevant to the patient and the financial resources available from insurance, family savings or compensation may well influence placement. In urban Australia, generally regarded as solidly in the first world, commital of young patients to a nursing home after several weeks unconsciousness is not uncommon. Finally, the potentially self-fulfilling nature of a PVS diagnosis may, by its influence on the level of support that a patient receives, distort perceptions of capacity for emergence.

Some estimates of the frequency of emergence from prolonged unresponsive states have been formulated. Najenson *et al.* (1978) reported on the recovery of communicative capacity in 9 of 15 patients who had been in "prolonged traumatic coma" for periods ranging from 3 weeks to 5 months. Levy *et al.* (1981) noted that 3 of 23 patients who remained in a vegetative state one month after the onset of non-traumatic coma subsequently regained consciousness. All three of them were described as being severely disabled and two died within a year. The authors concluded that the longer the coma lasted, the less were the chances that a patient would regain independent function.

Of more recent reports of series of patients in a vegetative state, Andrews (1993a) observed that 11 of 43 who remained vegetative at 4 months subsequently regained consciousness (at intervals of up to 12 months). The 11 patients included cases in whom the vegetative state was a consequence both of traumatic and non-traumatic episodes. In an economic analysis of a large series of patients passing through the Établissements Helio-Marins at Berck (HMEB), the major French referral centre for comatose and vegetative patients, Sailly (1994) indicated that, of 179 successive patients diagnosed as vegetative, 24% regained consciousness but 21% of these remained severely disabled. Whilst the intervals after which the return of consciousness was first observed in these patients were not specified, the average duration of residence in HMEB suggested that these intervals were likely to have been of the same order as those observed by Andrews. A report of the application of PET to a group of comatose and vegetative state patients in Milan included the information that 2 out of 10 vegetative patients had recovered consciousness after 2 months (traumatic) and 4 months (non-traumatic) (Tommasino *et al.* 1995). Each of the preceding groups of patients had been residents in institutions which had a specific interest in caring for patients in prolonged coma and vegetative states. Individual instances of the return of consciousness have been reported, both in medical journals and in the "lay" press. Given the dismissive attitude of many neurologists and neurosurgeons towards the latter category of report, cases from the two sources will be summarised separately.

9.2 INDIVIDUAL CASES OF EMERGENCE: MEDICAL LITERATURE

Two well documented cases of complete recovery from a vegetative state were those reported by Shuttleworth (1983) and Falk (1990). Shuttleworth's patient, a 23 year old female, remained in a vegetative state for 7 weeks after carbon monoxide poisoning but subsequently resumed an independent life and was described as being "gainfully employed". Falk's patient, a 60 year old university professor, who not only remained in a vegetative state for at least 8 weeks after prolonged cerebral hypoxia, but presented the "typical" features of a vegetative state on CT scan, subsequently resumed and maintained a full complement of professorial responsibilities. Whilst a succession of instances of the return of consciousness after considerably longer periods in a vegetative state have been reported, there do not appear to have been others who achieved the remarkable degree of recovery observed in these two patients. As all reports of recovery refer to patients who remained under more detailed observation, either in an institution or in their home, and as the indefinite maintenance of vegetative patients under conditions of specialised care would be the exception, it is not too surprising that reliable statistics on the prevalence of vegetative patients *failing* to evince any signs of returning consciousness whilst under close observation are unavailable. Similarly unquantifiable is the extent to which cases of other patients who may have regained varying degrees of consciousness have not been reported in the literature.

Neither potential authors nor editors of medical journals are likely to continue to publish further single case reports of emergence unless they have some special feature such as breaking the existing "record". Nevertheless, a selection of cases from the "mainstream" medical literature illustrates the time scale of returning consciousness that has been observed in institutionalised patients. The widely publicised case of Childs and Mercer (1996a) was an 18 year old female who sustained a traumatic brain injury and was first observed to manifest some inconsistent signs of consciousness 15 months later. Over the following years, a gradual improvement occurred in her communicative capacity. A 43 year old man in a vegetative state as a result of anoxic brain injury was first observed to be attempting to talk after 17 months. Further, gradual improvement occurred after this (Rosenberg *et al.* 1977). Twenty-two months after anoxic brain damage, a 36 year old male patient of Snyder *et al.* (1983), diagnosed as being in a PVS, became "alert, attentive and able to follow simple commands". An 18 year old female remained in a vegetative state for 30 months after traumatic brain injury but then showed signs of gradually returning consciousness (Arts *et al.* 1985). Whilst all of these patients continued to have severe motor disabilities, commonly quadriplegia, and required assistance to communicate with others, all were considered by their medical attendants to have regained cognitive capacity. An instance of emergence that attracted much attention because of its circumstances was that of Carrie Coons. Having been regarded as in a PVS for 6 months she became the subject of the first successful right to die petition in New York State (Steinbock 1989). However, shortly before cessation of tube feeding was scheduled to occur, Mrs Coons regained sufficient consciousness to demur over the removal of the tube. Her arousal was said to have occurred in response to "aggressive efforts by the nursing staff to stimulate and feed her" (ibid). On the following day the judge vacated his earlier order for tube removal. A disconcerting case of a remitting vegetative state in a 69 year old man who passed through successive periods of awareness and unawareness raises some difficult questions about management of the vegetative state, in particular concerning the procedures to be followed in making the diagnosis (Thomasma and Brumlik 1984).

9.3 EMERGENCE IN THE NON-MEDICAL PRESS: A CLUSTER OF CASES

The response of some medical practitioners to newspaper reports describing the emergence of patients from vegetative states has been to question the original diagnosis, to reject the claim for return of consciousness, to disparage the subsequent state of the patient as representing an unacceptable life quality or, quite frequently, some combination of all three of these. However, the detail and the quality of reporting of issues relating to vegetative states were enhanced in response to the intense community interest engendered in the U.K. by the sanctioning by the House of Lords of the withdrawal of hydration and nutrition from Tony Bland. This case was followed by a succession of similar cases and the evolution of responses by English courts to requests for withdrawal of feeding of PVS patients will be discussed in Chapter 15. In consequence of the public interest which these cases involving cessation of feeding of vegetative patients aroused, reports of patients awakening from a vegetative state became much more newsworthy. Reports often included direct quotations attributed to medical practitioners eminent (or aspiring to be so) in the context of recognition of the PVS.

The first 6 of the 8 cases whose stories are summarised below were published in English newspapers in the period from January, 1996 to April, 1997, apparently stimulated by the Bland case. Recognition of their emergence had been spread over a longer period than the 16 month reporting period. In that sense, their "clustering" reflected an editorial perception of what would sell newspapers. In the absence of any indication of the proportion of families prepared to forgo privacy, or of the tenacity of reporters in identifying them, no inferences can be drawn about the possible frequency of other, similar but unreported cases. Publication of instances of emergence tailed off, as did that of court cases involving cessation of feeding, presumably reflecting editorial assessments of waning interest by readers. That the latter cases continued unabated in following years can be confirmed from court reports of hearings which failed to enter the media but no ongoing source of information on "emergences" is available. What follows is a summary of reports in the English press together with available medical comments on the patients concerned.

A significant feature of the published reports of these patients is that 6 of the 8 were identified by name. As the medical histories of some of them were also reported, in much more detail, in the *British Medical Journal* there was considerable potential for the identification of those patients, already named in newspaper reports, and correlation of identity with their detailed medical histories as written up in the *Journal*. Recognising this most unusual situation, the editor of the *Journal* noted that:

> "This paper made us think hard about the issue of getting consent from patients for publication of identifiable information about them" (Smith 1996: 16).

He pointed out that the media had already gathered details about many of the patients but that any release of information about a specific doctor – patient relationship, without the consent of both parties, had always been considered as completely unacceptable. In deciding whether the circumstances of the cases of vegetative patients could be sufficiently important to justify publication of identifiable medical information without consent, the editor acknowledged that:

> "Minimizing the danger of just one patient being misdiagnosed as being in a vegetative state might to some people justify breaching patient confidentiality" (ibid: 16).

However, after taking into account, both the breach of trust involved in not safeguarding the confidentiality of the patient – doctor relationship and the more extensive right to privacy, the editor decided to impose a requirement for agreement to publication by relatives.

The case of Anita Bailey was published in January, 1996 following an episode in Leeds

> "when an attempt to stop the feeding of (another) brain damaged woman was halted at the last moment after she pressed a button to show she wanted to live" (Anon. *The Standard Recorder* 1996).

Anita Bailey was said to have been diagnosed as being in a PVS following a motor vehicle accident. Later transferred to the Royal Hospital for Neuro-disability (R.H.N.) at Putney, she was said to have first evinced some sign of awareness a year after the accident, in response to the slamming of a door. Mark Newton, already referred to in Chapter 4, had remained apparently unconscious for 6 months after a diving accident when he regained the capacity to communicate and disclosed that he had been aware of events going on around him. Four years after emergence, he had recovered sufficiently to be undertaking a course at Portland College, Nottingham

(Fletcher 1996). Dr Vivienne Nathanson of the British Medical Association, when interviewed about his case, made the point that:

> "It may be that some patients who appear to be in a vegetative state may also have a degree of awareness and it is vital that nothing is done in a hurry. The biggest diagnostic tool we have in assessing persistent vegetative state is time" (ibid).

The Guardian carried a report by its legal correspondent in March, 1996 of an unnamed former businessman who had become aware of his surroundings and began to communicate with hospital staff after having been regarded as in a PVS for 7 years following an anaesthetic error during a routine operation (Dyer 1996a). One week later, the *British Medical Journal* carried a report by *its* legal correspondent, who had already filled the same role for *The Guardian* (Dyer 1996b). The *Journal* noted that the health authority responsible for care of this patient had discussed asking the High Court to sanction withdrawal of hydration and nutrition "though it dropped the idea when his wife opposed it". The Journal report continued:

> "His condition had been diagnosed by Professor Bryan Jennett, emeritus professor of surgery at Glasgow University, a world authority on the condition, and another specialist" (ibid).

Contacted by *The Guardian*, Professor Jennett was quoted as saying: "It's very alarming if he's waking up. I saw him and didn't think there was any doubt it was PVS" (Dyer 1996a). In discussing this case, *The Guardian's* legal correspondent, noted that the High Court had, to that time, approved the withdrawal of hydration and nutrition from a further 8 patients in a PVS since the House of Lords had sanctioned this course of action for Tony Bland (ibid).

The story of Geoffrey Wildsmith was reported by the English press as it progressed during 1997. Following head injuries sustained in a train accident he was said to have been regarded as unconscious by the medical staff at the first hospital at which he stayed for a period of 15 months (Appassamy 1997). Writing later, his mother claimed that she had seen reactions to her presence from Geoffrey during this time but had been told that these were not anything intelligent, but just reflexes. Several months after his transfer to the R.H.N., Geoffrey Wildsmith was deemed to be conscious and had learnt to communicate with others effectively using a buzzer. Andrew Devine made one of the most forceful media impacts of any person emerging from a vegetative state when his story was published in March 1997. The context again was that of the Tony Bland case and the special relevance of Andrew Devine was that he also had been a victim of the Hillsborough disaster when a number of spectators had been crushed at a football match (Ferriman 1997, Bowcott 1997). Keith Andrews from the R.H.N, where Andrew Devine had been treated told the media that, although there had been signs that he was becoming aware during 1994, it was not until 1996 that he began to communicate consistently. Andrews also indicated his belief that this was a case of genuine improvement (albeit after an unprecedented period of 5 years) rather than an original misdiagnosis. He also stressed that, in his experience, such a late recovery was very rare (Ferriman 1997).

In the month following publication of the Devine case, an interview with Professor Tom McMillan was reported in the London media and further details were subsequently published in the journal *Brain Injury* (Fraser 1997; McMillan 1998). McMillan, Professor of Neuropsychology at the University of Surrey, described the use of a buzzer communication system which he had designed. In 1995 he had been asked by the Official Solicitor to examine a 24 year old woman who had been in a road accident. Of five doctors who had examined her, McMillan said three had believed that she was so disabled that she was "unable to think or feel", one had thought she had expressed a wish to die and one just didn't know. Having seen the patient on 16 occasions and repeated a set of questions, McMillan had been able to demonstrate that the patient's responses, communicated by means of the buzzer, were statistically consistent. As a result of this testing, a court application by her medical attendants to withdraw hydration and nutrition had been withdrawn three days before the scheduled hearing. The stimulus for release of information two years after the event was a court decision in the preceding month that hydration and nutrition could lawfully be withdrawn from the 29 year old woman, Miss D, already discussed in Chapter 8 "even though she did not fit established medical criteria for persistent vegetative state" (Fraser 1997). McMillan published a postscript to this case (titled *Neuropsychological assessment of a potential 'euthanasia' case: a 5 year follow up*) in *Brain Injury* in 2000. The patient was said to remain dependent on others for all care but was feeding orally and talking. He noted that "as before, she consistently reported a wish to live" (McMillan and Herbert 2000).

Two cases of emergence described in some detail in the English press after the 1996/97 "cluster" illustrate features shared with other cases. The first report in *The Times* described a medicolegal case in June, 1998, involving another patient, Catherine Roberts, whose parents reportedly had been told that if she did not die after a brain haemorrhage, she would remain in a PVS (De Bruxelles 1998). Her mother said that:

> "We accepted what the doctors told us. When they say your child is going to be a vegetable you don't think they can make a mistake" (ibid).

When the nasogastric tube placed in the 26 year old student fell out, it was not replaced. Two months later, medical advice had been to cease the intravenous fluids which had been the only form of support following the loss of her nasogastric tube. After the planning of Catherine's funeral in consultation with the vicar, and on the day before all support was to be withdrawn, she was observed by her mother to respond.

> "The day before they were going to remove the tube I thought there was something different about her. She opened her eyes and blinked. I said 'If you can hear me Catherine, blink' – and she blinked. This time I did not tell the nurses. Instead I told her that if she could understand me to poke her tongue out. She did and then I told her I loved her. When she mouthed it back, my heart leaped. The feeding tube was put back in and she has made steady progress ever since then" (Lakeman 1998).

In June, 1998 a substantial out-of-court settlement was agreed between Catherine's parents, acting on her behalf, and the Frenchay NHS Healthcare Trust which had been responsible for her care. The family solicitor described the basis for the settlement as being that the NHS Trust had been negligent in that:

> "They failed to come to come to a proper diagnosis, and they failed to provide Catherine with the proper care that she required" (De Bruxelles 1998).

A spokesman for the Trust indicated that:

> "The Trust is pleased that this complex and difficult case is settled".

As of June 1998, Catherine Roberts, notwithstanding her remaining disabilities, was undertaking a social sciences course at the Open University (Lakeman 1998). Finally, Gregory Dygas who had sustained severe brain damage in the course of an asthmatic attack was said, subsequently to have been vegetative (Petty 1999). However, after a five month placement in a Traumatic Brain Injury Unit near Sheffield, a specialist nurse at the facility told a reporter that he was not in a vegetative state "despite previous pronouncements" (ibid).

Several features recur in this series of cases. The most striking (and typical of similar case histories in other locations) is the strong support provided by highly committed family members – in some cases, by a single individual. In any case, family acquiescence with medical advice to curtail, or discontinue, support would have precluded the reported outcomes. The opinions of the two medical specialists (Andrews and Jennett) most cited in relation to vegetative states that the two patients who had been regarded as unconscious for the longest periods had not originally been misdiagnosed cannot readily be ignored. The group of patients were probably atypical in not having been transferred at an early stage to nursing homes without opportunity for cognitive rehabilitation. Their families continued with attempts to communicate. It is probable that a majority of individuals diagnosed as PVS will be transferred at an early stage to a nursing home regime of minimal maintenance unlikely to be conducive to the detection, or the encouragement, of any subtle, early indications of emergence. It is interesting to compare these instances of late emergence with data from the International Coma Data Bank which suggests better prospects for long term improvement in the conscious state of vegetative patients who had been discharged from hospitals than has usually been inferred (Levin *et al.* 1991). Fifty-eight percent of patients in a vegetative state following trauma improved in level of consciousness within 3 years of their injury.

9.4 RECOGNITION OF EMERGENCE

The time of transition from being diagnosed as unconscious to recognition of returning awareness in the preceding group of patients was usually not clear cut. If attempts at *communication* with people diagnosed as vegetative are to be successful, active participation by two individuals, namely the patient *and* an observer, will be required. Disagreement between observers on the question of whether a specified patient is, or is not, capable of communicating is not uncommon. Families of individuals who have subsequently shown improvement in conscious status after being diagnosed as in a vegetative state often claim to have perceived signs of awareness considerably in advance of any acknowledgement of this by medical specialists. For example, recalling the patients described above, the claim of Geoffrey Wildsmith's mother that she was told that she was reading too much into her son's responses (Appassamy 1997), and the remark of Catherine Roberts' mother that:

> "At one stage we saw her blink. But we were told we were only seeing what we wanted to see" (De Bruxelles 1998)

are both illustrative and typical.

Whilst the experience and perceptions of the families of vegetative patients who have subsequently improved have frequently been dismissed disparagingly in the general medical literature, journals more specialised in the field of rehabilitation after brain injury have increasingly tended to place a considerably greater value on their claims. Two U.S. rehabilitation specialists writing on *The care and rehabilitation of the patient in a persistent vegetative state* (both subjects that have been dismissed as futile and meaningless by some commentators on vegetative states) observed that:

> "The physician who examines such patients once or twice may conclude that they are truly in PVS, and may discount family members' or staff claims as 'wishful thinking' or inability to differentiate reflex activity from responses initiated at a cortical level" (Whyte and Glenn 1986: 40).

They noted that stimuli with emotional significance to the individual are those most likely to elicit responses from them. It followed that

> "family members and others with whom the patient has a close relationship may be able to obtain a response when others have failed" (ibid: 42).

Two U.K. authors from a head injury rehabilitation unit described two patients with severe brain injuries who exemplified the point that "stimuli with personal relevance provoked strong responses and presaged further behavioural change" (Watson and Horn 1991: 421). Whilst they remained uncertain whether the stimuli had served only to disclose previously unrecognised improvement or had actually facilitated some degree of improvement, their experience exemplifies the association between committed family members and the return of capacity to communicate. A correspondent, writing from a rehabilitation centre in response to Andrews' 1996 report of misdiagnosis of the vegetative state, made the point that any clinician confronted with the task of diagnosing the PVS should interview "at least one nurse who knows the patient well" and "at least one relative who has been close to the patient" (Wade 1996: 943). Nevertheless, it is clear that there remains considerable reticence on the part of some neurological specialists to accept possible evidence bearing on emergence from vegetative states unless and until it is tendered by a fellow medical graduate. For instance, in expressing his reservations about a report of "alleged recovery" of many "supposedly vegetative" patients from a Coma Recovery Institute in New Jersey, Bryan Jennett (1993b) referred to that report dismissively as a "paper from two nurses in a nursing journal".

Apart from the question of whether persons who are familiar to a patient are more likely to detect and/or to elicit signs of returning consciousness, the means employed in attempting to communicate may also influence the outcome. The buzzer system of Professor Tom McMillan, mentioned above, was used to apply a statistical analysis of a patient's response to questions (Fraser 1997). McMillan described numerous repetitions of the test set of questions in the course of his 16 very short interviews with a patient over the course of 2 days. Techniques which require a patient to provide statistically consistent responses by means of a buzzer have not yet gained universal acceptance. Thus, Cranford expressed doubts about the touch-sensitive buzzer system used by Andrews *et al.*, when they demonstrated that 40% of the patients referred to the R.H.N. had previously been incorrectly diagnosed as vegetative. In commenting upon these results, Cranford (1996) indicated that he would view the buzzer system with scepticism until it had been validated, for example, by its use in other rehabilitation units and by the provision of videotapes of its use for others to examine. Another approach to testing for any returning, or persisting, consciousness has been developed at the R.H.N., and was presented at a conference of the British Psychological Society in December, 1997. It involved systematically stimulating each of seven sensory modalities. A semi-quantitative score of responsiveness to these stimuli was said to provide "an early warning that a patient is about to emerge" (Wilson and Gill-Thwaites 2000).

There have been recent indications that the use of specialised scanning techniques may permit the early detection of signs of emergence from a vegetative state. Owen *et al.* (2002) used PET to study covert cognitive processing in patients with a clinical PVS diagnosis. Two patients who were observed to manifest "clear and predicted cerebral blood flow responses to face recognition" made a significant recovery some months later. Different observers who select different goals will place different values on identical outcomes. Increasing emphasis has been placed on the post-vegetative condition by some commentators as reports of patients who have regained consciousness after being diagnosed as in PVS continue to appear. In discussing futility and the withdrawal of hydration and nutrition from PVS patients, Mitchell *et al.* (1993) stressed the results of a study which found that no patient who remained vegetative beyond 3 months became independent of nursing care. Cranford (1996) speculated that most people would find an outcome in which returning consciousness coexisted with major neurological impairment "more horrifying than the vegetative state itself" and, perhaps, an even stronger reason than that state itself for stopping treatment. A final comment on the subject could be that of Bryan Jennett, addressing a 1996 meeting on PVS:

> "When doctors have talked about patients 'recovering' from PVS, they have only meant that patients have seen a tiny improvement. These patients have not taken up their beds and walked" (Ferriman 1996).

This serves to emphasise the need to identify *what* is to be regarded as an acceptable outcome and this should be a judgement for the affected individual *not* for others, irrespective of their technical expertise.

9.5 RECAPITULATION

"*Emergence*" was selected as the title for this Chapter because the *only observable* feature which differentiates PVS patients from others with very severe brain damage is the ongoing loss of detectable capacity for consciousness. "*Emergence*" as used here connotes the appearance of indications that a patient has regained some level of conscious awareness. In this sense, it is considerably more specific, and constrained, than another term "recovery". "Recovery" from PVS could be construed as anything from "emergence" as defined above to return to neurological normality. Apart from this imprecision, the use of "recovery" to describe patients who have improved after sustaining a severe brain injury has been vigorously attacked by some neurosurgical authors as inaccurate and delusory.

With increasing recognition that emergence from PVS can occur, much attention has focused on individuals who have done this. A common extension of the argument that life in a PVS would be unacceptably bad has been to assert that life in a cognitive but totally dependent state following emergence from a vegetative state would be even worse. Consequently, the measure of withdrawal of hydration and nutrition that has often been adopted for patients in a PVS has been advocated also for those who have regained consciousness but remain totally dependent on others.

Acknowledgement that a number of patients can, and do, regain consciousness after attracting a diagnosis of PVS was forthcoming predominantly in the 1990s with earlier descriptions of PVS often indicating that *any* return of consciousness was excessively rare. It is not possible to distinguish between changes in the *actual frequency* with which patients emerged from PVS (perhaps as a result of improved management) and changes in the *ascertainment* of emergence by others as a basis for this apparent increase in reports of emergence. The strategies that have been developed at institutions such as the R.H.N., as described in this and the preceding Chapter could have had the dual effect of facilitating emergence and of facilitating its recognition by others. Certainly, there appears to have been a sea change in the attitudes of many medical professionals so that observations made by families, nurses and paramedical personnel are no longer routinely dismissed as wishful thinking or self delusion but constitute a valued adjunct to medical management.

Reliable estimates of the frequency with which patients might be predicted to emerge from a PVS after various intervals are lacking and are likely to remain so. The proportion of patients remaining in a vegetative state, other than for short intervals, after brain injury is likely to be quite small compared with the percentages of the starting population who either die or regain consciousness in the early months. Further, major attrition of starting populations is likely as patients are transferred to nursing homes or domiciliary care and can no longer be traced. The differing levels of care likely to be provided in different placements will further complicate attempts to estimate percentages of emergence (and in so doing are likely to interfere with attempts to assess the value of interventions intended to accelerate emergence). Attempts to estimate the frequency of late emergence from published reports of cases are no more likely to be successful. Individual case reports that conflicted with the paradigm of permanent unconsciousness were acceptable to medical journals until the universal application of that paradigm was disproved. Lay media are interested in cases of emergence when this is topical news as, for example, were the cluster published in the English press in 1996/7 in the wake of the public interest generated by the Bland case and its early successors. However, the interest of either medical or lay press in a subject is unlikely to be sustained once a number of reports have been published.

CHAPTER 10

A PERSPECTIVE OF DISABILITY

> "They are not, as those in the 'Right to Life' movement would have us believe, 'handicapped' or 'disabled'. These are not patients with diminished capacity. They are unable to give or, what is far more important, perceive love on even the most primitive of levels ... rather, they are nonmentative organ systems, artificially sustained like valued cell lines in cancer laboratories" (Armstrong and Colen 1988: 39).

Some would deny vegetative patients inclusion within the spectrum of disability in the terms quoted above from a lawyer who represented the families of PVS patients in two major U.S. cases. In proposing to infer something about the likely interests of PVS patients by extrapolating from general attitudes of people with disability, I recognise that some authorities would maintain that the concept of disability, because of implications about interaction with others attached to it, is irrelevant for these "non-persons". If the proposition is accepted that the term "disability" be restricted to those retaining levels of communicative function, and inferentially of cognition, in excess of those usually conceded to patients diagnosed as vegetative, a chapter on disability becomes quite superfluous. I have not found this proposition reasonable because of its arbitrary nature and of the arrogance with which it is sometimes presented. Two goals of this Chapter will be to draw attention to the inaccurately negative assessment of the lives of individuals with disabilities, in general, by the non-disabled and to assert that patients in vegetative states cannot be partitioned off from the general spectrum of disability as uniquely different objects.

As outlined in Chapter 1, the terms "vegetative", "persistent vegetative state" and "permanent vegetative state" will be used in this text with the same connotation that has been applied to them in any article to which reference is made. Use of the abbreviation "PVS" will be confined to "*persistent* vegetative state". It has been indicated also that the incorporation of unconsciousness as the essential feature of the PVS has been enshrined in definition of the condition. However, as examined in Chapter 8, misdiagnosis of PVS in patients who further examination has shown to be conscious has certainly not been rare.

It is notable that the *recognition of misdiagnosis* has been reported principally from specialised institutions the staff of which have had the most extensive experience of caring for patients diagnosed as vegetative. Apropos of this, Andrews *et al.* (1996) have reported that the frequency of detection of misdiagnosis among patients referred to the Royal Hospital for Neuro-disability (R.H.N.) increased over the years preceding their report on this subject (2 in 1992, 1 in 1993, 4 in 1994 and 10 in 1995). Apart from suggesting that diagnostic accuracy was not increasing in the catchment area of the R.H.N., this increase implied, and was explained by Andrews *et al.* as

> "probably due to the team's increasing sensitivity owing to the accumulation of experience over several years coupled with the development of more effective assessment measures" (ibid: 15).

I believe that it would be naïve to anticipate that any group of patients *diagnosed* as in a PVS could not include an unknown number who have retained or attained some level of consciousness and so, in the terms of the definition of PVS, represent misdiagnoses. Most patients diagnosed as in a PVS do not have the opportunity for prolonged admission to highly specialised facilities. Some of these are "warehoused" at an early stage after diagnosis and so are afforded minimal opportunity for reassessment, let alone rehabilitation.

The likely existence of a substantial cohort of patients who are erroneously considered to be completely unconscious, and regarded as being in a PVS, is relevant to the proposition to be advanced in this Chapter. That proposition is that the most suitable analogy with which to attempt any estimate of likely attitudes of those patients who, whilst diagnosed as in a PVS, have any level of consciousness will take account of others who, whilst neurologically similar, have been able to communicate *their* attitudes. What of those who have been diagnosed as in a PVS and who are completely unconscious? Assuming them to be currently devoid of attitudes, what is likely to be the most appropriate approach to forming an opinion about their interests? Possible responses could be to ascertain their previously expressed attitudes (if known), to note the attitudes of their families and medical attendants ("If *I* was in his position, I would want…") or to take account of what has been learnt from patients who were previously in, or close to, a PVS.

When considering questions of "interests" relating to individuals who have been diagnosed as vegetative, it is frequently asserted that they are beyond the stage at which the concept of "best interests" can retain any meaning. In response to this, I consider that their description, in derogatory terms, as in the quotation leading this Chapter or as identified persons, such as Tony Bland have been described in court (See 10.8 and Chapter 15) provide the most persuasive case that they *retain* interests that are susceptible to damage by denigration. The content of this Chapter is, I suggest, of direct relevance to those patients who have been accorded a diagnosis of PVS, but who have had some level of consciousness *irrespective* of whether this has subsequently been recognised. If one realistically accepts that the clinical distinction between those PVS-diagnosed patients who have some unrecognised level of consciousness and others who have absolutely none will often not be made, I suggest additionally that this content has some relevance to *any* patient diagnosed as in a PVS. Its most significant feature is the inaccuracy in estimation of life with severe neurological disability that is usually formed by the non-disabled.

The question of what a PVS patient *might* wish, in relation to treatment, has been approached almost exclusively in a negative context, most notably exemplified by withdrawal of hydration and nutrition. More positive aspects, such as whether active measures to increase the possibility of emergence may be desired, are less frequently discussed. Much of the published discussion about patients in vegetative states has revolved around the question of the type of treatment these people would want for themselves, assuming that they were able to make a judgement and to communicate it to others. However, as patients in the vegetative state are excluded, by definition, from the exercise of either of these capacities, alternative approaches to answering the question on their behalf are required. The two types of approach most commonly adopted when decisions about withdrawal of support are to be made for a PVS patient have been attempts to reconstruct the patient's previously expressed wishes and the use of a substituted judgement. To implement previous wishes, a formal advance directive is most useful but, because of the relative infrequency of such directives relating to wishes for management if the writer is diagnosed as vegetative, this is not usually practicable. The alternative of relying on a substituted judgement about the decision the patient would wish to be made on his or her behalf by a family member or close friend is based on recognition of the patient's right to autonomy *and* an assumption of the legitimacy of allowing that right to be exercised by another. Whilst the right to autonomy is generally unchallenged, the same cannot be said of its transfer. As one advocate of the recognition of patient autonomy has forcefully pointed out, a second person has no more right to make such decisions *in the name of patient autonomy* than he or she has to vote on the patient's behalf (Ellman 1990). Patient autonomy and the available decision-making approaches will be considered in Chapter 15. The present Chapter will examine a more practical aspect of substituted decision-making, namely the track record of non-disabled individuals in making decisions for others who are disabled.

10.1 ASSESSMENTS BY THE NON-DISABLED OF THE WISHES OF THOSE WITH A DISABILITY

Opinions about what patients in vegetative and related states would be likely to wish for themselves have been derived either from surveys of non-disabled people or from what the author of the article, if placed in a similar situation, would wish for him- or her-self. As such, conclusions remain open to the objection that the impressions of non-disabled people about the lives of others who are disabled tend to be inaccurately negative. This objection was recognised by the U.S. Secretary for Health and Human Services in responding to the 1989 Oregon Health Care Plan within the framework of the *Americans with Disabilities Act* (Secretary Health and Human Services 1994). The Oregon Plan was based on surveys of the perceptions of the general population of the State about the relative severity of the impact that various medical conditions would have on their life. The Secretary observed that people without disabilities systematically undervalued the quality of life of those with disability and concluded that the Oregon surveys tended to quantify stereotypical assumptions about people with disabilities.

Attitudes developed specifically towards vegetative state patients have considerable potential to influence the way in which people living with *other* forms of disability are regarded and so to shape perceptions of them within the general community. For example, in response to two decisions of Scottish courts (one sanctioning the withdrawal of food and water from a woman diagnosed as in a PVS and another the withholding of cardiopulmonary resuscitation (CPR) from a 23 year old patient with severe brain damage, in the event of a cardiac arrest) the United Kingdom organisation "SCOPE" (formerly the Spastics Society) expressed concern that questions about distinctions between those lives which were "worthwhile" and others which were not considered to be so would increasingly be voiced (MacDermid 1996). One surveyed group of people with disabilities (among whom cerebral palsy was the commonest disability) was selective to the extent that Weinberg (1984) regarded them as better educated, wealthier and more independent than would be expected among a random sample. Fifty percent of this group indicated that they would not opt to undergo "curative surgery" for their condition, assuming that such treatment was available and without risk. A girl whose sole limb was half an arm felt that she was already whole and refused to use a prosthesis. Weinberg identified societal beliefs that strength, independence and appearance were essential aspects of self-worth as responsible for shaping attitudes of others towards people with disabilities and advocated the challenging of these beliefs and the adoption of other values. Even respondents who were comfortable coping with their disabilities, nevertheless felt that the able-bodied public treated them as socially inferior.

10.2 PERCEPTIONS OF NON-DISABLED MEDICAL ATTENDANTS ABOUT PEOPLE WITH SEVERE NEUROLOGICAL DAMAGE

A number of studies which have examined the attitudes of health care workers towards individuals with severe neurological disability have revealed that staff perceptions of patients can influence patient behaviour. In a study comparing the psychological status of patients with spinal cord injuries with the impressions of the staff attending to them, it emerged that 6 of the group of 7 staff members whose assessment of the patients in their charge most accurately resembled the patients' own views about themselves were those who had been newly appointed to the health care service (Bodenhamer *et al.* 1983). The longer a staff member had been working with patients with spinal injury, the more likely it became that he or she would become insensitive to the reactions of the patients. The exceptions to this trend were staff who had received special training that placed emphasis on developing a greater awareness of patient feelings, responses and social consciousness. In commenting upon right to die cases involving conscious, non-terminal people that had come before U.S. courts, a disabled author noted that there was scant evidence that anyone had sought an explanation, other than the presence of a disability, for the patient's distress (Gill 1992). The author, Carol Gill regretted that disability and quality living were regarded as antithetical by many non-disabled commentators. She complained that the voice of the disabled community was "less often heard and rarely heeded". She asserted that many non-disabled thought that "if permanent disability is the problem, death is the solution" and drew the implication that many regarded it as "natural, reasonable or proper" for a disabled person, but not for a non-disabled person, to die. A study comparing views of patients about their care with the views of their physicians was undertaken with chronically ill, elderly patients who were competent at the time of questioning but who were likely to have anticipated further deterioration in their condition. Whilst most of the patients presumed that their physician's views would accurately reflect their own wishes (in relation to the initiation of CPR in response to a hypothetical cardiac arrest occurring in the course of progressive dementia), the study found that physicians did no better than chance alone in predicting the wishes of their patients (Seckler *et al.* 1991).

As an alternative to grouping vegetative patients among the disabled, Jennett and Bond (1975) have pointed to similarity between the status of patients who were "vegetative" and those who were dead. They considered that:

> "For the present argument the vegetative state is equivalent to unconsciousness: for the person affected this is presumably no different from death" (ibid: 484).

Jennett published a study in 1976 reporting the views of non-disabled individuals about their own preferences for management in the event that they were subsequently diagnosed as having entered a vegetative state. One surveyed group consisted of experienced health professionals in San Francisco, while the other contained medical students from Glasgow. Both groups believed that a "vegetative survival" would be worse than death and over 40% thought that to regain some conscious awareness of their plight would be even worse than vegetative survival. Both groups also thought that relatives would be less likely to admit this than they would themselves (ibid). Jennett cited the findings of his survey again in 1993 and reaffirmed his confidence in their significance (1993a). Without questioning the accuracy of these responses as representative of the assessments that non-disabled individuals would typically form in relation to those who are living with severe disability, I would question their *relevance* to the views of those with severe disabilities. In particular, some indication of the satisfaction of severely disabled individuals with their existence and their wishes in relation to its continuation would be more useful.

Commentaries on people in minimally responsive states retaining or regaining some observable awareness have often proposed that their predicament is worse than that of PVS patients. For example, Ronald Cranford (1996) asserted that:

> "Reasonable people may differ in their views of the quality of life of these conscious individuals, but I would speculate that most people would find this condition far more horrifying than the vegetative state itself, and some might think it an even stronger reason for stopping the treatment than complete unconsciousness" (ibid: 6).

Such patients, with most of the neurological features of PVS but with awareness that is detectable by an observer, include some who regain consciousness after a period in a vegetative state. To the extent that Cranford was expressing what he believed to be the likely views of many non-disabled individuals, his statement may well have been an accurate representation. It is reasonable to anticipate that a non-disabled individual will assess any disabled state unfavourably in comparison with his or her own existing status. However, the question of whether *affected patients* generally find the minimally responsive state as horrifying as Cranford proposed remains a separate issue. Cranford's statement represents a prediction of the views of a class of severely disabled people by the non-disabled and, as noted above, such assessments have been notoriously negative and inaccurate. Commenting specifically on Cranford's statement after emergence of a patient from PVS, Keith Andrews aptly pointed out that:

> "This is a case of an able-bodied person making a judgement of what it is like to be in that condition" (Lawrance 1996b).

10.3 FAMILY VIEWS ABOUT SEVERELY DISABLED MEMBERS

Family views about the likely wishes of patients diagnosed as in a vegetative state have generally been regarded as providing as accurate an indication of these as it is possible to obtain. Court proceedings to determine whether it would be permissible to withdraw hydration and nutrition from patients in, or approximating to, a PVS have frequently included requests from the patient's family for such withdrawal. Requests to English courts for withdrawal of support from vegetative patients have invariably been endorsed and/or initiated by the National Health Service Trust directly responsible for funding the care of the patient at the centre of the appeal, in association with the patient's family. The family's views on patient management generally carry considerable weight, both because other family members are usually expected to be most familiar with any previous wishes expressed by the patient and also because a family member is likely to be the patient's legal guardian. Nevertheless, it has been clearly indicated, in English court hearings that, whilst the family will be *consulted*, the decision to withdraw support will be made by the medical attendants.

Despite one's intuitive belief that other family members would provide the most accurate account of the patient's wishes, objective studies of the subject have suggested otherwise. Older children and physicians have been reported to rate the quality of a parent's life lower than the patient's own assessment (Zweibel and Cassel 1989). Gill (1992) noted that:

> "Any therapist who has worked with disabled people has heard tragic stories of harm inflicted by loving, well-meaning family members making decisions on their behalf. The consciousness of such recollections reminds us that loving someone with a disability does not naturally confer insight or even immunity from prejudice" (ibid: 51).

Taking account of the stresses imposed on the family of any patient in, or near to, a PVS it is reasonable to anticipate that family decisions about the patient will inevitably reflect the foreseeable impact of those decisions on both the patient and the family. Some insight into the factors influencing family decision-making may be gained from the reported comment of Tony Bland's father on the occasion of the emergence of Andrew Devine, who like his son, had also been in a PVS after the football stadium catastrophe at Hillsborough:

> "Andrew's condition is not something I would want for Tony and it's not what I would want for us. I could never have reconciled myself to seeing him in that state forever" (Greaves 1997).

10.4 PATIENT VIEWS

No differences between handicapped and normal individuals were detected in a study of the life satisfaction of "non-normal" persons, reported in a clinical psychology journal. No differences in frustration with life were apparent between the two groups and there were some indications that the group with handicaps were less suicidal, more religious and more oriented towards the "generalised other". They tended to feel that their lives were more difficult (Cameron *et al.* 1973). Published assessments of the likely wishes of people in vegetative or minimally responsive states appear to have been entirely constructed on the basis of analogies with the views of non-disabled individuals attempting to visualise what it would be like to be so disabled. As the validity of this analogy appears rarely to have been questioned, it is legitimate to consider the relative accuracy of alternative analogies. The closest analogy is that in which the views of people in minimally responsive or locked-in states (both of which permit some communication) are ascertained as a means of construing the most likely preferences of others with a comparable degree of neurological deficit but lacking any communicative capacity (and so inevitably meeting the diagnostic specifications required for designation as vegetative). Two independent reasons could be offered for regarding the views of people in these two groups as providing the most reliable analogies. In the first place, many of the commentators who have promoted extremely negative opinions about individuals in vegetative states have often simultaneously asserted that people who have recovered, or retained, some observable capacity for awareness are in an even worse predicament. Admittedly, this is a very subjective assessment, but it at least suggests that these patients would be highly suitable as a test group because they would not be expected to present an unrealistically optimistic account of their situation. Secondly, some minimally responsive persons who have provided information about insights into their current situation have actually emerged following a period during which they were considered to be in a vegetative state and so should have the closest possible impression of it.

Whilst the evidence noted above from studies of disabled patients and their medical attendants and families indicates a consistent tendency of the latter groups to have a more negative view about the disability than that of the affected individual, it might be argued that extrapolation to near-vegetative patients from studies based on patients living with other, lesser disabilities would not be justified because the former group does not fall within the spectrum of "disability". However, a sizeable number of personal accounts of the response of people close to, or previously in, vegetative states have become available during the last 10 years. These have taken the form of communications in medical periodicals and of verbatim accounts in the lay press. Many of the latter appear to have been of a good evidentiary standard. Consequently, I do not believe that the arbitrary exclusion of these patients from the category of "disability" and the dismissal of their accounts is sustainable. Of accounts in medical journals, one of the best descriptions of the subsequent attitude to life of patients who have emerged from PVS is that provided by Andrews from the R.H.N. Andrews' (1993a) report on 11 patients who regained consciousness, having been regarded as being in a PVS for 4 or more months, specifically commented on patients' attitudes:

> "Only one patient showed obvious distress at his condition. He had been a professional and fully appreciated his poor physical recovery. All the other patients were able to take pleasure from environmental changes within the limits of their cognitive ability" (Andrews 1993a: 1598).

An account of an individual case has been provided by Childs and Mercer (1996a), writing in the *New England Journal of Medicine*. An 18 year old woman who started to emerge from a diagnosed PVS 15 months after trauma was reported, five years after her injury, to have an attention span of 15 minutes and to be severely disabled and totally dependent. However, it was noted that her mood was usually euphoric, that she enjoyed pampering, humour and making jokes and that there was no behavioural evidence of depression or despondency. I question the entitlement of others to impose contrary assessments of the value *to her* of her life.

First hand accounts of the attitudes of identified individual patients following emergence from PVS have appeared at intervals in the lay press. Reports of three such people published in the London *Times* and *Daily Telegraph* in 1996 illustrate the most common features. Francis Chateau, a 32 year old former journalist, was said to be extremely angry and unhappy because of his earlier treatment but, when interviewed, was glad to be alive (Cornwell 1996). Anita Bayley, a 23 year old former model also indicated that she was happy to have been kept alive (ibid). In another interview, her mother expressed surprise that someone whose quality of life had been so severely affected could be happy (Anon. *The Weekly Telegraph* 1996). The same report included reference to the case of Mark Newton, whose history has been summarised in Chapter 8, and observed that he was confined to a wheelchair but had embarked on a college course. A forceful illustration of the way in which this report reflected the perceptions of the non-disabled reporter, rather than that of the person with the disability was provided to me by a friend living with disability who stated emphatically that she would feel confined *without* her wheelchair. Ian Doughty, a 23 year old former carpenter, evinced the first detected signs of consciousness 14 months after a motor vehicle accident which had left him with a diagnosis of vegetative state. His father was reported as saying that Ian had a sense of humour, could remember friends and family and could undertake mental arithmetic. As his father told a reporter:

> "He is locked in a body he can't control but his mind is there" (Laurance 1996a).

In the light of accounts such as these, it is difficult to accept conclusions about the likely wishes of people with severe neurological disability that have been drawn from surveys of non-disabled individuals. The conventional contention that the generality of people who have massive neurological disabilities and remain close to a vegetative state regret the preservation of their lives is highly questionable. In evaluating surveys of the views of people without disabilities it is important not to conflate a preference for non-disability over disability with one for non-existence over a severely disabled and limited existence.

10.5 THE REMARKABLE JEAN-DOMINIQUE BAUBY

Without question, the most striking recorded testimony of a life accompanied by almost total physical incapacity tethered to an extremely limited capacity for communication with others is that of Jean-Dominique Bauby. The 42 year old Parisian Bauby, editor of *Elle* magazine, became comatose following a stroke. When his consciousness returned, he was speechless and unable to move any part of his body other than his left eyelid. Bauby remained in this condition until his death 15 months later. During that period, he set up the Locked-in Syndrome Association and dictated a book documenting his experiences and thoughts. The book, *The diving bell and the butterfly* (Bauby 1997), was produced with the help of his speech therapist (described by Bauby as his guardian angel) utilising a process in which Bauby selected each letter from a complete alphabet repeatedly read to him. After selection of almost 10,000 individual letters, his work, described by the reviewer in *The Daily Telegraph* as the most extraordinary book of the year (perhaps of any year), was complete. An editorial article noted of Bauby that:

> "His writing makes clear, that far from wishing to die, M. Bauby still revelled in life" (Editorial *The Daily Telegraph* 1997).

The quality of Bauby's book, of his life whilst "locked-in" and of the person himself can be hinted at, albeit most inadequately, by recounting several episodes from it. He envisaged himself as living in a cocoon and regarded his 92 year old father and 8 year old daughter as "outer links of the chain of love which surrounds and protects" him. In a thought provoking insight he perceived both his father and himself as "locked-in cases". Bauby senior was confined by his 92 year-old legs to his fourth floor apartment near the Tuilleries, whilst his son was "confined to his carcass" at Berck-sur-Mer. Notwithstanding his massive physical limitations, Bauby could still find humour in the reported description of him by two Parisian gossipers as a complete vegetable – "the tone of voice left no doubt that henceforth I belonged on a vegetable stall and not to the human race" (Bauby 1997: 90). The overwhelming importance of his residual contact with the outside world is emphatically brought out in his description of the absolute terror that seized him when an ophthalmologist began to sew his right eyelids shut (to prevent corneal ulceration) lest his sole means of communication – a left eyelid – were to be similarly treated. Bauby's assessment of this specialist:

> "The very model of the couldn't-care-less doctor, arrogant, brusque, sarcastic... already disinclined to chat with normal patients, he turned thoroughly evasive in dealing with ghosts of my ilk" (ibid: 61),

could profitably be circulated among many of the physicians who have written disparagingly of PVS patients. It would not be reasonable to claim that all patients in locked-in states and otherwise close to PVS could emulate him. However, his documented experience provides a compelling rebuttal of the argument of many non-disabled experts in relation to the disabled namely that to exist in these conditions would invariably be a fate worse than death.

10.6 TREATMENT PREFERENCES OF SEVERELY DISABLED PEOPLE

It is often maintained that the lives of people who are in, or close to, a PVS are so awful that initiatives to curtail them are preferable, an assumption often buttressed by a conviction that such patients would not appreciate any treatment. For example, Jennett and Bond (1975) maintained that

> "terms such as 'practical' 'useful' or 'worthwhile' to define recovery of this class of patients are usually euphemisms which conceal major and persisting disabilities" (ibid: 481).

The terms to which they objected patently represent relative assessments and it is reasonable to query *to what* they are relative. There are two alternative responses to this question. Should the patient's condition be compared with that before the onset of disability or with that when the disability was most severe? (for instance, during the first days in an intensive care ward). More correctly, with which of these two conditions is it likely that *the patient* will draw the comparison? Jennett and Bond evidently anticipated that patients will draw the comparison with their preceding status:

> "The patient, remembering only how well he was before his injury, is unlikely to share the satisfaction of his doctors (about any improvement in condition) when he finds himself left with serious permanent disability" (ibid: 481).

However, accounts noted above, and to follow, would suggest that, in most of the patients with whom the question of acceptance of disability has been explored after the acute stage, feelings such as resentment and despair were not prominent.

I suspect that Jennett and some of his colleagues have adopted an unduly mechanistic attitude towards individuals living with severe neurological disability. Thus, they write that:

> "The relief of symptoms is perhaps the most difficult aspect of assessment after brain damage because the patient often lacks insight and may even deny disability, especially in the mental sphere"(ibid: 482).

(Such a statement might tempt one to question *who* it is that lacks insight). The prevailing medical use of the term "*symptom*" connotes some item of information about a patient which can be appreciated, and is described, *by the patient* but is not necessarily directly observable by another. This has traditionally distinguished a symptom, elicited by questioning the patient, from a sign that can be independently documented by an observer. I take it from the context that Jennett and Bond were applying "*symptom*" in this conventional medical sense and, accordingly, I question whether they might have missed the most significant point. If a patient is not dissatisfied with life to any greater extent than most non-disabled individuals are from time to time, even though his or her condition appears appalling to some observers, this should occasion a positive assessment of the overall state. Any external assessment of a patient's attitude deserves to be treated with circumspection.

> "What people thought they would want often turns out to be very different from what they do want" (Kadish 1992: 873).

This conclusion, presented by Kadish, writing about construing the *current* wishes of patients who have become disabled, having previously left an indication that they did not wish to be treated should they become incompetent is completely consistent with the change in wishes of specific disabled individuals as exemplified by the people referred to above. Nevertheless, Kadish drew a sharp distinction between PVS and all other conditions:

> "When the patient is in a vegetative state that is known to be permanent... there is no basis for not respecting his earlier competent choice to die" (ibid: 871).

This concept of PVS as a condition *sui generis*, with well defined and understood features sharply separating it from all other conditions, has influenced most commentary on the subject. Given the rarity of reports of near-PVS patients expressing a wish to die, as distinct from one to continue to live and the improbability that a clear preceding statement of the patient's wishes will be available, Kadish's conclusion appears questionable. A challenge to the proposition that a majority of severely disabled and highly dependent individuals would prefer to have their support discontinued has been provided by a study of patients with motor neurone disease (amyotrophic lateral sclerosis, ALS) from a muscular dystrophy clinic.

> "Virtually all ALS patients and others with neuromuscular disease, when asked early on, indicate that they would rather die than use respiratory support. Virtually all change their minds during episodes of acute respiratory failure" (Bach and Barnett 1994: 138).

Individual reports are available relating specifically to patient requests for treatment (rather than only indicating whether the person was happy or unhappy). For instance, the Archdeacon of York commented in the London *Daily Express* upon the case of "Miss G" who was about to be the subject of an application to the High Court for an order authorising the withdrawal of her hydration and nutrition on the basis that she was in a vegetative state (Austin 1996). However, 72 hours before court proceedings were to commence, Miss G communicated her wish, by means of a signalling device, that she did not wish this course to be followed (as in the U.S. case of Carrie Coons). The surprising feature of her case was that, before the accident which disabled her, she had consistently indicated to her family that she would not wish to be kept alive in the circumstances in which she ultimately found herself. Archdeacon Austin also recounted the story of the 15 year old son of a friend who, although severely disabled following 5 months in a coma as a result of a motor vehicle accident, "enjoys life with all its limitations". Similarly, an article by a doctor in *The Daily Telegraph* observed that "what one considers intolerable changes dramatically with what one is obliged to tolerate" (Daniels 1996).

An insight into the status attributed to individuals with very severe neurological impairment, recalling Kadish's comment above, came from the ethicist Daniel Callahan. Whilst acknowledging the impossibility of completely dissociating the judgements that we would make in relation to ourselves from those we make on behalf of others who are incompetent to decide for themselves, Callahan (1995) draws a sharp distinction between people with advanced dementia and those in a vegetative state:

> "Even at the latest stage, however, the demented patient should clearly be distinguished from the (carefully diagnosed) PVS patient when all possibility of selfhood has almost certainly been lost" (ibid: 27).

The implication was that there exists a clear distinction between PVS and any other neurological disability. This sits somewhat uneasily beside Callahan's citation of Joseph Foley, writing on the experience of being demented, to the effect that, if communication is absent, it is therefore *assumed* that internal mental processes have stopped (my italics). The assumption inherent in making the "careful diagnosis" of PVS that was specified by Callahan was not discussed.

Opinions of others about the condition of disabled individuals may have an adverse impact on them. Thus, La Puma *et al.* (1988) have advocated that comatose patients be talked to. Jarmulowicz (1995) has expressed caution about discussing vegetative patients within earshot. Carol Gill, who is both partially ventilator-dependent and trained in assisting disabled people, was emphatic that the *perceptions* of attending staff and family around a disabled person about the quality of his or her life readily feed in, and if negative, are likely to initiate or aggravate depression (*Affidavit of Carol J Gill* 1994). If a disabled person gains the impression that others regard the measures required for his or her support as burdensome, there can be a relentless erosion of that individual's will to live which exceeds that arising from any physical illness alone.

Any consideration of the opinions of others about the worth of the life of a disabled person, should recognise the devastating impact of being discussed, as though in one's absence, on the assumption that awareness has vanished. Keith Andrews commented to *The Times* that:

> "Just to be lying there with everyone assuming you are unaware of what is going on must be very disturbing" (Laurance 1996b).

This followed the publication in the *British Medical Journal* of his report that 17 out of 40 patients diagnosed by others as in PVS had

> "functioning minds imprisoned in bodies so severely disabled that their efforts to communicate went unrecognised" (ibid).

An Italian neurosurgical group acknowledged that:

> "There always remains the lingering doubt that the patient might in fact have some mental activity, which we have simply failed to detect: this doubt is often kindled by claims by those caring for the vegetative wreck (*sic*) on a full-time basis that the patient actually makes himself understood in some uncommon or even eerie way" (Bricolo *et al.* 1980: 632).

10.7 QUALITY OF LIFE ISSUES

> "The phrase 'quality of life' was minted in 1957 as a political slogan in the USA and has featured in political discussions in Europe since the early seventies" (Stensman 1985: 87). (Richard Stensman, Departments of Rehabilitation Medicine and Social Medicine, Uppsala University, Sweden).

> "Quality of life is something I have, not something you tell me I have" (Laurance 1996b). (Interview with Keith Andrews, medical director of the Royal Hospital for Neuro-disability, Putney, U.K.).

> "Disability and quality living seem antithetical to many" (Gill 1992: 46). (Carol Gill, psychologist living with a disability, Chicago, USA).

Quality of life assessments by disabled people often differ substantially from the assessments made, on their behalf by others. As there is little stability in the assessments of the happiness of *non*-disabled people in the immediate past (for example, over the preceding 24 hours), but considerable stability in assessments over a longer period (for example, the preceding month) (Emanuel *et al.* 1994) it is reasonable to apply an extended time frame in attempting to assess the views of people with disabilities about their life. Disabled individuals rated functions which they lacked as being less important than did the non-disabled in a Swedish study (Stensman 1985). In interpreting his data and reviewing earlier studies, Richard Stensman emphasised that significant differences between handicapped and non-handicapped persons had not been detected. He speculated that the undiminished quality of life reported by severely disabled subjects might be explained as the result of an adjustment process. For example, the ability to walk was ranked very low (averaging 27th out of 30 possible abilities) by mobility-disabled persons, whereas a group of non-disabled individuals rated it at 11th out of 30. Stensman inferred that the actual loss of a function was of less importance than the *image* of that loss which prevailed in the mind of a non-disabled person, and contrasted this with the frequency of "predominantly negative attitudes that exist towards the disabled".

Quality of life assessment is an individual matter. However, assessments about people with disabilities made by others are much more common than those based on self-assessment.

> "Whatever our opinion of someone's quality of life, if that person disagrees then we must be wrong" (Andrews 1993b: 1600).

The comment by the mother of Anita Bailey (see above) that:

> "I'm really surprised that somebody whose quality of life has been so severely affected can be so happy" (Fletcher 1996),

also calls into question the notion that a person's "quality of life" can be accurately assessed by another, even a close family member, on a proxy basis. As two rehabilitation specialists have asked: "Whose quality of life is it anyway?" (Bach and Barnett 1994).

Medical attendants can, inadvertently, transfer their own non-disabled attitudes to patients in their care. Bach and Barnett (1994), reporting from a rehabilitation clinic in New Jersey, were explicit on this point:

> "Indeed it appears that there are hardly any limits that some physicians will impose on this self-determined right to make life and death decisions for their patients" (ibid: 137).

They were especially critical of the application by health professionals of their own perceptions of patients' quality of life and life satisfaction to rationalise the withholding of simple medical interventions that would both prolong life and improve its quality. As already noted, a study by Bodenhamer *et al.*, (1983) indicated that staff are likely to overestimate the distress experienced by patients. A formal study at the Mt Sinai Medical Center, New York of the accuracy of physicians' predictions of their patients' wishes concluded that they may find it difficult to leave their *personal* assessments of quality of life aside when asked to make decisions on behalf of patients (Seckler *et al.* 1991). This practice of transferring assessments has been rejected by authoritative commentators within the medical profession. For example, the chair of the board of the American Medical Association has been quoted to the effect that:

> "The medical profession will not tolerate being put in a position to judge the value of the lives of the patients we are trained to heal" (McDaniel 1996).

In an attempt to explain the negative tendency of many physicians when assessing patients' quality of life, Gill (*Affidavit of Carol J Gill* 1994) has suggested that a training which is primarily concerned with *curing* acute health problems is unlikely to equip one to deal with *incurable* conditions.

10.8 THE QUESTION OF INDIGNITY

Two aspects, which have often been associated with each other in discussion of PVS, and are likely to have influenced the attitudes of non-disabled commentators towards their own management preferences should they become disabled, are those of indignity and dependency. Jennett (1993a) has identified the "indignity of this state" as being influential in the formulation of a wish not to have one's survival in a vegetative state prolonged. Citation of "indignity" inevitably prompts the question of deciding what is "dignity" and how it is to be determined. Leaving this aside, a more immediate question is whether the dignity of individuals is diminished by their physical state *per se* or by the manner in which others deal with them. The latter may, of course, be a reaction to a disabled individual's physical state.

Gill, writing from the experience of working with severely disabled persons, concludes that:

> "Even individuals with inexorable terminal conditions frequently talk about the richness and value of their final days and their profound realization that physical weakness and reliance on others does not steal one's dignity" (*Affidavit of Carol J Gill* 1994: 5).

Examples of the erosion of the dignity of an individual by the attitudes of others (rather than by the disability *per se*) have been provided by Fisher (1993), quoting from the decision of the House of Lords in the case of Tony Bland. It would be difficult to argue that some of the expressions selected by the Law Lords, such as "grotesquely alive", "humiliating and degrading" and "an object of pity", could do other than diminish the regard that others have for the affected person. In discussing Ronald Dworkin's arguments for withholding treatment from a demented patient who appears to be enjoying life, but who had previously indicated a wish not to be kept alive if demented, Dresser highlighted the relevance of the subjective responses of those in contact with the patient:

> "The 'tragedy' and 'horror' of dementia is partially attributable to the ways in which others respond to people with this condition" (Dresser 1995: 34).

10.9 SOCIAL ISOLATION

The retarding effect of social isolation on recovery from head injuries has been well documented (Oddy *et al.* 1978). Preoccupation with the physical status of an individual can result in personality and emotional problems being overlooked by the attending physicians so that little attention is paid to the isolation imposed by the injury (Gill 1992). Conversely, attending to these problems may result in gains not otherwise attainable, a point made by Jennett and Bond (1975) discussing the assessment of recovery from severe head injury. Whilst stressing the notion of a "fixed disability" a more certain concept in 1975 than in 2001, given progress in recognising "brain plasticity", they concluded that success in social reintegration achieved many years after brain damage could be attributed to adaptation by the person to that fixed disability. More recent recognition of the capacity of the nervous system to undergo repair raises the possibility that this process will operate alongside social adaptation.

Social isolation as an issue was brought into focus by introduction of the *Americans with Disabilities Act* (ADA). The ADA precludes health care providers from applying criteria of eligibility for life-sustaining services that either screen out, or tend to screen out, persons with particular disabilities. The World Health Organisation definition of "disability" places it completely in the context of interaction between an individual and the world. On this basis, it has been argued that references in the ADA to improving the access of people with disabilities to the environment automatically excluded those diagnosed as vegetative because they lacked an environmental interface. Banja (1993) asserted that arguments for the applicability of the ADA in PVS cases are not sustainable because "accessing the environment" is not an option and held that the ADA does not require rehabilitation to be provided to people in PVS, only maintenance "to sustain biological life". If this point was accepted, withdrawal of hydration and nutrition is not contraindicated by the ADA because it is undertaken "in the name of humanity or to relieve suffering". The alternative position, namely that the ADA *does* apply to individuals, notwithstanding a diagnosis of PVS, has been presented by disability advocates. Avila (1994) from the National Legal Center for the Medically Dependent and Disabled has argued that to exclude patients diagnosed as vegetative from basic care necessary for life would be in breach of the ADA.

10.10 DEPRESSION

A common impression of the non-disabled is that anyone in a near-vegetative state should automatically be assumed to be totally dissatisfied with living and hence, if such a patient is depressed, this represents no more than a natural component of the disability rather than a medical condition requiring specific management. There is little evidence to support these assumptions, but much to belie them. Stensman (1985) noted that data published to the time of his writing failed to support a contention linking self-destructive behaviour with disability. A 1992 report by Katz *et al.*, on life-care planning for a group of patients with locked-in syndrome noted that a

> "depression scale, albeit crude in comparison with previously described scales in able-bodied populations, did not suggest that most of our subjects were severely depressed" (ibid: 407).

They emphasised that decisions should be made *with* rather than *for* these patients.

Acute depression after sudden loss of a function is a natural response seen, for example, after high spinal injury. Affected patients have often been reported to be suicidal but, with adjustment to their condition, this outlook usually does not persist (*Affidavit of Carol J Gill* 1994). A similar reaction sequence, and the need for medical attendants to recognise and manage it, have been described by Andrews in patients previously in, or close to, a vegetative state:

> "Some patients are distressed and I would not blame them... They go through a bereavement process about being disabled and it's our job to help them through that. We have got to give patients an opportunity to live before we give them an opportunity to die" (Laurance 1996b).

Gill has emphasised that one cannot assume that, simply because a person is physically ill, he or she is not also susceptible to the treatable psychiatric problems that affect many physically healthy persons. Any psychological support that would be offered to a physically healthy person should not be withheld from another with severe disability.

> "Incurable physical problems do not imply incurable emotional distress" (*Affidavit of Carol J Gill* 1994: 3).

As with non-disabled persons who reveal suicidal intentions, a wish to die expressed by a person with severe disability may sound unwavering but nevertheless be characterised by deep ambivalence. Gill (1992) has identified a selective attitude towards persons with disability in relation to expressed wishes to die namely that the desire for death in a non-disabled individual is categorised as "suicidal", whereas a similar wish of a severely disabled person (for example a request for disconnection from a ventilator or of withdrawal of feeding) becomes a "refusal of treatment". She has drawn attention to a common presumption that there is something "natural, reasonable or proper" about the death of a person with a disability.

10.11 DEPENDENCY

> "What do we make of a young man who remains totally dependent on others for all his needs but smiles all day and apparently enjoys watching simple activities and being part of a group" (Andrews, 1993b: 1601).

It is paradoxical that, in placing a high value on individual independence and inculcating apprehension about dependency, many fail to recognise the high level of *interdependency* which characterises first world communities. Apprehension about complete dependency and highly negative attitudes to it appear to be most important influences underlying requests by healthy persons for the withholding of treatment should they become severely disabled at some future time. Kitwood and Bredin (1992) have written that severely disabled individuals with dementia

> "are clearly dependent on others and have come to accept that dependence; whereas many 'normal' people, living under an ideology of extreme individualism, strenuously deny their dependency needs" (ibid: 274).

Dependency can evoke excessively protective responses from carers. Irving Zola, a disabled sociologist, has written of over-zealous concern by others about possible risks to disabled individuals as one of the major impediments to attempts by these people to undertake activities which would improve the quality of their life (Zola 1982). Concern about incurring an expensive legal liability can be an inhibitory influence in the management of people with severe neuromuscular disorders leading to "the dehumanizing indignity in safety" (Bach and Barnett 1994).

A preoccupation with dependency projected onto disabled individuals by the non-disabled may represent another way in which inaccurately negative perceptions of people with severe neurological disabilities can adversely affect their prospects. Zola (1982) has commented upon the adverse impact upon his own psychological and social independence of attempting to comply with someone else's definition of physical independence. Concern about the impact of the fear of dependency in the "achievement-oriented" U.S. society led a United States Catholic Bishops' Committee to query the extent to which "dependency" is conditioned by the reactions of others towards an individual with a disability (U. S. Bishops' Committee 1992).

10.12 RECAPITULATION

The argument has been advanced by some commentators that PVS is a unique condition such that it is not legitimate to regard affected patients as "disabled" and so eligible to be considered as would other categories of people with disabilities. This is not a position with which I agree. This Chapter has considered some general aspects of disability in relation to PVS patients in addition to specific information about this group.

A general conclusion which has repeatedly emerged from attempts to compare the attitudes of the non-disabled towards people with disability with the attitudes of disabled individuals themselves is that there is usually considerable undervaluing of the quality of life of the latter by the former. Surveys of non-disabled health workers have revealed a belief that a vegetative state is worse than death and also that retention of some awareness in a near vegetative state could be even worse than being vegetative. In responding to these propositions, I would not question their accuracy as reflections of the respondents' perceptions of what these disabilities would be like. Those perceptions are undoubtedly based on respondents' comparisons of the disabled status with their own current status. This is, of course, not necessarily the comparison that very severely disabled patients will automatically make. For instance, their predicament at the acute stage of their injury may constitute the baseline for comparison.

Attitudes of a number of severely disabled patients who had emerged from a vegetative state, or who were sufficiently incapacitated to be misdiagnosed as in a PVS have been reported. As a common perception among the non-disabled is that retention of awareness of one's condition would be an even worse plight than being vegetative, it is reasonable to conclude that the views of these patients would not be unrealistically positive. Notwithstanding this expectation, the assessment which the staff at the R.H.N. formed in relation to such people was that most of them took pleasure in their environment within the limits of their ability. While some such patients regretted that their life had been preserved, this was not the attitude of the majority.

Patients with severe neurodisability are as likely as anyone else to become depressed. A bereavement process is as characteristic of the early stages after brain injury as it is in any other group of previously non-disabled persons who suddenly experience disablement. The case for treating clinical depression in an individual with a severe disability is as strong as that applicable to the non-disabled. Prevention of depression, or reduction of its likelihood, requires attention to the attitudes adopted towards patients by those working with them. These can readily impact upon the individual with a disability and have an adverse effect.

CHAPTER 11

POSITIVE MANAGEMENT OR AN EXERCISE IN FUTILITY?

> "While there are advocates for prolonged programs for active rehabilitation, the reality in most countries seems to be that many rehabilitationists are reluctant to accept these patients until they are showing some signs of recovery and are therefore expected to benefit from rehabilitation. As a result most such patients either remain for long periods in acute care settings or are transferred after a few weeks to nursing homes. Because of this, some believe that many vegetative patients do not reach their full potential for recovery". (Jennett, 1997: 8).

Jennett has accurately summarised the experience of many patients who are diagnosed as being vegetative. Management of PVS is often approached very negatively. Papers canvassing acceptable criteria for the withdrawal of basic care, in the form of hydration and nutrition, from PVS patients numerically exceed papers which describe positive measures aimed at their successful management by at least an order of magnitude. The negativity permeating many approaches to PVS has been neatly encapsulated by a group of British psychologists and rehabilitation specialists in the following terms:

> "Definition of coma is more frequently achieved by describing what patients cannot do than by what they can do" (Shiel *et al.* 1993: 162).

The International Working Party on the Management of the Vegetative State concluded:

> "The Working Party was very aware of the lack of research information about the effect and outcome of rehabilitation and disability management programmes… Many patients have not had the opportunity of a disability management programme, whilst in some cases acute and even life-threatening medical treatment has been withheld or withdrawn (presumably, treatment of acute and life threatening conditions); these patients may therefore have died before their full potential was reached" (Andrews 1996: 797).

Bryan Jennett commented on the medical care of vegetative patients:

> "In some hospitals, there seems not much middle ground left between intensive care and relative neglect" (Jennett 1976: 595).

11.1 ATTITUDES TOWARDS MANAGEMENT OF PVS

Positive management and futility may be seen as two sides of the one coin in that, depending upon the outlook of an observer, an identical measure may be categorised as one or the other. Attitudes towards PVS patients appear to be conditioned to a significant extent by the medical speciality of the commentator. Neurosurgeons are, predictably and reasonably, heavily focussed on early treatment of the acutely disabled patient with the aim of remedying the remediable and averting aggravation of existing damage. Patients who survive the acute stage of a traumatic or ischaemic brain injury but do not regain consciousness soon thereafter may be regarded as treatment failures unlikely to benefit from later measures. However, rehabilitation specialists have not necessarily regarded such cases as closed. Andrews (1992a) has described PVS as one of the least understood conditions in rehabilitation medicine. On the question of whether *clinical advantage* is to be gained by active treatment of PVS patients, he pointed out that some of those addressing this point, including at least one of the judges in the Bland case, regarded such advantage as synonymous with recovery (Andrews 1993b). Andrews placed an alternative interpretation on "recovery", namely the possibility of preventing distressing complications and providing the optimal quality of life within the limits of the patient's disability. The question remains whether the maintenance of a patient with severe residual disability is a *worthwhile achievement*. The divergence between those advocating and practising positive aspects of management of people in vegetative states and others who maintain that continuation of the life of PVS patients is futile justifies separate consideration of the two approaches in this Chapter. The first part will outline some positive management strategies whilst the second will attempt to summarise arguments on medical futility as these relate to PVS.

11.2 A REHABILITATION APPROACH

The adoption of a more positive approach to PVS patients has been exemplified in the change of name of the *Hospital For Incurables* to the *Royal Hospital for Neuro-disability* (R.H.N.) (the principal specialised institution in the U.K. for PVS patients) (Cornwell 1996). The management of patients referred to R.H.N. with a PVS diagnosis in 1993 included the provision of specialised seating to ensure posture control, the control of any intercurrent infections and management of bladder and bowels, use of sensory stimulation and the establishment of an adequate plane of nutrition (Andrews 1993a). A 1992 British Medical Association discussion paper acknowledged the value of this approach to management. While regarding artificially administered food and water as medical treatments which could be withdrawn by a clinical decision, the paper noted that committee members had been particularly struck by accounts of improvements produced in some patients by "relatively simple methods", a description applicable to the measures described by Andrews (Dyer 1992). The discussion paper identified

> "a vital need to draw the attention of the profession to the urgent need for rehabilitation and stimulation of suspected patients (*sic*) in a persistent

> vegetative state as soon as is practicable after the patient's condition has stabilised" (ibid: 853).

Apart from measures relating to seating, management of bladder and bowels, nutrition, etc., there have been suggestions that some patients in coma may be capable of learning and that it might be possible to harness this capacity to avoid the adoption of postures likely to lead to contractures. A study by a group of British psychologists and rehabilitation specialists arrived at the provocative conclusion that learning was achievable independently of any lightening of coma, that is without any detectable change in arousal levels (Shiel *et al.* 1993). If correct, this conclusion implies either that the clinical means available for detection of consciousness were distinctly unreliable or that residual cognitive activity could occur in the absence of consciousness as this is usually conceptualised. The investigators in this attempt to achieve learning by means of an operant conditioning mechanism, raised the possibility that coma might entail an active inhibitory process rather than a purely passive one.

Repeated measurement of responses to various forms of sensory stimulation have been used both to assess the conscious status of PVS patients and to attempt to improve that status. A 1991 R.H.N. report describing significant improvement in arousal of patients in vegetative states following repeated multi-modal sensory stimulation led to the development of the Sensory Modality Assessment and Rehabilitation Technique (SMART) (Wilson *et al.* 1991). This incorporated assessment of arousal/attention, auditory response, expressive communication, visual response, tactile response, smell and taste. Of 30 successive patients diagnosed as in a PVS, 7 emerged during the course of a study using SMART and a further 6 had done so by the time that analysis of data had been completed (Wilson and Gill–Thwaites 2000). The SMART assessments provided a means of differentiating those patients who subsequently emerged from the remainder. It was noted that recovery was not a smooth, continuous process.

Once a patient who has been diagnosed as in a PVS has passed through the early stages without signs of emerging, the adoption of positive management measures becomes less likely and the attitudes of whoever is responsible for the patient's care become most influential in determining the future course. Andrews (1997) has commented that:

> "Life expectancy depends very much on the attitude of the family and clinicians – i.e. how long the patient is *allowed to* live rather than how long he can live" (Andrews' emphasis) (ibid: 594).

On the question of how long patients *actually* live, the International Working Party on the Vegetative State emphasised that there was an almost total lack of long term follow up studies of vegetative patients beyond 2-3 years. Given the paucity of reliable information on the long term clinical course and variable standards of management, generalisations about outcomes are of dubious value. Shewmon and De Giorgio (1989) have pointed out that the more severely affected patients are unlikely to survive for prolonged periods, irrespective of management procedures.

When the likelihood of improvement in the patient's state of awareness has become negligible, two Boston rehabilitation specialists suggested that "one does not of course abandon the patient, but rather changes the goals of treatment" (Whyte and Glenn 1986: 40). Emphasis changes from efforts at stimulating patients to "maintaining their health and keeping them comfortable" (ibid). The authors acknowledged their assumption, that the patients have some consciousness of their health and comfort, although irrefutable evidence on this point was lacking. They stressed that a level of sedation which would be of minimal relevance in impairing the conscious status of a normal individual could have profound masking effects on those with marginal responsiveness and that sensory stimuli with specific emotional significance to the individual would be more likely than generic stimuli to elicit responses.

11.3 AVOIDING COMPLICATIONS

If one accepts that patients in a PVS have, by definition, already sustained the most devastating disability, extending to loss of personhood, and so cannot sustain any additional complication, it may appear logical to withhold anything other than minimal maintenance. However, unless one accepts this proposition, the avoidance of complications remains an integral part of the provision of basic care. One reason, specific to PVS, for attempting to minimise additional disablement is that the emergence of patients from a vegetative state may be curtailed when contractures retard the patient's physical recovery. Apart from impeding, or even completely precluding, the regaining of mobility, contractures may eliminate the only potential for communication that a patient retains if that potential is dependent for its expression upon joint movement to trigger some form of sensing device. In their 1996 paper on misdiagnosis of the vegetative state, Andrews *et al.* commented specifically on this complication. Recounting the history of a patient whose original misdiagnosis had not been rectified until 25 weeks after admission to the R.H.N., they reported that he had been admitted to the R.H.N. with very severe joint contractures which required surgical release followed by an extended physical management program.

> "Only when he was satisfactorily seated was it identified that he had a slight shoulder shrug which could be used for communication purposes" (Andrews *et al.* 1996: 15).

Another reason for avoiding complications in PVS patients relates to their ongoing need for other specialist nursing. The complexity of this, and the additional time required to accomplish it, will impose a significant burden on the patient's attendants and increase liability to "burn out" (De Young and Grass 1987). Ted Freeman, a clinician with long experience of the domiciliary care of patients in, and close to, vegetative states has stressed the desirability of remedying impediments such as contractures and constipation and of adjusting sedating therapy as much as possible before attempting diagnosis (Freeman 1997b). Andrews made the point in an interview that many of the patients arriving for admission to R.H.N. come "with malnutrition, bedsores infections, bad teeth, poor muscle condition and depression" (Cornwell 1996). A third reason for preventing the development of physical complications in PVS patients, perhaps less specific than the two preceding ones, could be to avoid the affront to the community caused by presiding over the frequently preventable deformation of a patient. I question whether maintenance of a decent respect for patients in general is possible in the face of the coarsening of attitudes likely to be encouraged by neglect of any one group.

Discussion of the measures that should be provided to, or may be withheld from, patients diagnosed as in PVS has frequently been segmented into discussion of medical measures apart from others which are considered to represent basic nursing care. I am constantly impressed (negatively) by the artificiality of this distinction and the arbitrary manner in which it is argued. The distinction is grounded in a mindset envisaging a segregation of roles which has been overtaken now for some decades. Any consideration of a specific medical or nursing procedure in isolation from the circumstances in which it might be initiated or continued is questionable. However, courts adjudicating on withholding medical care as a general issue, consistently ignore the case for providing treatment for relief of symptoms when cure is not an option (Calvert 1988).

Provision of medical care does not require the continuation of measures that are disproportionate in the circumstances of the specific case. For example, an intensive care physician considering the case of Helga Wanglie, an 86 year old ventilator-dependent PVS patient, drew attention to a 1990 report from the Society of Critical Care Medicine, which was considered to represent a broad, mainstream consensus:

> "The PVS patient should be removed from the ICU (Intensive Care Unit) unless it is not possible otherwise to meet the patient's nursing care needs. A PVS patient should not be maintained in the ICU to the exclusion of a patient who can derive benefit from ICU care" (Rie 1991: 25).

11.4 NUTRITION

The question was raised in Chapter 6 of whether inadequate nutrition could contribute to the brain atrophy often observed in vegetative states. It was suggested that the reversal of atrophy reported in anorexia patients following resumption of eating inevitably raised questions about the value of adequate nutrition in PVS patients. In a monograph, *Brain repair*, Stein, Brailowsky and Will cited a literature review to the effect that 160 to 240% increases in protein intake were necessary to maintain a normal level of metabolism in patients with head injury. Failure to achieve this level of intake would lead to muscle wasting (Stein *et al.* 1995: 112). Having noted an earlier report from another clinic that people with brain damage admitted to the rehabilitation unit averaged only 85% of their ideal body weight, Andrews estimated that up to 80% of PVS patients transferred to the R.H.N. were suffering from undernutrition as assessed by their body mass index (Andrews 1993c). He added that this finding was not surprising as it could require up to 3 hours/day of nursing time to feed a patient via a nasogastric tube. Compounding this limitation was the greatly increased nutritional requirement after severe head injury (he estimated that up to 350% of the normal resting metabolic expenditure could be required to maintain a positive nitrogen balance). Two rehabilitation specialists from a Tel-Aviv brain trauma intensive care unit have reported on the prolonged catabolic state that occurs in patients manifesting post-comatose unawareness. They described the success of a high caloric nasogastric tube feeding regimen in forestalling complications such as bedsores (Sazbon and Groswasser 1991). Whilst the information available about the increased metabolic requirements of patients with head injuries implies that augmentation of dietary intake would be beneficial, few randomised, controlled trials have been conducted to test this hypothesis. A Cochrane review update in 2001 suggested that adequate early feeding of patients with head injuries may be associated with a trend to fewer infections, better survival and less disability (Yanagawa *et al.* 2001). It was concluded that further trials of nutritional support were required in order to detect any "modest but nevertheless clinically important" treatment effects.

11.5 ORAL VERSUS TUBE FEEDING

Presentation of the issue of tube feeding of vegetative patients, especially in the course of court proceedings, has often given the impression that this is a highly technical and intrusive procedure. As discussed above, tube feeding of PVS patients is likely to be time consuming in terms of nursing resources if the intention is to avoid the patient entering, or remaining in, negative nitrogen balance. Whilst there have not been detailed studies of tube feeding complications in PVS patients, a comprehensive study of 253 tube fed patients (90% with nasogastric tubes) with a variety of medical conditions provides some indication of the complications to be anticipated. The commonest complications, disturbances of bowel function, most often profuse diarrhoea affecting 6% of patients, could usually be eliminated by appropriate adjustment of the feeding formula. Less frequent complications, mechanical or metabolic, were generally alleviated by tube repositioning /replacement or by formula adjustment, respectively. The authors concluded that enteral tube feedings were economical and safely tolerated by most patients in the study (Cataldi-Betcher *et al.* 1983).

The published experience of long term nutritional management of patients who were comatose, vegetative or demented emphasises the desirability of substituting gastrostomy for nasogastric feeding, and also of resumption of oral feeding in place of either form of tube feeding. In describing the experience of feeding PVS patients at the R.H.N., Tudor wrote:

> "Many come to us on nasogastric tube feeding. Imagine being awake, possibly aware but mute; the most immediate thing you see is a nasogastric tube in front of your eyes. This tube may feed you, but with it you have difficulty trying to speak or even swallow your saliva. Your appearance is not pleasing either to yourself or your relatives. Hence we advocate the insertion of a fine bore Percutaneous Endoscopic Gastrostomy as soon as possible" (Tudor 1993a: 39).

The removal of a feeding tube from any patient who has swallow and gag reflexes, is capable of swallowing semi-solid food and can eat sufficient to maintain weight was advocated in a report from a U.S. coma recovery program (De Young and Grass 1987). A 1994 article by Leff *et al.* with the eye-catching title *Discontinuing feeding tubes in a community nursing home* could easily be misconstrued by a reader familiar only with the mass of articles arguing the pros and cons of withdrawal of hydration and nutrition from PVS patients. However, this article differed from them in that removal of nasogastric and gastrostomy tubes from demented patients was *followed by their replacement by oral feeding*. Concerted efforts at weaning off tube feeding, based on "diligent nursing care and a desire to help residents achieve their highest level of function" were successful in half of the cases (Leff *et al.* 1994). Attempts at oral feeding were undertaken with the patient in an upright position with environmental distractions minimised and having been appropriately cued. Once a patient consistently consumed more than 75% of the orally offered food, the feeding tube was removed. Whilst concurring with the decision, in the Cruzan case, specifically that "tube feeding is a technological intervention comparable to mechanical ventilation", Leff *et al.* drew attention to a substantial divergence in practice in relation to withdrawal of the two forms of technology. Whereas most patients in receipt of artificial ventilation will undergo weaning trials to assess their capacity to breathe naturally if the ventilator is to be disconnected, patients from whom removal of feeding tubes is to be undertaken are much less likely to be afforded a trial of weaning to determine their capacity to accept food and fluids orally. Leff *et al.* observe that

> "the presence of the tube and its use may create the impression that it is crucial for the maintenance of life" (ibid: 132).

Much of their experience with demented patients in a nursing home would appear to be applicable to PVS patients.

11.6 NUTRITION AND NEURONAL MULTIPLICATION

Many earlier reports of the adverse impact of subnutrition on cell division in the developing brain have acquired a new relevance with recent demonstrations of the retained capacity for multiplication of cells in the mature brain (Winick *et al.* 1970). A 1999 perspective article in *Science*, entitled *Brain, heal thyself*, summarised the situation in the following terms:

> "It is time to lay to rest the dogmatic assumption that the central nervous system (CNS) of adult mammals cannot repair itself. Obviously, CNS injuries such as stroke, trauma or neurodegenerative processes do not fully reverse themselves spontaneously. Recent work suggests, however, that the mammalian CNS has a much greater potential for producing new neurons and repairing damaged regions than previously thought" (Lowenstein and Parent 1999: 1126).

It is reasonable to infer that this capacity for repair, involving mitosis of progenitor cells, remains as highly susceptible to interference from poor nutritional status as neuronal mitosis in the course of brain development has been shown to be. The implications for patient management would likewise seem reasonably clear. Suboptimal nutrition is likely to preclude realisation of potential for recovery.

11.7 SEDATION AND RECOVERY FROM BRAIN INJURY

Drugs with sedative activity, either as their principal action or as a side effect, are frequently used in the management of patients with severe brain injury to control complications such as seizures and muscular spasticity and to facilitate nursing during periods of agitated behaviour. Their use, as a management aid, often continues indefinitely. Divergence of opinion exists between those responsible for patient management and rehabilitation as to whether complete rest, facilitated by sedation or, alternatively, early intervention with stimulation is the optimal course. Intensive sensory stimulation has been claimed to interfere with recovery and possibly, as discussed in Chapter 5, to lead to habituation with resulting impairment of responsiveness. On the other hand, it is argued that the early introduction of stimulation, involving a range of sensory modalities can assist the re-establishment of neurological function.

Retardation of recovery of neuronal function by sedatives is suggested by some experimental findings. Thus, following sensory impairment produced in rats by damaging defined parts of the cerebral cortex, daily exposure to diazepam (Valium) for 3 weeks resulted in an indefinite delay in the sensory recovery that occurred in control rats which had been subject to similar brain injuries but had not received diazepam. The researchers, Schallert *et al.* (1986), concluded that

> "important mechanisms serving recovery of function may be vulnerable (to the effects of diazepam) during a short period after brain damage" (ibid: 104).

The nature of the vulnerable mechanisms was not determined, although the release of neurotransmitters, or an effect of the drug on receptors for transmitters, within neurones, was suggested. Schallert *et al.* commented, in discussing the results of administration of diazepam, that recovery of sensory function could also be blocked using phenobarbital. They speculated about the existence of a "critical period" after brain damage in which the recovery process is vulnerable to disruption by sedative drugs.

11.8 CARERS – THE FAMILY ROLE

> "Most traumatic brain injuries shatter more than one life" (Winslade 1998: 92).

It is a truism that severe brain injury to one of its members affects subsequent functioning of a family to an extent that is probably unsurpassed by any other medical condition. The appearance of the patient often remains, to all intents and purposes, as it was before the episode or accident, but communication may no longer be possible, or only practicable to an extremely limited extent. The stress of having a family member diagnosed as in a vegetative state over a period of years can be most disruptive for all forms of interpersonal relationship within the family.

Nevertheless, the family of a patient diagnosed as being in a vegetative state is often in a unique position to assist that individual.

> "Community-based rehabilitation recognizes that in the secure, loving environment of his/her own home, the person with a brain injury and the family, provided with support and guidance, can effectively augment or supersede hospital-based rehabilitation" (Freeman 1997a: 143).

As stressed by Freeman, a pioneer of community-based rehabilitation of patients with brain injury, an effective input from family members requires that *they* receive support.

The significance of the members of the family of a patient in the vegetative state can lie both in their persistent advocacy on behalf of their family member and in their capacity to establish some means of communication which is peculiar to that patient and family. As regards advocacy, Andrews (1993a) observed that most of the patients referred to him had relatives who were determined that everything possible should be done to help recovery. He was unable to determine whether these families were typical of patients in vegetative states or a self selecting subset whose persistence had effected the transfer of their family member to the R.H.N. Two American nurses emphasised the point that the family always retains primary responsibility for a coma recovery program's implementation (De Young and Grass 1987). Falk (1990) acknowledged the role played by his family in the remarkable recovery of an Israeli professor from a reliably diagnosed vegetative state. The mother of a patient who recovered cognition after two months in a vegetative state expressed her appreciation that the hospital had allowed her to use ideas from "coma" books (Sibson 1995).

A correspondent to the *New England Journal of Medicine* referred to the powerful bond that may exist between mother and daughter and raised the question of its being a positive influence for recovery from brain injury (Schwaber 1996). The International Working Party on the Management of the Vegetative State concluded that:

> "The family and other carers are often the first to identify changes in cognitive function, especially when there is gross limitation of motor responses, because of their more sensitive interpretation of the patient's facial expression and body language, associated with the greater amount of time parents spend with vegetative patients" (Andrews 1996: 800).

In accepting that eye tracking by a patient was often the first sign of emergence from a vegetative state, the Working Party added that the response to members of the family, and to some members of staff may be more consistent than to other members of staff. Nevertheless, it has been common historically for medical attendants to discount the perceptions and role of the family. Whyte and Glenn (1986) commented that a physician may conclude, on the basis of one or two examinations of a patient that the family is indulging in "wishful thinking" and is incapable of differentiating reflex activity from responses initiated in the cerebral cortex.

An ongoing family commitment to support the disabled member will inevitably require major changes in lifestyle of the other members. The British press accounts of the family of Andrew Devine who began to emerge from a PVS 6 years after the Hillsborough disaster illustrate this. Andrew's parents had modified their house and his father had quit his job as a police inspector to care for him (Hopkins 1997). The economic and social impact on a family of having a member who is vegetative will vary with the available health care system. In discussing the general situation of the families of patients with chronic illness, three members of the Hastings Center suggested that the burdens imposed on the family are "artifacts of the social and cultural context in which they live" (Jennings *et al.* 1998). Improved community facilities, it was pointed out, could substitute for some aspects of family care. One example of a possible adverse impact on the family was highlighted in a letter to the *British Medical Journal* from a general practitioner one of whose families included a young man who had been in a PVS for 3 years. While acknowledging the value of specialised regional centres for vegetative patients, he stressed the "devastating physical, emotional, social and financial" effects on the family if they had to re-locate to remain in contact with their son following his admission (Anon. 1992). A frequently expressed alternative solution for the families of PVS patients was that attributed to the professional carers responsible for a young woman in PVS:

> "They also feel her parents would benefit from Ms T's death as they could then attend to their own lives" (Brody 1988: 33).

11.9 CARE OF THE CARERS

Management of a patient in a vegetative state should recognise the role of his or her family and, as a natural extension of this, the need for support of these carers. Whilst primary responsibility for embarking on any form of coma recovery program is likely to rest with the patient's family, the immediate impact of instituting that program, and of the general care of the vegetative patient, is likely to devolve upon the nursing staff. As already noted, burn-out occurs frequently among nurses working with comatose patients. Factors such as the lack of significant improvement, or the slowness of that improvement, and the monotony of the nursing regime are likely to contribute. Whilst the occurrence of burn-out in association with coma recovery programs has not been documented, it has been proposed by the staff of one program that nurses should be reassigned away from the care of comatose patients every two to three days (De Young and Grass 1987).

11.10 ACTIVE INTERVENTION TO INTERRUPT THE VEGETATIVE STATE

Apart from the adoption of positive approaches to the clinical management of PVS patients, which may extend through to attempts to achieve "coma arousal", there have been a number of instances in which much more aggressive (arguably experimental rather than therapeutic) efforts have been made to arouse affected individuals to a level of observable consciousness. The most striking approaches have been those that entailed electrical stimulation of different structures within the nervous system. Instances of the use of electrical stimulation as a means of restoring vegetative patients to a conscious state have been reported intermittently over a span of 30 years. They have shed more light on the nature of vegetative states than they have benefited individual patients.

One of the earliest reports on the electrical stimulation of a patient in a PVS by Hassler *et al.* (1969) was published 3 years before the naming of the condition but the clinical description of this patient, with alternating periods of apparent wakefulness and sleep unattended by external evidence of awareness, anticipated that event. Reflecting the diversity of nomenclature that prevailed before 1972, the title of the Hassler report referred to "apallic syndrome" whilst the text, in different places, described the patient as manifesting "akinetic mutism" and being in "coma vigil". The 26 year old patient, whose condition was believed to be of traumatic origin, had electrodes implanted deep within the cerebral hemisphere (in basal ganglia and thalamus). After repeated stimulation over two days, there was an increase in spontaneous movements and the patient had a more wakeful and purposeful appearance. Continued repetitive stimulation produced further improvements until, on the nineteenth day, movements of the patient's arm broke off the electrodes and the experiment was discontinued. No further improvement was observed after this.

Another report of the use of intra-cerebral electrodes from Hassler in 1977 raised the possibility that PVS often resulted from a non-specific loss of cortical activation and was associated with damage to structures other than the cortex. A number of Japanese clinicians have applied electrical stimulation to PVS patients. In 1989, Momose *et al.* reported an increase in cerebral glucose metabolism, unaccompanied by any observable clinical improvement, in response to electrical stimulation of the spinal cord of a vegetative patient. Kanno *et al.* (1989) reported that 8 out of 23 patients diagnosed as being in a PVS showed good clinical improvement, accompanied by an increased blood flow to many parts of the brain, after electrical stimulation of their spinal cord. They noted that the subset of patients who had responded tended to be younger than the overall group and not to have bilateral diffuse low density areas on CT scan of the brain.

Tsubokawa *et al.* (1990) applied electrical stimulation deep within the brain (to the mesencephalic reticular formation or the thalamus) of PVS patients over a period in excess of 6 months. They reported that 3 out of their 8 patients subsequently regained the ability to communicate and, recalling the results of Kanno *et al.*, they identified a responsive subgroup. Selection of patients to be treated was recommended on the basis of prior examination of their EEG. Although repeated stimulation of patients was required over an extended period to provide substantial improvement on the prolonged coma scale, strong arousal was noted immediately in response to stimuli. They speculated that the requirement for long term stimulation implied that this treatment produced its effects by gradually increasing blood flow and metabolism. A further report on electrical stimulation of the brain from the same group at the Nihon School of Medicine focused on the variety of pathological lesions grouped together under the term "PVS" (Katayama *et al.* 1991). It was suggested that some individuals diagnosed as vegetative, who were not immediately identifiable, did not have gross brain damage. On the basis of the divergent responses observed after attempts at electrical stimulation, Katayama *et al.* proposed "that the PVS in certain subgroups of patients may be attributable to dysfunctional brain activity which is potentially reversible" (ibid: 121). Clarification of the nature of this dysfunction might help to establish the manner in which deep brain stimulation had assisted recovery of some patients from a PVS. A recent report from Nihon University has provided further evidence that electrical stimulation may offer an opportunity to benefit a subgroup of PVS patients. Seven of 20 patients treated with deep brain stimulation emerged from PVS and became responsive to verbal commands (Yamamoto *et al.* 2002).

A series of PVS patients reported from Bordeaux in 1993 were subjected to continuous long-term quantitative EEG recording over a period during which they received thalamic stimulation from implanted electrodes. It appeared that continuous EEG monitoring might reveal the most appropriate times at which to apply stimulation (Deliac *et al.* 1993). In 1998, the medical correspondent of *The Sunday Times* described the use of a "pioneering electronic pacemaker" at Cambridge and the success achieved in 13 of 25 patients with a similar treatment by a Bordeaux neurosurgeon, Francois Cohadon (Rogers 1998). Professor Roy John, director of a brain research laboratory at New York University, was quoted as saying

> "I have seen patients who can speak and move under electro-stimulation but who go back into coma if the stimulation is turned off" (ibid).

The likely existence of subgroups within PVS, suggested by trials of electrical stimulation and inaccessible to conventional clinical investigations, could be significant in at least two ways. First, it further strengthens the case for regarding PVS as a disparate collection of conditions sharing some clinical features in common rather than as a single well defined entity. This has significant implications for medical and legal recommendations promulgated as generally applicable to PVS patients. Secondly, it raises the prospect of identifying in advance a subpopulation of "PVS" patients who may benefit from one form of treatment.

The use of pharmacological agents in PVS has been discussed by some authors but has not been submitted to extensive formal trial. Nevertheless, as their administration does not require the extensive technical expertise and risk involved in the implantation of electrodes deep within the brain, it is more likely to have been used in individual patients on an *ad hoc* basis. The underlying rationale has been to increase the activity of neurotransmitter agents responsible for normal interaction between neurones. Apart from the experimental use of these agents in the management of patients with severe head injuries on a one-off basis, examination of their actions in patients diagnosed as being in a PVS has been reported from Japan (Higashi 1978) and the Netherlands (van Woerkom *et al.* 1982). In neither case was there clear cut evidence of benefit, although van Woerkom *et al.* suggested that there may have been an acceleration of the recovery process in those patients in whom this was already spontaneously occurring. A recent study of the use of bromocriptine produced some promising results but the need for further investigation was stressed (Passler and Riggs 2001). An example of the use of pharmacological agents in an individual case was provided by the patient of Childs and Mercer (1996a) in whom emergence from PVS began 15 months after injury.

> "Research that lacks direct benefits to subjects too cognitively impaired to consent to or to terminate their participation forces us to face squarely the difficulties in balancing individual autonomy and the need for society to obtain information leading to treatments and cure of dementing diseases" (De Renzo 1994: 547).

This assessment of research into Alzheimer's disease applies equally to PVS. The ethical validity of undertaking experimental procedures to assist recovery of subjects incapable of informed decision-making, or of indicating a wish to withdraw from the experiment, requires comment. The procedure of providing electrical stimulation to PVS patients remains highly experimental, although, to the extent that previous studies raise the possibility of direct therapeutic benefit to some patients, it becomes more readily acceptable to recruit additional participants. To justify including PVS patients and other cognitively impaired individuals in experiments requires that no more than minimal risk is entailed in the experimental procedure and that existing types of therapy are unsatisfactory. It is essential to involve next-of-kin in the decision process (Karlawish and Sachs 1997) but any consent to participation in a highly experimental procedure on behalf of a patient perceived to be in a hopeless situation requires careful examination to ensure that it has not been influenced by unrealistic expectations.

11.11 THE INFLUENCE OF PROGNOSTIC NEGATIVITY

The strongly negative impression that is conveyed by the term "persistent vegetative state", may exert an unduly negative impact on subsequent patient management which might contribute to the highly variable longer term survival rates of PVS patients that have been reported from differing institutional settings. A practitioner from a Philadelphia rehabilitation institute reported that he had seen only "a handful of deaths" over 5 years among more than 100 vegetative patients in its specialised coma-care facility (Whyte 1994) whereas the M.S.T.F. cited a much higher death rate within institutions in general. Another physician cited a five-year survival rate of 81% among a cohort of 27 persons who had been diagnosed as locked-in syndrome for more than a year, and again contrasted the poorer survival M.S.T.F. figures (Haig 1994). He suspected that:

> "Many of the patients in the studies cited by the Multi-Society Task Force may have died as a result of a conscious or subconscious neglect by care givers or a decision by their families not to have them treated" (ibid: 1380).

Andrews has observed that considerable difficulties can be created for those treating brain injuries in the acute phase by excessively negative prognoses that lead to families losing faith in the medical profession. He commented on the accentuation of those difficulties "by the number of patients who recover after their family have been requested to allow the organs to be used" (Andrews 1993c: 113).

Apart from avoiding the adverse influence of prognostic negativity on patient management, mediated indirectly by its impact on medical and nursing attendants, a *direct* influence on the patient should not be dismissed out of hand. The precept of not discussing *any* patient's condition with others in the presence of that patient unless he or she is included in the conversation can be overlooked with patients regarded as being permanently unconscious. A limited amount of data and many anecdotal reports exist bearing on the possibility that patients who are unconscious as a result of intra-cranial injury may nevertheless be affected by conversations in their presence. Mitchell and Mauss (1978) observed 9 unconscious patients who had pressure-controlled ventriculostomy drainage systems in place (to allow the egress of cerebrospinal fluid from around the brain and spinal cord and prevent excessive increase in pressure). They reported that conversations between others across a patient increased the rate of ventricular fluid drainage if the patient was the subject of the conversation. However, conversations on general topics did not have this effect. The small number of patients in their study requires caution in interpretation but, in the absence of published conflicting studies, the conclusion of the authors is worth noting:

> "It lends credence to the assumption that hearing and possible processing of external stimuli remains long after observable response is absent" (ibid: 10).

If negative discussions can have an adverse impact on progress, it might be suspected that a positive attitude in talking about a patient's condition could have a beneficial influence. La Puma *et al.* (1988) have advocated talking *to* comatose patients "because they are especially vulnerable and because some may recover".

11.12 ESTABLISHING COMMUNICATION

Any attempt to communicate with an apparently unconscious patient raises the question of whether, and how, one would assess that contact had actually been established. Attempts to establish whether some apparently vegetative or unconscious patients could be aware of inputs from others have been intended both to test for undetected capacity to receive information and to improve any nascent capacity for response. An early example of concerted attempts to communicate with patients in a vegetative state following traumatic brain injury evaluated communication skills by methods developed in an Israeli rehabilitation hospital by Najenson *et al.* (1978). Of the patients who were considered to have regained some capacity to communicate, all but one continued to suffer from dysarthria (motor limitations to articulating speech). It was suggested that such problems would be likely to conceal any returning capacity to formulate (as distinct from articulating) attempts at conversation initiated by attendants. This team persisted with attempts to communicate with their patients for a longer period than typically occurs and it was concluded that 6 of their group of 15 patients showed complete recovery of semantic function.

The rationale of attempts in an American brain injury rehabilitation service to "access the remaining awareness capability present in vegetative patients" was based on avoidance of neural habituation, that is, a failure to respond to a given stimulus because of previous repetitive exposure to similar stimuli (Wood 1991). To minimise the risk of habituation, reduction of the level of background stimulation was advocated,

> "eliminating unnecessary paging systems, creating a 'quiet' environment as far as staff activities and movements are concerned and regulating the way in which staff communicate with patients, using key words and slow delivery of such words to facilitate understanding" (ibid: 408).

A group of British rehabilitation specialists and psychologists expressed a more ambitious goal in their report title: *Can patients in coma following traumatic head injury learn simple tasks?* (Shiel *et al.* 1993). Their results suggested that patients in coma following severe head injury *can* nevertheless remain capable of simple learning. The strategy used to examine this entailed the use of "backward chaining", a technique in which a selected task is broken into a series of components and the subject is then cued through each component by means of verbal and physical prompts from the observer. A completely counter-intuitive observation, namely, the absence of any consistent relationship between the depth of coma and the capacity to learn the trial task, suggested that ability to learn was *not* just a consequence of the lightening of coma. In interpreting this backward chaining procedure, Shiel *et al.* considered that it was most likely to represent operant conditioning in which an association between a stimulus and the response to it is inculcated into the subject. If this conclusion is correct, its significance for implications about brain function would depend on the interpretation placed on an operant conditioned response, namely whether it is only a passive reflex or, entails an active cognitive component. Shiel *et al.* did not explore this issue although, interestingly, they cited the proposition that, rather than being a passive state as generally assumed, coma might be regarded as an active inhibitory process. This unorthodox interpretation from the perspective of experimental psychologists recalls some of the suggestions already associated with deep electrical stimulation of the brain of vegetative patients.

Most recently, the feasibility of establishing communication with some patients in a vegetative state was canvassed on a BBC2 *Horizon* programme. As this was subsequently reported in the London *Sunday Telegraph* under the disconcerting headline *Treatment offers hope for 'human vegetables'*, Professor Paul Schönle from a clinic at Lac Konstanz in Germany described the use of an electrical brain scanner on patients unconscious for more than a year (Macdonald 1996b). Semantic processing, as evidenced by electrical responses to comprehensible, but not to nonsensical, conversation had been demonstrated in some individuals. Schönle indicated a belief that his techniques might permit identification of patients who, although meeting all of the clinical criteria for diagnosis of PVS, retained a capacity for high-level brain function and could benefit from intensive rehabilitation efforts. Andrews observed that Schönle's research represented the "cutting edge of rehabilitation research" which might give even those in PVS some chance, he commented that:

> "What we are now seeing is that now people are taking an interest in the vegetative state, there are a lot more developments coming forward" (ibid).

11.13 THE ISSUE OF FUTILITY

> "Many clinicians view futility the way one judge viewed pornography: they may not be able to define it, but they know it when they see it" (Truog *et al.* 1992: 1560).

> "Rather than being a discrete and definable entity, futile therapy is merely the end of the spectrum of therapies with very low efficacy" (Lantos *et al.* 1989: 81).

> "The Council finds great difficulty in assigning an absolute definition to the term futility since it is inherently a value-laden determination" (American Medical Association Council 1999: 940).

Discussion of futility, whilst it is frequently undertaken as an isolated exercise, has often been initiated in examining grounds for resource allocation. The frequency with which the PVS has been incorporated into discussions of futility in medical practice probably exceeds that applicable to any other condition. To conclude this Chapter, I will briefly address those aspects of futility which have most frequently been introduced into discussion of PVS. These centre principally on the goals of providing ongoing care to patients, the question of whether those goals can be regarded as futile and the distinction between futility of specific procedures and futility of the continued existence of the PVS patient to whom they are applicable.

Considerable ambiguity exists in the application of the term "futility". As acknowledged in introducing this Chapter, it is inevitable that an identical approach may be considered as a positive management initiative by one observer and as futile by another. It is essential as a prerequisite to making this distinction to identify the goals of therapy. The next stage is to estimate the likelihood of achieving them. Several potential goals exist in management of a vegetative patient. They include the prevention of complications (such as contractures) which would curtail the extent of any possible improvement, the application of measures that have been reported to assist in re-establishing communication, the augmentation of any returning awareness and the maintenance of the patient in the best possible physical condition. As regards the likelihood of goal attainment, maintenance of physical condition should be the most readily attainable, given appropriate quality of nursing care. Consequently, it could not be described as futile for not achieving its intended goal. Andrews (1995) has pointed out in discussing the withdrawal of tube feeding from patients with brain damage,

> "I would argue that tube feeding is extremely effective because it achieves all the things we intend it to do" (ibid).

The likelihood of attaining the goal of regained awareness will decrease with time but, in view of the reports of very late emergence from PVS that have appeared in the last decade, a possibility for improvement should be considered to persist for longer than previously acknowledged. Prevention of complications, which would impede any improvement in the patient's conscious state, might be regarded as becoming a futile goal as time passes. On the other hand, it can be argued that, to the extent that this goal is achieved, it will materially assist and simplify attainment of the goal of maintaining the patient's condition. Apart from direct effects on the patient, preventable complications are likely to impact adversely on nursing personnel. The possible negative impact, on nursing staff, of the deterioration of a PVS patient's condition has been advanced by some commentators as a reason for withdrawing hydration and nutrition. Alternatively, one might adjust the patient's care so as to minimise complications and, consequently, their adverse impact on carers. Maintenance of physical condition and minimisation of complications could be argued *not* to be futile *either* as worthwhile goals *or* on the basis of likelihood of their successful achievement. Emergence from PVS is clearly not futile (in the sense of not being *worth* achieving) as a *goal* unless one considers that persistent major disability renders it so; however the diminished *likelihood* of its occurrence after an extended period may render its *achievement* increasingly futile.

The assessment that a particular treatment is futile for a patient may differ with the assessing clinician. Different values may be attached to any goal and different estimates of the probability of its attainment are likely. An identical goal may be patently futile in the circumstances of one patient but well worth seeking for another. Additionally, designation as "futile" seems frequently to have been transferred from the specific management goal, to the *life* of the individual patient. In the case of PVS patients, it is often asserted that "treatment" (unspecified) is futile. However, I believe that the term futility cannot retain any meaning unless its use is confined to consideration of a *specified* goal. It is as meaningless to apply it indiscriminately to *any* treatment provided to an individual as it is to apply it to the *life* of that individual. Specific components of treatment of a PVS patient may become futile. For example, the lack of any progress after a certain period of time in a coma arousal program may prompt a decision about "the futility of continuing with the program" (De Young and Grass (1987). The distinction between the futility of any *specific* measure and the futility of *treatment of a patient* has been drawn succinctly by Tomlinson and Czlonka (1995). In discussing decisions that cardiopulmonary resuscitation for a particular patient would be inappropriate (or futile), they have made the point that:

> "A futile CPR policy can in practice slop over into a futile *treatment* policy, without due regard for the relevant differences between CPR and other treatment modalities" (authors' emphasis) (ibid: 30).

In effect, the assessed futility of *one* form of treatment may be translated into futility of *every* form of treatment.

There has been a tendency to invest "futility" with the status of a well defined, quantifiable, even legally definable entity. In an article in the *New England Journal of Medicine*, aptly entitled *The problem with futility*, Truog *et al.* (1992) raised the question of "futile in relation to what?". They also emphasised the significance of probability in assessment:

> "Futility has been conceptualized as an objective entity independent of the patient's or surrogate's perspective, but differences in values and the variable probabilities of clinical outcomes undermine its basis" (ibid: 1563).

Youngner (1988) has referred to the "categorical ring" of the word "futility" and noted that, apart from physiological futility and absolute incapacity to postpone death, all definitions of futility involve value judgements. The expression "physiological futility" refers to clinical measures that have as their goal the attainment of physiological effects, which offer no benefit to the patient. An example would be the apocryphal caricature of the intensive care unit which aims to ensure that every patient dies in fluid and electrolyte balance.

Grubb (1997a) has drawn attention to some legal implications of the concept of medical futility that emerged from the decision of the House of Lords in the Bland case. While not attaching a precise meaning to the term, this concluded that if a treatment is considered to be futile it may automatically be regarded as not being in the patient's "best interests" with all of the implications of that phrase. This goal of a legal definition of futility has been advocated by Mason and Mulligan (1996). Specifically utilising PVS as the example, these authors advocated the introduction into the U.K. parliament of a "Medical Futility Bill". "Persistent" was to be replaced by "permanent" for legal purposes, removing the ambiguity that the former implied and "futile" was defined in terms of treatment which could not *improve* the patient's condition.

11.14 WHO DETERMINES FUTILITY?

Once the questions of *what* futility is, and *how* it is to be assessed are resolved, the further question remains of *who* is to determine it. A common starting point for resolving this, as for example in a 1991 position paper of the American Thoracic Society, has been that a medical practitioner cannot be compelled to provide a patient with treatment which he or she considers to be of no value to that patient. The Society's assessment of futility in the case of a permanently unconscious patient was based, not on the failure of treatment to ensure survival, but on the *judgement* that the survival which ensued would have "no value" for such a patient. The position paper, in a specific reference to patients who are "permanently unconscious" indicated that if a patient had explicitly specified in an advance directive that he or she would regard such an existence as being of value,

> "health care providers may provide life-sustaining interventions out of respect for the patient's prior expression of autonomy" (American Thoracic Society 1991: 482).

However, a life-sustaining medical intervention could be withdrawn without reference to patient or family if it is judged to be futile, this being assessed by the low likelihood of "meaningful survival", not the most value – free terminology.

In a progression from the preceding "default" position that a medical practitioner *need not* undertake measures necessary for survival of a patient considered to be permanently unconscious unless that patient had specifically indicated a wish for those measures, Angell (1994) has categorised such a wish as "idiosyncratic" (again, one senses that values are creeping in). Her article, in the same issue of the *New England Journal of Medicine* as the report of the M.S.T.F. on PVS, proposed that the burden of establishing the nature of the patient's wishes should be shifted to those sharing the patient's previously expressed "idiosyncratic" view. In Angell's view

> "we should instead presume that patients in a persistent vegetative state would *not* want to be kept alive indefinitely – a presumption buttressed by public opinion polls" (author's emphasis) (ibid: 1525).

The relevance of opinion polls of *non-disabled* individuals to the views of those living with disability has been questioned in Chapter 10, on the basis of their frequent divergence from the wishes of *disabled* individuals.

Two issues which are likely to be influential in decisions about whether a course of patient management is assessed as futile in a particular case, although neither constitutes a component of futility as discussed above, relate to the "burdensomeness" of that course and to its resource implications. In relating the potentially burdensome nature of any procedure to a decision about its futility it is necessary to establish some proportionality between the extent to which it is likely to be burdensome and the likelihood that it ultimately will prove to be futile. This requires specific consideration of *what* treatment measures are in prospect. To illustrate the need for evaluation of the nature of the specific therapeutic measures that are proposed, consider the range of measures which might be provided for a PVS patient. These could include initiating cardiopulmonary resuscitation (CPR) after a cardiac arrest, connection to a ventilator in response to decrease or cessation of spontaneous respiration, administration of antibiotics for an infection (or prophylactically), provision of hydration and nutrition and undertaking basic nursing care of bowels, bladder and skin. The intensity or potential intrusiveness of the specific measure would progressively decrease as one proceeded down the above list. Aggressive interventions would intuitively appear much more difficult to justify than less intrusive measures. While the first two measures on the above list (CPR and ventilator) are highly intrusive, the remaining three (apart from the infrequent possibility of a severe hypersensitivity reaction to an antibiotic or a complication from a nasogastric or gastrostomy tube) are not.

When factoring in the likely intrusiveness or "burdensomeness" of a particular measure for a specific patient in order to decide on its use, the necessity for its initiation or continuation to achieve the desired goal should also be taken into account. In contrast with the above listing of measures according to their level of intrusiveness, their order is altered when they are ranked in terms of their necessity for attaining the goal of maintaining the patient. Thus, whilst spontaneous resumption of cardiac action must be vanishingly rare if the need for CPR has been accurately diagnosed, the possibility of resumption of spontaneous respiration in response to weaning a PVS patient from a ventilator is not. Patients, whether in PVS or not, frequently survive infections in the absence of antibiotics. The measure which offers absolute certainty of outcome, namely failure to achieve the goal of maintenance of the patient is, of course, withholding of hydration and nutrition.

11.15 FUTILITY AND RESOURCE ALLOCATION

An issue which is likely to come to attention, together with futility, when making decisions on the initiation or continuation of a particular therapy is resource allocation. This issue should not bear directly upon the decision of whether the application of specific resources to achieving a particular goal in *the individual* PVS patient is futile. However, the possibility that such an application may preclude using those resources in the interests of *another* individual for whom the outcome is likely to be better could, in general, be a very legitimate consideration in allocating limited resources. This issue of whether the use of a specific treatment measure for the benefit of one patient is likely to deprive another patient of the opportunity to receive that treatment has been advanced as the basis for a moral distinction between withholding and withdrawing therapy. Sulmasy and Sugarman (1994) have proposed that if a measure is effective for a patient, its initiation establishes a claim to its continuation whereas Harris (1994) has argued that having first access to a treatment does not alter the balance of the argument about entitlement – if a second patient is more likely to benefit, then he or she has the greater entitlement. The particular relevance of the difference between withholding and withdrawing to the question of futility is that, whenever withdrawal of treatment that is already being administered is contemplated, there is likely to be more information available for making an assessment of its potential efficacy for the patient who has been receiving it. Whilst a majority of commentators express the belief that withholding and withdrawing are ethically synonymous, it is notable that accidental interruption of tube feeding of PVS patients, thereby transforming the issue from one of withdrawing to onc of withholding, has had some impact on English courts. The concurrent transformation of the issue from one of commission (removal of a feeding tube) to one of omission (not replacing the displaced tube) has also been regarded as critical by some.

Apart from the relative burdens likely to be imposed by the two measures and the feasibility of still attaining the goal in the absence of either measure, the relative availability of the resources required for ventilation and tube feeding may influence decisions. Limitations on the number of ventilators, and in the staff needed for their supervision are much more likely to arise than are those associated with tube feeding. Considered solely from the perspective of resource allocation, it is difficult to envisage how the latter could legitimately be argued to constitute a limiting factor in developed countries other than in conditions of severe social disruption.

Brett and McCullough (1986) having stressed that, notwithstanding a patient's autonomy, a physician cannot be obliged to provide therapy regarded as useless, proposed as a guideline that:

> "Decisions in individual cases should not ultimately be made on the basis of economic considerations unless the society has developed formal guidelines for the use of the medical resource in question" (ibid: 1350).

Whilst such guidelines are well defined in most communities in relation to access to resources such as transplantable organs, it seems unlikely that they would be instituted in the foreseeable future, primarily on resource allocation grounds, in relation to procedures as basic as nursing care and tube feeding. Whilst a physician is entitled to decline to provide treatment requested by the patient or family if the physician considers the requested treatment to be futile, Brett and McCullough considered that such a refusal should be accompanied by the offer of *alternative* treatment. Furthermore, the obligation to offer supportive care should endure in the event that a request by patient or family for treatment is refused as futile. The Appleton Consensus on guidelines for decisions to forgo medical treatment considered supportive care to be a "decent minimum of basic health care" (Stanley 1989). A question to be addressed is whether the provision of food and water, irrespective of the way it is administered, is part of a decent minimum.

11.16 IS MAINTENANCE WITHOUT RECOVERY A FUTILE GOAL?

Is maintenance of a PVS patient's condition, *as distinct from achieving recovery*, futile? Is any procedure aimed primarily at a goal of maintenance of a patient's condition, without improvement inherently "burdensome" irrespective of whether it imposes significant disadvantage on the patient? The poll on which the Oregon Basic Health Care Act was based opted to classify a treatment as burdensome whenever a patient remained disabled after its application. This classification held irrespective of whether the treatment had ever been intended to eliminate the disability and restore normal function (National Legal Center for the Medically Dependent and Disabled 1994). If this position is to have general applicability, rather than being devised specifically for patients with the level of disability prevailing in PVS, I believe that the argument becomes patently unsustainable. For example, many young patients who suffered permanent paralysis of their respiratory muscles during the poliomyelitis epidemics of the first half of the twentieth century had to face indefinite existence in an "iron lung". Such treatment offered no prospect of improvement as a goal, but, notwithstanding its possible negative psychological impact, it was not generally accepted as futile. Presumably, this reflected the dichotomy between treatment with an iron lung (technically futile) and the worth of a life lived in an iron lung (worthwhile). Currently, individuals with irreversible renal failure who, for any reason, are unable to receive a renal allograft will need to undergo dialysis three times a week for the remainder of their lives. Again, there is no possibility whatsoever of improvement from this therapy but, nevertheless, few would dismiss it as futile for that reason. Presumably, again, a life on dialysis is generally regarded as worthwhile and acceptable. The argument that a goal of maintenance without improvement is futile in the case of a PVS patient but not in the other instances can only be sustained if some estimate of the negative value (i.e. futility) of the PVS *life* is introduced into the assessment.

The case for futility of specified procedures when applied to a patient in a PVS, but not to others with precisely the same goal, can only be consistently presented if one is prepared to attach different values to different lives. This argument has been advanced, albeit not so explicitly. For instance, Schneiderman *et al.* (1990) have maintained that nutritional treatment which fails

> "to restore a conscious and sapient life.... is futile for the simple reason that the ultimate goal of any treatment should be improvement of the patient's prognosis comfort, well-being or general state of health" (ibid: 950).

While conceding the right of a patient or his or her family to opt for treatment which can only yield what are described as "qualitatively poor results", Schneiderman *et al.* propose that:

> "Other sorts of qualitatively poor results fall outside the range of the patient's autonomy and need not be offered as options. The clearest of these qualitatively poor results is continued biologic life without conscious autonomy" (ibid: 952).

Developing a similar argument to that of Schneiderman *et al.*, Mitchell *et al.* (1993) have contended that the provision of food and water to a patient in a PVS produces a physiological effect but does not "ultimately result in either short - or long-term benefits of the kind consistent with our humanity" (ibid: 73). They have argued that provision of food and water should be undertaken *solely* to maintain life until consciousness returns and "not at all" to maintain total medical dependence in a state of permanent unconsciousness

> "which clinical data indicates is certain beyond twelve months post-trauma".
> "When the clinical prognosis is certain, though not absolute, we believe there already exist sufficient moral reasons to make feeding the permanently unconscious optional" (ibid: 73).

Leaving aside the question of validation of "permanent" and "certain", the coupling of one sentence specifying "not at all" with a succeeding one in which "certain" and "absolute" are treated as separate, but undefined, attributes and the provision of nutrition for PVS patients is "optional" inevitably introduces considerable ambiguity about precisely *what* position Mitchell *et al.* were advocating. Their subsequent argument substitutes an obligation *not to maintain* for *no obligation to maintain*. Human compassion "demands" an end to the "significant burdens and suffering borne by both the family and the health care team and to a lesser extent, society" (ibid: 74). Such an argument that an imperative exists for suspending support on the grounds of ending suffering by others, rather than the patient, invites the response that a case may exist for *continuing* with provision of hydration and nutrition *for the benefit of others* (Stanley 1989). For instance, this latter point of view was aired in the course of the Appleton consensus, namely that such treatment of the PVS patient for the benefit of parents or close relatives was reasonable. Both arguments exclude *patient's* interests from the decision.

The possible resource implications of maintaining support for PVS patients should be considered at a population level. Mitchell *et al.* (1993) asked in their opening sentence:

> "Why do we persist in the relentless pursuit of artificial nourishment and other treatments to maintain a permanently unconscious existence?" (Ibid: 71).

This question was bracketed with reference to "huge numbers" of PVS patients, (a contention not in accord with available epidemiological data), so linking the issue of maintenance versus recovery with that of resource allocation. One consideration with clear resource implications, often factored into general considerations of futility, is the anticipated life expectancy of PVS patients. The length of time for which a patient is likely to live may be crucial in any decision as to whether an available treatment is worthwhile. A high probability that such survival will be very short may suffice to convince family and doctor that a form of treatment (especially if burdensome) should be considered futile. On the other hand, the prospect of a long survival could fuel resource arguments against providing the treatment.

While much of the literature devoted to discussion of non-medical aspects of PVS acknowledges that these patients, (subject to provision of food and water) are not dying, a recent major statement from the American Medical Association Council on Ethical and Judicial Affairs (1999) has chosen to put aside this distinction. In discussing medical futility in end-of-life care, the Council opens with the statement that:

> "Use of life-sustaining or invasive interventions in patients in a persistent vegetative state or, who are terminally ill may only prolong the dying process" (ibid: 937).

Subsequent recommendations by the Council left the issue of whether treatment should be provided in the case of any individual patient more open with futility being recognised as essentially a subjective attribute. Whilst acknowledging the need for futility to be taken into account in decision making, it was also recognised that:

> "To impose an objective definition of futility would inevitably cause some patients to receive treatment or to die according to judgements with which they disagree" (ibid: 938).

11.17 RECAPITULATION

The continued support and attempted rehabilitation of a patient diagnosed as in a PVS may appear as an instance of positive management to one person but as a futile exercise to another. The goal of ongoing management of patients in a PVS has been proposed as the prevention of complications and the attainment of an optimum quality of life within the limits of disability. The positive physical measures specified as prerequisites for encouraging cognitive improvement have included management of the patient's posture, bladder and bowels, and nutrition as well as the control of infections. The urgency of addressing these requirements as soon as the patient's acute condition has stabilised is emphasised as an aspect of positive management.

Whilst ensuring the maintenance of the patient's physical condition in order to optimise the chances of cognitive improvement, positive management is likely to include measures specifically intended to provide a range of sensory stimuli. The intention of these is to augment the level of the patient's awareness and, by means of repeated assessment of sensory capacity, to detect any improvement. Specific procedures are likely to include the use of specialised equipment to facilitate communication and the inclusion of the patient's family in this process. The administration of sedatives should be restricted as much as possible to avoid the risk of masking improvements in awareness.

All of the preceding measures may be regarded as futile by some writers and the PVS has often been used as an example in discussions of futility. Whilst the definition of futility varies, it may usefully be considered in two parts. A therapeutic goal may be futile because of the very slim chance that it is achievable or it may be regarded as futile because the goal, even if it is achieved, is judged to be of insufficient worth. The question of whether the maintenance of a patient in a PVS is a futile goal, being heavily value laden, is likely to elicit differing responses. If the goal of maintenance and prevention of deterioration is considered not to be worthwhile, the approach to positive management summarised above can also be dismissed as futile. However, if this goal is regarded as having worth, the chances of achieving it are likely to be sufficiently promising to exclude futility.

CHAPTER 12

THIRST

> "The sensation of thirst is basic to our very existence. Its gratification is universally held to be one of the pleasures of life; it cannot be ignored and, if water be lacking, the sensation comes to dominate our thoughts and behaviour" (Fitzsimons 1972: 469).

As emphasised by Fitzsimons in his classic review of the subject, cited above, thirst is a central feature of existence. Unlike many other types of neurological function which entail cognitive participation and consequently differ considerably between species, the neurophysiological basis of thirst appears to be essentially similar among species. The relevance of the thirst sensation to PVS is twofold. In the first place, thirst is an example of sentience, albeit concerned with awareness of the person's *internal* environment rather than awareness of his or her surroundings, the topic of Chapter 5. As noted below, thirst has usually been regarded as a "visceral" sensation associated with the relatively primitive limbic system in the brain. In view of the centrality of the concept that a complete loss of all capacity for sentience is a definitional feature of vegetative states, any inferences that can be drawn concerning retention or loss of the thirst sensation by affected patients are likely to be relevant to an improved understanding of these conditions. It is of interest that, whilst a substantial literature exists describing the neurophysiology of thirst, this is rarely cited in discussion of the capacity of patients with brain injury of the types commonly associated with vegetative states to remain subject to thirst. As will be pointed out in this Chapter, citations relating to the absence of thirst in a vegetative state have invariably been to a small group of papers containing very limited data.

The second connection between thirst and PVS arises from the increasingly common practice of ceasing to provide food and fluids to patients in vegetative states. Humane considerations presumably require that, before one can argue in favour of this course of action, it must be possible to exclude with confidence any persistent susceptibility of vegetative patients to thirst. Unless thirst can be excluded beyond reasonable doubt if withholding of fluids is to be used as a means of ending the PVS patient's life, the elimination of the sensation of thirst by pharmacological intervention becomes an issue. This Chapter is concerned with experimental and clinical information necessary for defining the minimal neuroanatomical requirements for existence of the thirst sensation on the basis of which some assessment can be made of the likelihood of their retention by a PVS patient.

Whilst it is possible to identify much of the neuroanatomical and neurophysiological basis for thirst, it is not feasible to specify which of those structures and functions are likely to be intact and operative in the "typical" patient diagnosed as being in a PVS. The heterogeneity among such patients has already been referred to. In relation to the capacity to experience discomfort, Andrews' (1993b) opinion that very few of the PVS-diagnosed patients he had seen were so deeply unconscious as to permit confident exclusion of any such capacity has also been noted. This observation is consistent with the original acknowledgment by Jennett and Plum (1972) of the likely existence of a "spectrum" of cases.

The question of the extent to which patients diagnosed as in a PVS, may nevertheless retain some conscious capacity arose in Chapter 8-10 as did that of the extent to which *unrecognised* misdiagnosis of PVS (defined as *complete* unconsciousness) may occur. Certainly, Andrews' assessment, in view of his extensive clinical experience, would suggest that *very few* of those diagnosed as in a PVS (with the clinical diagnosis not in dispute) are *totally* unconscious. For the purpose of considering whether any patient diagnosed as in a PVS is completely insusceptible to discomfort of external (Chapter 5) or internal (this Chapter) origin, one might question why a majority of these patients would not remain susceptible. That only a small number of patients, previously diagnosed as in a PVS have recovered sufficient capacity to describe their recollections of that state tells us little about whether a few or many of those who failed to recover and to recollect resembled them. These descriptions, by nature of the patients' circumstances, have not been subject to the laws of evidence. On the other hand, the general presumption that *some* (often taken to be *all*) people diagnosed as being in a PVS are totally insusceptible to any discomfort lacks any direct evidence and has ultimately to be based on a belief in what PVS is theoretically conceived as being. In the absence of direct evidence to bolster that concept, I propose that the case to be presented in this Chapter for retention of a capacity for thirst merits consideration in relation to *any* person so diagnosed, rather than to some subgroup.

12.1 THIRST IN THE CONTEXT OF PVS

The case for insusceptibility of PVS patients to thirst has generally been stated without attempt to present biological data and has had, in my opinion, a distinctly circular format. For instance, a 1990 statement from the Council on Scientific Affairs and the Council on Ethical and Judicial Affairs of the American Medical Association (A.M.A.) resolved the issue of the possible susceptibility to thirst of patients diagnosed as in PVS in a "definitional" way, so obviating any necessity for reference to a source of data. Thus, it was pointed out that, *by definition*, the capacity of PVS patients to experience discomfort associated with starvation and dehydration after removal of a feeding tube had been lost (American Medical Association Councils 1990). An article on PVS from the Institute of Medical Ethics (1991) published in *The Lancet* in the following year, stated, when discussing withdrawal, that "there is no remaining neurological mechanism to make pain or suffering possible" citing the A.M.A. Councils' paper as its source for this information, so reinforcing the earlier claim without adding any data to support it. (ibid: 97).

The 1993 American Neurological Association statement on PVS, while endorsing withdrawal of food and fluids, did not refer to the possibility of PVS patients experiencing thirst (American Neurological Association 1993). The most frequently cited article on PVS, the M.S.T.F. Statement (`1994b), indicated that "patients in a PVS cannot experience thirst or hunger" and provided a single reference to support that position. That reference was to an article entitled *The sloganism of starvation* by Ahronheim and Gasner (1990) (the latter author being a legal officer with the New York office of the Right to Die Society) published under the *Viewpoint* heading in *The Lancet.* Mention was made of that article in Chapter 1 when considering some semantic aspects of PVS. As *The Lancet's* editorial classification of it as *viewpoint* implies, it did not present any new data but merely set out the views of its authors on the subject of withdrawal of food and fluids. Of the four reports cited by Ahronheim and Gasner actually presenting data on thirst sensation during dehydration, two related to studies of terminally ill patients (Printz 1988; Billings 1985) whilst the others dealt with reduced thirst sensation in normal elderly subjects (Phillip *et al.* 1984; Miller *et al.* 1982). These reports, and others, will be examined below together with the validity of extrapolating from observations on dying individuals to PVS patients.

In contrast with the slim referenced basis for the M.S.T.F. statement on the lack of capacity of PVS patients to experience distress when food and fluids are withheld has been the subsequent profuse citation of the statement itself on this point. A more guarded statement, which could be read as conceding some doubt on the subject, came from the 1997 Aspen Neurobehavioural Conference, when considering the issue of distress after withholding food and water. This was that "patients in vegetative states are_thought to be incapable of experiencing pain and suffering" (Giacino *et al.* 1997: 87) In summary, it is suggested that the statements and reports on PVS which are commonly regarded as the most authoritative, which have been most frequently cited by other authors and which have had the greatest influence on thinking and practice, have been based on remarkably few published reports of data that has survived critical peer review. Contrary to the paucity of peer-reviewed reports concluding that PVS patients *can not* experience thirst, solid data *does* exist which bears on the question of the capacity of PVS patients for thirst and this will be considered within the framework outlined below.

12.2 SOURCES OF INFORMATION ABOUT CAPACITY FOR THIRST

Whereas pronouncements about thirst in PVS patients have been based on analogies with terminally ill and elderly subjects, little attention has been paid to the substantial literature describing experimental investigation of thirst in animals. This suggests, with considerable precision, which structures in the central nervous system must be non-functional to eliminate thirst. This Chapter will draw attention to clinical reports of abnormalities of thirst sensation in patients with discrete, anatomically localised brain lesions and to studies of fluid deprivation in young, healthy subjects before focusing on results of experimental investigation of thirst in animals.

The validity of, and scope for, extrapolation from animal experiments to clinical situations such as PVS will be determined by the specific subject under investigation. Whereas it is difficult and probably unreliable to draw inferences about human cognitive function from studies in animals, the apparent inter-species conservation of the neurological basis of thirst renders this a more suitable subject for extrapolation. Another feature of thirst, namely the highly localised nature of the neuroanatomical structures responsible for mediating this sensation, permits precision in producing experimental lesions of small structures within the brain. Whilst the equivalence of the structures responsible for initiating thirst sensation in humans and other species is not in dispute, the imputed role of the cerebral cortex in this process appears to have been the basis for statements which discount any susceptibility of PVS patients to thirst. However, worthwhile experimental data from animal studies is available which questions the *essentiality for*, as distinct from the *normal participation* of, the cortex in thirst.

Whilst the terms of definition of PVS, by excluding capacity for communication, specifically preclude the otherwise obvious approach to ascertaining whether a patient not in receipt of fluids and food is aware of thirst, namely that of asking the person, other approaches remain possible. It is feasible to draw some inferences about thirst capacity in vegetative states from consideration of the following:

1. basic neuroanatomy and neurophysiology of thirst,
2. accounts of the effects of experimental dehydration provided by healthy volunteers,
3. observation of patients with complete adipsia (loss of thirst sensation) and of elderly patients with reduced thirst sensation (hypodipsia),
4. accounts of the effects of dehydration on patients in the terminal stage of illness given by the subjects themselves and by their medical attendants, and
5. information on thirst-associated behaviour in animals after precise placement of experimental lesions in the brain.

12.3 BASIC NEUROANATOMY AND NEUROPHYSIOLOGY

Any inferences drawn about the degree of loss of a specified neurological function that a patient is likely to have sustained will be dependent on the accuracy of information available about both the severity of lesions and their anatomical location in that patient. How accurately and with what degree of neuroanatomical detail can the structures in the *normal* brain responsible for the function of interest be identified? How precisely can the lesions in the brain of that patient be located? This approach has been used, in a rather informal manner, to specify loss of consciousness and sentience by individuals in vegetative states. The types of conclusions about conscious status drawn in this manner have been criticised in Chapter 4 because of their vague nature. However, substantial differences exist between the extent to which the neuroanatomical structures mediating thirst and consciousness can be confidently specified. Whilst understanding of the neuroanatomical basis of thirst remains subject to some deficiencies, a major reason for it exceeding that of consciousness is the greater feasibility of investigating thirst in animals. Undoubtedly the higher degree of complexity of neurological structure and function entailed in consciousness, and especially the involvement of many parts of the brain rather than several well-localised structures have also been important contributory factors. The difficulty in extrapolating from animal observations to humans is also likely to be much greater for consciousness than it is for thirst.

It has been known since the mid-twentieth century that a number of nuclei in the hypothalamic region at the base of the brain are involved in mediating thirst (this subject has been reviewed briefly by Martin and Reichlin (1987)). The established understanding of the neuroanatomical basis for sensing thirst and then initiating drinking behaviour has centred on the hypothalamus as the critical area. Traditionally, the cortex has been held to be responsible for no more involvement in thirst than "facilitatory influences on the hypothalamus" (American Physiological Society 1963: 182). Interacting with the neurones in the hypothalamic nuclei to mediate both thirst itself and thirst-initiated behaviours is the limbic forebrain (a term which includes hippocampus, amygdala and septum). These structures, which have together been described as the "visceral brain", are responsible for such *routine* activities as regulating body temperature and others characterised as "vegetative" functions in the original description of PVS (Jennett and Plum 1972). In terms of the evolutionary conservation of its neuroanatomical location in proximity to those structures and its basic role in regulation of the "internal environment', thirst may be regarded as a vegetative attribute *par excellence*. As was suggested by Jennett and Plum those parts of the brain responsible for vegetative functions are believed to remain intact in PVS patients. The brain centre mediating thirst is located in a structure that is phylogenetically one of the oldest parts of the central nervous system. Descriptions of the neuroanatomical lesions in PVS patients have confirmed the original clinical inference that the hypothalamus (including the thirst centre) remains intact.

12.4 DEHYDRATION IN HEALTHY VOLUNTEERS

Studies of the consequences of depleting body water in healthy, young male subjects have been concerned primarily with characterisation of changes in their metabolism of electrolytes and water, but have also included accounts of the symptoms experienced by the subjects during the various procedures. A 1941 study from Michigan compared two types of dehydration (Nadal *et al.* 1941). It was observed that dehydration resulting from simple water deprivation was accompanied by thirst, whereas dehydration resulting from abnormal salt loss was not. A later study undertaken on US Army personnel entailed partial or complete deprivation of water and food for several days. The lead observation on reactions of those subjects was that "thirst appeared early and regularly" (Winkler *et al.* 1944). It was observed that thirst could be quenched by ingestion of an amount of water much less than that which had been lost. Whilst the age and (non-neurological) physiological status of individuals in vegetative states is variable, as is the underlying neuropathology, the body fluid balance of a substantial number of younger persons with a history of severe brain injury followed by a vegetative state would resemble that of these healthy volunteers much more closely than that of the terminally ill or elderly patients with whom they have frequently been equated in commentaries which have dismissed any possibility of retention of thirst sensation in PVS.

I am not aware of any published formal studies of the existence of thirst sensation in normal individuals who are asleep. However, I believe that the experience of being awakened in response to thirst is not rare. Whether the arousing stimulus was perceived as thirst whilst still asleep or whether an individual is aroused by changes in body fluid concentration and then becomes aware of thirst is not clear. The degree of precision with which one can specify the features of unpleasant experience during a state of altered consciousness, such as sleep, might be impaired notwithstanding the persistence of discomfort.

12.5 ADIPSIA AND HYPODIPSIA

A number of reports exist of the effect of well localised brain injuries on thirst in otherwise healthy patients. Adipsia, the absence of a capacity for thirst, and hypodipsia, a reduced capacity for thirst, can both occur after brain injury. Patients with these conditions have been most instructive in localising those parts of the brain critical for thirst and comparison of their lesions with those produced in experimental animals has supported extrapolations about thirst from animals to humans. Complete inability to experience thirst (adipsia) is rare, but study of affected patients has provided the most precise confirmation of the anatomical location of the neurones normally mediating thirst. The patient of Hays *et al.*, (1963) a 40-year-old bank auditor, required hospitalisation on two occasions on account of spontaneous dehydration. Lacking the capacity to experience thirst, he had failed to compensate for fluid loss. Significantly, he also showed clinical signs of impairment of other hypothalamic functions (responsible for other "vegetative" activities) in addition to occult hydrocephalus. It was inferred by Hays *et al.* that enlargement of the third ventricle of his brain accompanying the hydrocephalus had compressed the hypothalamus, underlying the floor of that ventricle, and so damaged his thirst centre.

Another adipsic patient reported by Spiro and Jenkins (1971) lost the spontaneous desire to drink after recovering from a subarachnoid haemorrhage. This loss was accompanied by other indications of hypothalamic dysfunction, most noticeably a persistently low body temperature. It was inferred from this combination of symptoms that she had a residual lesion in the anterior part of the hypothalamus. Given the small size of the thirst centre and the close proximity to it in the hypothalamus of other centres fulfilling "vegetative" functions, together with the random nature of brain injuries following trauma and vascular accidents, patients with hypothalamic lesions may be expected to manifest a multiplicity of symptoms. A third patient, described by Conley *et al.* (1976), was unable to appreciate the sensation of thirst. In the absence of any demonstrable neurological lesions elsewhere, it was inferred that she had a very localised lesion restricted to the thirst centre in the hypothalamus. All three of these patients were subject to recurrent episodes of dehydration, precipitated, in the absence of thirst, by failure to maintain an adequate water intake.

Hypodipsia, or a reduced capacity for thirst, is more common than adipsia and case reports have been cited to support the contention that patients who have been diagnosed as vegetative will not be susceptible to thirst when fluids are withheld. Two reports of hypodipsia were cited by Ahronheim and Gasner (1990) in their paper *The sloganism of starvation*. In one of these studies, 7 healthy elderly, but active, men were compared with 7 healthy young men. Following a 24 hour period of water deprivation, the older men were less thirsty than the younger group as assessed by their consumption of freely available water during the following hour which was approximately 50% of that of younger men (Phillip *et al.* 1984). The other report described 6 elderly patients with past histories of cerebrovascular accidents who required recurrent hospitalisation for dehydration. When hospitalised, it was found that their spontaneous daily water consumption was inadequate to compensate adequately for fluid loss (Miller *et al.* 1982). Neither report specifically explored the nature of the thirst sensation which had initiated drinking (albeit of volumes inadequate to replenish their water deficit) by the elderly subjects.

Comparison of the location of the brain lesion in adipsic patients with the types of lesion most commonly found in vegetative state patients strongly suggests that concurrent damage to the thirst centre would certainly not be a typical occurrence in patients diagnosed as vegetative. Any lesion to the thirst centre would be likely to be accompanied by other indications of hypothalamic damage. The markedly divergent locations of the lesions required to ablate thirst sensation and those which are considered characteristic of PVS should raise doubts about the claim that patients in a vegetative state no longer retain any capacity for thirst and may also prompt further questions. Which additional neurological functions, apart from those mediated by the hypothalamus, are likely to be required if a susceptibility to thirst is to be retained after injury to the brain? What is the likelihood that those functions will remain intact in patients diagnosed as vegetative? To what extent is an intact cortex, in addition to an intact hypothalamic thirst centre, required if a patient in a vegetative state is to remain susceptible to thirst? Which additional neurological functions, apart from those mediated by the hypothalamic thirst centre, are required if the natural response to thirst, namely drinking, is to occur and to be apparent to an observer?

Considerable information relevant to answering these questions, has been obtained from experiments with animals and this subject will be considered later. At this stage it may be pointed out that the prerequisites for a person to drink in response to experiencing thirst will include peripheral motor function to achieve swallowing and also the neural structures required to co-ordinate the complex individual muscular components of this action. However, in addition to these motor functions, neither of which is required exclusively for responding to thirst, animal studies point to the existence of a second hypothalamic centre that is responsible for *initiating the action of drinking* in response to stimulation of the thirst centre. If an observer is to be in a position to ascertain whether a patient is subject to thirst, it would be necessary that the capacity either to communicate this information to others or to respond to thirst by attempted drinking remain intact. Attempts at drinking would require that *both* the hypothalamic centre responsible for initiating drinking *and* the more peripheral neurological structures required to accomplish the actual mechanics of drinking remained functional in addition to the thirst centre itself.

12.6 DEHYDRATION IN TERMINALLY ILL PATIENTS

> "The ethical situation is not that the patient is failing to drink and therefore will die, but that the patient is dying and therefore does not wish to drink" (Lennard-Jones 1999: 39).

Terminally ill patients are extremely unlikely to be in a normal physiological state of fluid balance. Young patients in a PVS, if properly cared for, should be. Dying patients frequently have little interest in eating and drinking and will not benefit from maintenance of fluid balance by administration of fluid, either intravenously or by tube into the gastrointestinal system. This is encapsulated in the above quotation from a British gastroenterologist discussing withholding fluid and nutrients from dying patients. The reported experiences of dying patients, insofar as they are concerned with experiencing thirst and wishing to drink in response to it, have been used in attempting to infer the possible impact of withdrawal of fluids from patients diagnosed as vegetative. To infer that an otherwise healthy young patient in a PVS will be as indifferent to fluid deprivation is a dubious exercise given the substantial physiological differences between the two classes of subject. Before considering the manner in which reports of terminally ill people have been used as a basis for interpreting vegetative states, and especially their relevance to the heterogeneous group of patients commonly classified as vegetative, I would emphasise the need to distinguish between one person who is dying *with* dehydration and another who is dying *from* it. Notwithstanding the rather imaginative use by some commentators and courts of "terminal" to refer to PVS patients who may have been in a stable state for years and are likely to remain so (given the provision of food and water) for further years, the physical condition of many vegetative state patients (apart from that of their central nervous system) is very different from that of most terminally ill and dying patients. The different status of the two groups was neatly summed up in the title of one *Hastings Center Report* article on PVS, namely *Not dead, not dying* (Wikler 1988).

One of the earliest and most frequently cited articles on optimal fluid management of dying patients is that of Joyce Zerwekh (1983) from a Seattle hospice. Zerwekh maintained not only that there was no valid indication for the administration of intravenous fluids to a dying patient, but that this could be disadvantageous for the patient by increasing gut and bladder content and secretion into the respiratory tract. A short report from a London hospice in 1984 specifically addressed the question of whether maintenance of electrolyte and fluid balance during the last 48 hours of life improved patient comfort. Of 22 patients not in receipt of intravenous or nasogastric fluids, who had incidentally been subjected to venepuncture on one of the last two days of life, 12 had essentially normal electrolyte levels and the remaining 10 were abnormal, but none of the patients in either group was distressed (Oliver 1984). This accords with common experience of terminally ill patients. It is quite unexceptionable to agree with the proposition that a dying patient who declines to eat or drink should not be subjected to hydration by a gastric tube or an intravenous line. However, as encapsulated in the title of the *Hastings Center Report* cited above, the typical patient in a vegetative state is *not* in the process of dying and will have a fluid and electrolyte status very different from that of a terminally ill patient. It is most unlikely that the response of the thirst centre of the physically healthy vegetative patient to dehydration will resemble that of a cachectic, dying patient in whom many regulatory mechanisms are likely to have ceased to function in a normal manner.

During the writing of this monograph, I had the opportunity on a number of occasions to visit a person, incapable of oral feeding, who had decided, very reasonably, that the pain which she had experienced from prolonged (jejunal) enteral feeding outweighed its nutritional advantages. Following removal of her jejunostomy tube she remained fully conscious for close to two weeks, before accepting sedation, and reported considerable thirst during that interval. Patients who are within days of dying will almost certainly have major systemic physiological aberrations. An editorial in the *Journal of the American Geriatrics Society* on the question of whether dehydration was painful for the terminally ill made the point that dehydrated terminally ill patients commonly have mixed depletion of salt and water resulting from abnormal gastrointestinal or renal fluid loss. Whereas "pure water deprivation .... is characterized early in its development by intense thirst", the writer pointed out that *hypo*natremic dehydration (in which both salt and water are depleted) need not have this effect (Billings 1985: 809). Withdrawal of fluids from a PVS patient, in the absence of abnormal losses of electrolytes from gut or kidney, will certainly produce *hyper*natremic dehydration characterised by an increasing concentration of extracellular body fluid resulting from deficiency of water alone rather than from a combined deficiency of water and salt.

Two papers published in 1994/5 suggested that a considerable degree of variation exists among dying patients as regards thirst sensation. In an American study reported from Rochester, by McCann *et al.* (1994), 62% of terminally ill patients reported that they were either not experiencing thirst or had only experienced it initially during their terminal illness. McCann *et al.* noted that symptomatic relief could be obtained in the remaining 38% of patients who complained of thirst by the administration of much less fluid than was required to prevent dehydration as assessed by biochemical assays of body fluid. Musgrave *et al.* (1995) reported from Jerusalem on the sensation of thirst in 19 cancer patients during the last 24 hours of their life. All patients were receiving intravenous hydration. Six of the 19 experienced mild, 8 moderate and 4 severe thirst. However, little correlation could be demonstrated between the individual patient's fluid and electrolyte data and his or her thirst sensation. A Canadian report on the symptoms reported by terminally ill cancer patients failed to establish any association between thirst and fluid intake (Burge 1993).

12.7 EXPERIMENTAL STUDIES OF THIRST IN ANIMALS

An advantage of animal experimentation for investigating thirst mechanisms, when compared with clinical reports, is that lesions can be placed in the brain with precision so that structures adjacent to that which it is intended to damage can be left intact. This contrasts with having to rely on inferences drawn from observation of patients with poorly defined, spontaneous lesions. Whilst animals are unavailable for interview so precluding any direct account of symptomatology, it has been possible to assess thirst sensation in experimental animals by observing responses the linkage of which to the thirst sensation has previously been experimentally validated. There is a greater capacity to monitor thirst *sensation* in an animal with a well defined lesion not affecting structures required for the *response* to the sensation of thirst than there is in a PVS patient in whom damage compromising any of those structures may completely preclude any observable response to dehydration by the patient, irrespective of whether thirst is being experienced.

The two goals of attempting to evoke thirst sensation by stimulation or to interfere with it by producing localised lesions in the brain, have underpinned animal experiments which have provided much information about the precise location and function of the thirst centre in the hypothalamus. Some attempts to stimulate thirst have utilised direct stimulation of the cells responsible for thirst sensation using electrical stimuli similar to those applicable to any type of neurone. Others have employed the stimulus of change in body fluid composition which would be effective only with that specific type of cell. Electrical stimulation of neurones suspected of involvement in thirst provides a non-specific stimulus whereas a stimulus that specifically elicits thirst, such as the micro-injection of minute quantities of hypertonic saline into the brain will evoke a response only in those neurones specialised to detect hyperosmolarity (that is, an increase in the concentration of body fluids). The alternative approach of attempting to interfere with thirst sensation has entailed the precise placement of small lesions in regions of the brain that are thought to be involved in thirst.

Water-seeking behaviour by an animal is the only means of detecting its thirst. The water-seeking behaviour of experimental animals in response to electrical stimulation of the thirst centre in the hypothalamus has been observed closely to resemble the behaviour of intact, thirsty animals. Consequently, it has generally been inferred that the occurrence of this behaviour in response to an experimental manipulation affecting the hypothalamus may be interpreted as indicating that the animal *has actually experienced thirst* as a result of that manipulation. It could, however, be objected to this interpretation that, whilst the subsequent behaviour of the animal after stimulation of its thirst centre *appears* to be identical with that of an intact animal when it is thirsty, the experimental animal is not actually *experiencing* thirst as a result of stimulation but that the stimulus has merely evoked an act of involuntary drinking in the absence of thirst. If this was so, there would in effect be a short-circuiting of the process so that the *response* to thirst occurred *in the absence of the sensation* itself. If this was the case, inferences about the capacity of people, who are unable to communicate, to experience thirst could not be drawn from animal studies. This objection amounts, in effect, to dismissal of the animal's observed response as being of a "*reflex*" nature, unaccompanied by any sensation. This explanation has been invoked, I believe often on inadequate grounds, to exclude possibilities of other types of sensation in human subjects. Before any response which is indistinguishable from that observable in a healthy, mature person can be dismissed as "only reflex", when it occurs in another subject not fitting that description, at least two prerequisite conditions are mandatory. Comprehensive and accurate knowledge of the structures and processes involved in producing the "sensation", as distinct from the "reflex response" must have been obtained. There must also be proof that those structures and the processes which normally mediate sensation are inactivated or inoperative in the individual under consideration. It is disconcerting to reflect that responses consistent with discomfort in animals incapable of other forms of communication with an observer are, quite rightly, not dismissed as purely "reflex" whilst similar types of responses by human subjects without capacity for communication may be.

An experiment reported by Andersson and Wyrwicka (1957) strongly supports the contention that animals that have their thirst centre electrically stimulated *do* have thirst and initiate water-seeking behaviour in response to that sensation rather than doing so reflexly. In their experiment, goats were prepared by conditioning to respond positively with readily observable motor reactions to *natural* thirst. Preparation of these goats entailed withholding water from them until they became thirsty. Water was then provided, but only to the accompaniment of a complex conditioning stimulus. The individual motor patterns that developed in association with thirst and the provision of water were reinforced by repeated training. In the experiment proper, the hypothalamus of each goat was electrically stimulated. In each case, the goat responded with the individual motor-conditioned reaction which it had acquired in association with *natural* thirst. These observations of Andersson and Wyrwicka strongly support the contention that the responses observed after electrical stimulation of the thirst centre of animals are a consequence of thirst caused by that stimulation rather than a direct response to the stimulus itself, without the animal needing to experience thirst. The validity of extrapolation to humans of data obtained by observation of the responses of animals to experimental stimulation of the thirst centre is supported by this observation.

Two questions arise when considering the role of the cerebral cortex in thirst. Which parts of the brain other than the hypothalamic thirst centre have to be activated if an animal is to experience thirst? Which *other* parts of the brain need to be intact if the typical actions associated with seeking water are to be elicited by thirst and to be apparent to an observer? In order to explore the first question experimentally, it is necessary to resolve the second. Unless one can identify those structures required *to mediate a response* to thirst, and to confirm that they remain functional, it is impossible to infer lack of thirst sensation on the basis of lack of response. There is a centre responsible for *initiating* the characteristic motor response to thirst in the rat quite discrete from the thirst centre. Both centres are in the hypothalamus. The production of a motor response by rats wishing to drink can be prevented if a lesion is produced in the initiating centre in the lateral hypothalamus. However, rats which have been conditioned to press a lever when they wish to eat and drink continue to do so after placement of that lateral lesion which has inactivated the centre required for the response to thirst but *not* the thirst centre itself. These observations have confirmed the discrete anatomical location of the hypothalamic neurones responsible for the experience of thirst and the initiation of a response to that experience (Baillie and Morrison 1963). As already indicated, this raises the possibility that a randomly lesioned human brain could retain the capacity for thirst in the absence of ability to initiate water-seeking behaviours. That is, the absence of water-seeking behaviour following injury to the brain, even in an individual who retains the peripheral motor capacity to respond to thirst, need not necessarily signify the absence of thirst. A variety of lesions, apart from those specifically affecting neurones responsible for initiating a response to thirst, could also preclude any *response* to thirst. Any interference with the motor function required for drinking, or with parts of the nervous system responsible for co-ordinating that activity would produce a similar outcome in an individual who was, nevertheless, experiencing thirst.

> "Dehydration is commonly seen in patients with impaired consciousness whose thirst mechanism is undamaged but who are unable to ask for water" Hays *et al.* 1963: 227).

A point that was made in Chapter 5, when considering whether a PVS patient whose cortex is assumed to be disconnected or destroyed could remain subject to pain, is also applicable to thirst. The issue is whether normal participation by the intact cortex in thirst sensation can be assumed, in the absence of additional evidence, to be synonymous *with an essential requirement* for cortical participation if thirst is to occur. Given that an intact hypothalamus is *mandatory* for the experience of thirst, subject to the possibility, to be raised below, of relocation of this function, a contingent question is whether it is also *sufficient* for this. This question is highly relevant to the vegetative patient given the strong dismissal, in various authoritative statements on PVS, of the possibility that any of these patients could retain sufficient cortical function to experience thirst. Thirst and hunger have been shown to persist in cats and sheep in which the normal connections between the cortex and the remainder of the nervous system had been surgically sectioned (Fitzsimons 1972). The absence of any reports to the effect that anencephalic infants have to be artificially hydrated, rather than spontaneously wishing to drink, like their normal counterparts, when fluid is made available and the anencephalic infant's general condition permits the activity, suggests that a normal, functioning cortex is not mandatory for the experience of thirst in human subjects.

The propositions that normal function of the cerebral cortex *may not be essential* for thirst sensation and that the cortex *can* be involved in thirst sensation in a normal individual are not incompatible. Discussion of the possibility of thirst in vegetative patients invariably assumes that the cortex is implicated in thirst sensation *normally* and therefore that it must be so in any individual with a brain injury. However, it would not be inconsistent with recent changes in perception of plasticity in the nervous system to suggest that, following injury to the cortex or to its connections with the hypothalamus, processes confined anatomically to the latter can suffice to mediate thirst sensation without cortical participation. Experimental demonstration of the capacity for relocation of thirst sensation in animals following selective damage to the brain has been available for many years. Thus, Teitelbaum and Cytawa (1965) described the initial occurrence of adipsia in rats in which experimental lesions had been produced in the lateral hypothalamus. However, this was followed by the gradual recovery, over the course of a month, of the capacity for spontaneous drinking. This recovery of thirst sensation, and consequently of water-seeking behaviour, was shown to be dependent on the compensatory assumption of additional functions by the cortex. Thus, if cortical activity was experimentally depressed in rats which had previously sustained a lateral hypothalamic lesion but which had subsequently regained capacity for thirst, such rats once again became adipsic. It was concluded that:

> "Cortical activity may facilitate and maintain recovery from lateral hypothalmic lesions by enhancing the activity of depressed but intact tissue adjacent to those lesions" (ibid: 63).

This experiment demonstrated that partial transfer of responsibility for initiation of water seeking in response to thirst sensation from hypothalamus to cortex was possible in a lesioned brain.

12.8 RELIEF OF THIRST SENSATION WITHOUT CORRECTION OF DEHYDRATION

The efficacy of procedures to mitigate thirst, should it occur, during the one to two weeks elapsing between withdrawal of tube feeding and the patient's death, has been canvassed in discussion of withdrawal of hydration and nutrition from PVS patients. Inclusion of this aspect of management in articles which have already categorically denied the possibility of any awareness, sentience, thirst sensation etc. on the part of the patient in a PVS has not seemed illogical to some authors. Measures suggested as a means of alleviating any (allegedly non-existent) thirst sensation have included that of introducing small quantities of water into the patient's mouth. Another procedure, which seems generally to have eluded formal discussion, apart from occasional mention during court hearings, is to sedate and tranquillise the patient – seemingly an odd, if not oxymoronic, course of action in an insentient patient. (This practice will be considered in Chapter 13).

Given its subjective nature, it is not surprising that the precise location of thirst sensation is not clear cut. Thirst sensation is most commonly referred peripherally to the oropharyngeal region (mouth and throat), but certainly extends more widely. Robertson *et al.* (1982), in reviewing the mechanisms responsible for regulating osmolality of body fluids, described thirst as:

> "A deep-seated sensation of desire for water. When fully stimulated, it is one of the more powerful behavioural drives experienced by humans" (ibid: 341).

Careful oral hygiene, including maintenance of moisture in the mouth, is an important aspect of the care of dying patients and some accounts of thirst sensation in the days immediately before death imply that thirst can be completely alleviated by the frequent introduction of small amounts of water or ice chips into the patient's mouth. As already discussed, the physiological condition of younger PVS patients especially those who have received good nursing care, is likely to be much closer to that of subjects of similar age *without* brain injury than to debilitated individuals dying as a result of a prolonged illness or of old age. Study of young experimental subjects experiencing hypernatraemic dehydration has revealed that thirst appeared early but could be relieved by ingestion (not mouth washing) of less fluid than represented by the deficit (Winkler *et al.* 1944). As already discussed, comparison of the consequences of water deprivation in healthy subjects of different ages suggested that the ensuing thirst could be alleviated with lesser quantities of water in older subjects (Phillip *et al.* 1984).

There are two components to the relief of thirst following ingestion of water - a sensory stimulus provided by the act of swallowing the fluid itself and the correction of body fluid hyperosmolality after the ingested water has been absorbed. The relative contributions of these two processes to relief of thirst have been experimentally separated by protocols which allow for the occurrence of only one of them. Thrasher *et al.* (1981) surgically constructed gastric fistulae in dogs which enabled fluid to be administered directly into the stomach, without swallowing or, alternatively, fluid to be taken by mouth and swallowed but then diverted away from the stomach by means of the fistula so that it could not be absorbed. Swallowing of as much water as desired by a previously dehydrated dog, accompanied by diversion of that water away from the stomach, produced rapid relief from thirst. This was accompanied by inhibition of secretion of the hormone vasopressin from the posterior pituitary gland, a process which is regulated by hypothalamic neurones. However, the dog's satiety was short-lived and a dog which had not had an opportunity to absorb the swallowed water soon became thirsty and drank again when water was offered. In the other part of this experiment, dogs which received adequate water replacement via the fistula, that is directly into the stomach without swallowing, experienced ongoing relief of thirst. Thus, swallowing provided genuine relief from thirst sensation but rehydration was required if that relief was to persist other than for a short interval.

Several earlier experiments in healthy animals, which were cited in Fitzsimons' review, failed to support the existence of any physiological mechanism for relief of thirst by merely introducing water into a dehydrated animal's mouth. Oral moistening did not alleviate thirst in horses with oesophageal fistulae (Fitzsimons 1972). Furthermore, the production of permanent dryness of the mouth by surgical removal of the salivary glands failed to alter the volume of fluid ingested when this was freely available. It would seem very doubtful whether any physiological mechanism exists whereby the presence of fluid in the mouth can alleviate thirst sensation other than momentarily.

12.9 RECAPITULATION

Why consider thirst? The two reasons for inclusion of this Chapter derive from the intrinsic nature of thirst as a primitive sensation responsible for regulation of body fluid balance that is triggered by changes in the subject's *internal* environment and from the repeated assertion that any patient who is in a PVS will not be susceptible to thirst when fluids are withheld. Statements in medical and general literature about the lack of capacity for thirst by patients in a PVS appear, virtually without exception, to have been based on analogies with terminally ill patients who have declined food and fluids. They have been buttressed by some most emphatic statements categorically excluding any risk of thirst on the part of the former group. However, both in terms of its evolutionary conservation and its neuroanatomical collocation with functions such as body temperature regulation, thirst could reasonably be described as a "vegetative function" *par excellence*.

This Chapter has approached the subject from the perspective of what is known about the physiological basis for thirst. Quite a lot *is* known. An attempt has been made to draw some inferences from information readily available about thirst in experimental animals and patients with lesions specifically and exclusively affecting those parts of the brain responsible for initiating thirst.

Data about the neuroanatomical basis of thirst gleaned from animal experiments can be extrapolated to human patients much more readily than that relating to consciousness because it is more feasible to document thirst, compared with consciousness, in an animal and because the structures responsible for thirst are much more restricted in their location in the brain. Furthermore, it is practicable to achieve very precise localisation of thirst-associated structures within the brain, either by minute, accurately placed, lesions or by stimulation with concentrated saline (which evokes thirst) administered through a micropipette. Experimentation utilising animals with specific brain lesions supports the propositions that thirst sensation *can* be generated without cortical participation (which does not exclude a cortical contribution in an intact brain) and that the sensation of thirst can be assuaged only by ingestion of fluid (rather than by moistening of the mouth).

Complementing information about thirst that has been provided by experimentation with animals have been a number of reports of patients with adipsia, a medical condition in which the person loses the capacity to become thirsty. Patients with this rare condition have been found to have a lesion affecting the thirst centre in the hypothalamus and, sometimes, also to have symptoms attributable to lesions in adjacent parts of the hypothalamus. Of relevance to inferences about preservation of the thirst centre in any patient who is in a PVS, the functions likely to be impaired if a lesion in that centre affects surrounding parts of the hypothalamus include those vegetative functions which *by definition* have been identified among the positive features retained by patients in a PVS. On these grounds, and also on the basis of the usual description of lesion location in PVS, damage to the thirst centre is likely to be a rare occurrence in these patients.

As discussed in Chapters 4 and 5 dealing with consciousness and sentience, subjective symptoms will only become accessible to an outside observer if the subject either can describe them or can respond to his or her perception of them in a characteristic, observable manner. Preservation of the thirst centre in a patient who is in a PVS, and incapable of communication, will only be *detectable* if that patient also retains a second hypothalamic centre responsible for *initiating* drinking as well as the capacity to control and coordinate the musculature responsible for that action. Loss of any one of these capacities will effectively preclude ascertainment of retention of a capacity for thirst by an observer.

The outstanding flaw in the analogy between terminally ill patients and those in a PVS arises from the probability that fluid balance in the tissues of the former will be sufficiently abnormal that failure to ingest fluid may not stimulate the thirst centre in the way that it would in an individual with normal fluid and electrolyte balance (which is likely to be the case in many patients in a PVS). Additionally, the thirst centre of some elderly subjects appears to become less sensitive to increases in body fluid concentration, with consequent reduction in the capacity for thirst (hypodipsia).

CHAPTER 13

WITHDRAWAL OF HYDRATION AND NUTRITION FROM PATIENTS IN VEGETATIVE STATES

Cessation of the provision of fluids and food has been advocated as the course to be followed in response to a diagnosis of PVS. The argument for cessation has generally been posited in the form that the administration of fluids and food by means of a nasogastric tube is an invasive process that requires medical input and that the burden it imposes on the patient is disproportionate in comparison with the benefit it confers. As discussed in Chapter 11, tube feeding of a patient diagnosed as in a PVS is dismissed as futile, and not conferring benefit, in the terms of this argument because it will not *cure*. Acceptance of tube feeding as "a medical procedure", rather than as "basic care", which would be used to categorise feeding by mouth, places it in a category where its initiation or continuation is regarded as primarily a question for medical judgement.

The withdrawal of hydration and nutrition has been intensively discussed in relation to PVS patients although it has been a common practice when nursing patients with other medical conditions who are no longer able, or who decline, to accept food and fluid by mouth. Whilst this discussion has centred on PVS, arguments initially formulated to underpin the withdrawal of food and water from PVS patients have been applied increasingly to patients with other disabilities and withdrawal of hydration and nutrition has been seen as an intermediate measure in a very broad spectrum of treatment cessation ranging from withholding cardiopulmonary resuscitation to curtailment of routine physiotherapy. The concept of withholding treatment has often been argued to apply equally across this entire spectrum without any differentiation between the extremes and, as a consequence, the legitimacy of withholding has also been considered to have equal applicability.

This Chapter will initially consider the place of withdrawal of hydration and nutrition in relation to withdrawal of other procedures. This will be done both to place this procedure in a historical context and also to provide some background to the analogies that have been drawn between withdrawal of different modalities in the course of discussions of proportionality of their specific benefits and burdens. The issue of whether a withdrawal is to be classified as an act or an omission will then be examined, solely because it was invested with considerable significance in deciding the English test case of *Airedale NHS Trust v Bland*. Another distinction which has been drawn by some authors and courts is that between initially withholding hydration and nutrition and commencing it but subsequently withdrawing it. This subject merits inclusion because, notwithstanding the frequent assertion that the two processes are morally equivalent, English courts have, when considering the case for *replacement* of a dislodged or blocked feeding tube, adopted procedures at variance with those undertaken when the issue was one of *removal* of a functioning tube. Another distinction namely that drawn between care and cure will be discussed in response to the frequency with which "treatment" and "cure" have been conflated by commentators and courts when considering PVS. This will lead into a related issue, of which much has been made, namely the distinction between "medical" and "nursing" procedures. As will be apparent in discussion of this distinction, I consider it to be a tendentious contrivance but, as much influential writing on PVS has emphasised its importance, it can not be ignored. The final topic in this series of alternatives will be a comparison of the implications of oral and tube feeding. This subject is (or should be) inevitably brought into contention if one accepts the argument that tube feeding, as a "medical" procedure may be withdrawn whereas "basic care', which is generally envisaged as including the traditional method of feeding, may not be. In applying the "medical treatment" contention as the *justification* for cessation of feeding (rather than explicitly nominating the intention of ending the patient's life) there has been a propensity to ignore the capacity of some patients, albeit diagnosed as in a PVS, to take food and fluids by mouth. If the former justification is used and tube feeding, a "medical procedure", is to be withdrawn on the basis that it is "medical", it would be reasonable to offer a "nursing" alternative, namely feeding by mouth, to patients capable of participating in this.

The remainder of the Chapter will consider some of the events that may follow cessation of hydration and nutrition. These are often deftly omitted from accounts of withdrawal with the statement that "the underlying condition is taking its natural course". The Chapter will conclude with an account of the increasing trend in the United Kingdom to place decision-making about withdrawal exclusively in the hands of the medical attendants.

13.1 FROM VENTILATOR DISCONNECTION TO WITHDRAWAL OF HYDRATION AND NUTRITION

Clinical practice relating to cessation of *other* procedures has influenced attitudes towards cessation of tube feeding of patients in a vegetative state. The use of a ventilator (frequently, but inaccurately, described as a respirator) has been the procedure most commonly selected as analogous to tube feeding for the purpose of discussing withdrawal although any requirement for the former by patients who have entered a vegetative state usually applies for only a limited early period. The issue of ventilator withdrawal has been the central feature of some influential U.S. PVS court cases. In the most widely known of these, that of Karen Ann Quinlan, disconnection of the ventilator was sought by the family, opposed by the doctors and approved by the court. In the most effective demonstration that could be conceived of the potential difference between the consequences of cessation of respiratory support and cessation of feeding, Karen Ann promptly resumed spontaneous respiration and maintained it for another decade. In contrast, in the case of Helga Wanglie, the doctors sought ventilator disconnection, the patient's husband opposed it and the court rejected the application (Angell 1991).

U.S. court cases concerned with PVS patients have evolved from applications for ventilator disconnection to others seeking approval for withdrawal of hydration and nutrition. Reviewing this trend in the light of the data collated in the 1991 supplement to Meisel's book *The right to die*, Cranford noted that tube feeding had *not* been the primary issue at stake in any of 14 appellate court decisions relating to withdrawal of support from PVS patients which had been handed down in the U.S. during the period 1976-1985. However, during the period 1986-1991, all but one of the appellate court decisions about PVS patients involved withdrawal of hydration and nutrition (Cranford 1991). The question of why there were no applications solely for ventilator disconnection during the second period remains of considerable interest. Although many people who are subsequently diagnosed as being in PVS have passed through an early period of ventilator dependency, the continuation of this dependence is certainly not a feature of "typical" PVS cases. It is not immediately clear whether PVS patients who were ventilator dependent during the 1986-1991 period were submitted to disconnection without referral to an appeal court, whether they were maintained on ventilatory support until this was no longer required or whether some or all of them subsequently became the subject of court applications for withdrawal of tube feeding instead.

The validity of any analogy between ventilator use and tube feeding and the cessation of either procedure depends upon the legitimacy of comparing withdrawal of two forms of treatment one of which commonly leads to death whilst the other, always does so. Arguing the case against proposals for cessation of tube feeding of patients in a PVS, Dolan (1994) asserted:

> "The fact that we can, under certain conditions, turn off a respirator or stop chemotherapy does not in itself say anything about the permissibility of cutting off food or turning off the heat in the dead of winter" (ibid: 63).

Secondly, the relationship of the burden imposed by the medical technology or procedure to the benefit conferred by it in the two instances requires attention. Both the benefit and the burden associated with any specific procedure are likely to vary with the circumstances of the individual patient. For instance, assessment of benefit would take account of factors such as the extent to which the patient's condition might be improved, symptoms relieved and life expectancy extended. Estimates of burden could be influenced by the likely extent of any discomfort attributable to the procedure and by the patient's likely capacity to experience that discomfort. As a general guide to burden, the invasiveness of the intervention, which will tend to correlate with its level of "high technology" is likely to be significant. It has been suggested that persons requiring either a ventilator or tube feeding are pathologically identical in that they have lost the capacity for spontaneous respiration or of swallowing respectively, both of these functions being necessary to support life. The argument ran that it was inconsistent to sanction withdrawal of a ventilator but to oppose removal of a feeding tube "since air is as necessary to life as food" (Pollard 1991). In responding to this argument, it seems reasonable to question whether "pathological identicality", even if that concept is accepted as accurate, suffices to supplant the difference in likelihood of death following the two types of withdrawal as the most important consideration in the interests of the patient.

Ventilator disconnection and cessation of tube feeding differ (apart from the variation in degree of certainty of outcome) in the tactics adopted when undertaking the two procedures. I believe that this difference certainly weakens any analogy. Withdrawal of a ventilator is likely to be undertaken intermittently and gradually with increasing periods of disconnection, a process which a New Zealand judge observed in approving it, was somewhat disconcertingly described as "terminal weaning" (*Auckland Area Health Board v Attorney-General* 1993). A similar approach of terminal weaning is also the strategy adopted when patients are being disconnected from a ventilator with the intention, not of allowing them to die, but of gradually achieving the resumption of spontaneous breathing. Irrespective of the circumstances, the patient retains access to air if respiration resumes. Withdrawal of hydration and nutrition contrasts tactically with terminal weaning in that cessation of feeding is abrupt and ongoing (either effected by physical removal of a tube or by permanently stopping its use). The intention of testing whether the technological aid can be replaced by the natural function, which may be present in weaning from a ventilator, appears invariably to be lacking when food and fluids are withheld from a patient with a PVS diagnosis. Reports of withdrawal of hydration and nutrition from vegetative patients do not refer to attempts to test for residual or regained capacity to swallow food placed in the mouth, as would be done in *weaning* from tube feeding as distinct from *terminating* it. If the intention of removing the tube was *primarily* to eliminate any burden that it imposed on the patient, as is often asserted, ascertainment of the feasibility of reintroducing the less burdensome process of taking nutrition by mouth would be indicated. Withdrawal of ventilator support leaves open the opportunity that a patient may spontaneously regain capacity to breath whereas cessation of the possibility of feeding by *any route* extinguishes any capacity to survive.

The common use of sedation during the discontinuation procedure precludes *detection* of any regained capacity to accept food by mouth, even if specific tests for this were to be applied. It will certainly impair any capacity of a patient to receive food orally if this were to be tested. Sedation may reduce any discomfort experienced by the patient as a consequence of cessation of feeding: it will certainly remove any capacity on the part of the patient to indicate that discomfort to others. If a more accurate analogy with ventilator disconnection were to be sought, it would become necessary to specify that continuing requirement for *artificial administration* of food be confirmed by observation of a continuing inability on the part of the non-sedated patient to accept food orally. Alternatively, if the procedure of ventilator disconnection were to be adjusted in order that it became entirely analogous with the *practice* of withdrawal of hydration and nutrition, it would be necessary not only to remove the machine from the patient but also to deny access to any air that could be inspired naturally, without a requirement for artificial assistance. Intermediate strategies, such as placement of an intravenous line to supply fluids to patients in a PVS whilst the capacity to ingest food by mouth is tested do not appear to have been often contemplated when the decision is taken to cease feeding a patient diagnosed as vegetative. Even the temporary administration of intravenous fluids as a means of allowing further time for a court to consider a request for discontinuation of hydration and nutrition after a nasogastric or gastrostomy tube has been dislodged from a vegetative patient has been opposed in court on occasion (*Frenchay Healthcare NHS Trust v S* 1994). A hypothetical case study in a critical care nursing journal placed ventilator disconnection and cessation of tube feeding in a common context by applying the two manoeuvres sequentially to the same patient:

> "The respirator was withdrawn with the expectation that, in the absence of ventilatory support, the patient's illness would lead to his death. As often happens, death did not occur, and the family is now faced with withdrawal of the next level of therapeutic support - artificial hydration and nutrition" (Daly 1990: 187).

Arguments for tube removal on the basis of burden should (and sometimes do) clearly state that the "burden" to be removed is not that of feeding via a tube but the perceived burden of continuing to live as a result of that feeding.

13.2 WITHDRAWING OPTIONS

Andrews has explicitly examined the intents and actions associated with various withholding options for PVS patients:

> "Supposing, then, we decide that it is not in the patient's best interest to continue living, how does society (whoever that is) wish the life to be ended?" (Andrews 1997: 594).

Of the five levels of withdrawal that he nominated, the procedures precluded by implementation of a 'do-not resuscitate' (DNR) policy in response to cardiac arrest would be the least likely to be required in an otherwise healthy young person in a PVS. This contrasts with the situation of a patient subject to brain injury as a consequence of a preceding cardiac arrest associated with coronary artery disease. It has been stressed in the literature that DNR orders should relate exclusively to specified procedures, but it is also clear that such orders readily metamorphose into *de facto* 'do-not-treat' orders. Commenting on a 1996 case before the English High Court, Ian Kennedy (1997) observed that the initial approach of seeking a "global" order stipulating non-treatment was regarded by the Court as inappropriate. DNR orders have sometimes been interpreted to equate with decisions to withhold *any* active medical treatment if not with decisions to provide supportive care only (Lipton 1986).

Andrews' next level was withholding treatment of *intercurrent* medical or surgical disorders. (These would be disease conditions arising after a vegetative state was already present). Commenting on the third option, that of not treating *ongoing* medical disorders (medical conditions the onset of which antedated that of a vegetative state), Andrews considered that few clinicians were willing to do this. The example of a case described by Ronald Dworkin illustrates a situation entailing cessation of treatment of a continuing condition. The guardian of Joseph Finelli, a patient who sustained major neurological damage during a heart transplantation operation, recommended that his immunosuppressive therapy be discontinued, an omission virtually certain to lead to death because of rejection of the heart by his immune system (Dworkin 1993: 231). The fourth level identified by Andrews (1997) was withdrawal of tube feeding whilst the fifth was euthanasia. Having noted that the latter was illegal, he commented that:

> "Many argue that withdrawal of hydration and nutrition is in effect euthanasia, though in this case carried out without the patient's permission" (ibid: 594).

Four years after Andrews emphasised the likelihood of overlap between withdrawal of tube feeding and euthanasia, an editorial in the *British Medical Journal* also identified the overlap and advocated extension of the availability of withdrawal of hydration and nutrition to patients not in vegetative states (and not imminently dying). Following an English High Court ruling rejecting an application from a patient with motor neurone disease for access to physician-assisted suicide, the editorial pointed out that, had the patient been incompetent as a result of severe brain damage, her doctors could have withdrawn hydration and nutrition (Doyal and Doyal 2001). Invoking the precedent for withdrawal, it was argued that:

> "Once it is accepted that doctors should be allowed to make clinical decisions to end life passively on the basis of such claims (no medical 'benefit' or too 'burdensome'), active euthanasia in the best interests of such patients would be the next logical step" (ibid: 1079).

An additional level might be inserted between Andrews' third and fourth as described above. This would be the continuation of hydration and nutrition, but with the latter curtailed to a grossly inadequate level. Patients with severe neurological disability who are in, or near to, a PVS may become grossly underweight. Whether unintended, or subconsciously viewed as a compromise position between adopting an aggressive approach to maintenance of bodily condition and the cessation of feeding, an inadequate caloric intake will reliably suffice to achieve deterioration of the patient's condition and may accelerate death.

Advocacy for lumping together all of the first four of Andrews' levels of withdrawal as equivalent has not always been supported by court decision. For example, an English court ruled that a severely brain-damaged individual, 'R', need not receive antibiotics in the event of a life-threatening infection but should have a feeding tube inserted into his stomach (Laurance 1998). However, a more common approach has been to regard all medical procedures as equivalent in terms of "burden" effectively making a nonsense of any concept of attempting to calculate whether that burden is proportionate to the benefit conferred by a procedure. The distinction between tube feeding and other types of procedure appears to be observed much more in some European countries other than the U.K (see Chapter

15). Differentiation between withdrawal of procedures was also evident in a survey of the practice of Japanese physicians published in 1999. This revealed that, in the absence of a sound indication of a patient's previous contrary wishes, the numbers of physicians prepared to withdraw nutrition and hydration or to withhold antibiotics from a PVS patient were 4% and 30% respectively (Asai *et al.*1999).

The term "life support system" has been applied indiscriminately to procedures as disparate as connection to a ventilator, administration of an antibiotic and feeding by means of a tube. A consequence of this generic terminology is confusion about precisely *what* is to be withdrawn. For example, a newspaper report of one English case referred to being "given the right to have his life support system switched off" when what was in prospect was withholding tube feeding (Hall 1995). Perceptions of a non-medical reader could be substantially skewed by such a statement if "switching off" conveyed the impression of technologically advanced equipment that imposed considerable burden on a patient. Whilst a pump, which can be switched on or off, can be used to control tube feeding, this can also be achieved by means of gravity alone. The continuous propulsion of feeding by a pump may be less physiological than intermittent bolus administration and so less conducive to establishment of normal bowel function. However, the latter requires more nursing time which may be a more important resource consideration. An example of the impression created when "life support" measures are linked to technologically advanced equipment was provided in the recommendation of a draft paper from the 1998 Lambeth Conference of Anglican bishops. When a patient had no hope of recovery "and was being kept alive by life-support machinery, the family should be able to choose to withdraw nourishment and water" (Anon. *The Daily Telegraph* 1998). An indication of the differing perceptions of life support in different countries was given by the Archbishop of South-East Asia, who stated that:

> "Giving food and drink is Asian culture and to withhold it would violate our consciences" (Gledhill 1998).

13.3 ACTS VERSUS OMISSIONS

The subjects of this section and of the three which follow it all became of central importance in the Bland case which will be considered in Chapter 15. My intention at this stage is to examine more general aspects of each, using the Bland case in some places to illustrate these. The manner in which these subjects influenced the course of *Airedale NHS Trust v Bland* will be taken up in Chapter 15. The question of whether withholding or withdrawal of tube feeding from a PVS patient represents an act or an omission appears to have attracted a degree of attention in English courts disproportionate to its intrinsic significance because of its importance in criminal law. Surprisingly, the issue of *intention* which is also important in criminal law, has often been sidelined in considering the legality of withdrawal of tube feeding. I would question whether the act/omission distinction is as significant as the *intention* underlying the act or non-act. Requests to English courts in relation to PVS patients have usually taken the form of an application for the court to declare that the proposed action (or omission) is not illegal rather than directly seeking court approval for its performance. If the cessation of feeding were to be judged illegal, it would constitute either manslaughter or murder and the courts generally have examined such applications in the light of the law relating to these offences. As stated by Lord Mustill in his decision in the Bland case, the question of whether there has been an illegal killing "depends crucially on a distinction drawn by the criminal law between acts and omissions" (*Airedale NHS Trust v Bland* 1993: 885).

In commenting on the "Bland" decisions, Grubb (1997a) observed that intentional acts that cause death are always unlawful unless justified, for example, on the basis of self-defence and noted that:

> "The House of Lords, while unhappy with the simplistic nature of the distinction between acts and omissions, recognised reluctantly that it was part of English law" (ibid: 160).

Hence the judges agreed that a doctor's intentional *act* which caused the death of a patient would be murder. This would not necessarily be so in the case of an equally intentional *omission*. Nevertheless, the judges also acknowledged that a breach of a duty of care (as, for example, that owed by a doctor to a patient) could occur in circumstances in which hydration and nutrition were to be withdrawn. Lord Hope, the Lord President of the Scottish Court of Session which heard the case for withdrawal of nutrition and hydration from Janet Johnstone a patient in a PVS, noted that:

> "A deliberate omission which causes death may ….. expose the medical practitioner to the allegation that his conduct was criminal" (*Law Hospital NHS Trust v Lord Advocate*: 852).

Some neat semantic footwork was required for the court to sanction the exercise of the doctor's judgement in the case of Anthony Bland, namely that cessation of tube feeding, was not illegal, and that is precisely what eventuated. Whilst the removal of a nasogastric tube might appear to those without the benefit of legal training to be an *act*, Lord Browne-Wilkinson considered that:

> "Essentially what is being done is to omit to feed or to ventilate: the removal of the nasogastric tube or the switching off of a ventilator are merely incidents of that omission" (*Airedale NHS Trust v Bland* 1993: 881).

Having decided that an act would really be an omission, consideration was directed to the possible criminal liability of the doctors treating Tony Bland if they were reneging on a duty of care owed to him. Their Lordships decided that continued feeding (apparently by *any* route) was not in the patient's "best interests" and consequently that its omission would not represent an illegal failure of duty of care. Notwithstanding acceptance of a distinction between an act and omission in English common law, this issue continues to divide philosophers. In one such exchange, it was proposed that a sharp distinction existed between killing acts and non-actions that result in death, with the former always being morally wrong whereas the latter were sometimes permissible (Regan 1993). However, a letter in reply emphasised that the traditional *moral* distinction did not rest on whether outcomes resulted from acts versus omissions but on the *intention* of the person responsible for either (Fisher

1993b). Killing acts could be morally correct (for example in the course of self defence) and lethal omissions could be immoral (for example, failing to feed one's children). This interpretation recalls Lord Mustill's reservations noted above.

If a legal, in contrast to a moral, approach is adopted to resolving the status of an act versus an omission the argument about withdrawing hydration and nutrition from a PVS patient can rapidly become enmeshed in the technical details of nursing (or medical) procedures. For instance, leaving a feeding tube in place but ceasing to use it would be an omission, whereas physically removing the tube could not be other than a positive act even though its *consequence* would be the omission of further feeding. Successful court applications for cessation of hydration and nutrition have led, in some instances, to removal of a feeding tube but in others to its being left *in situ* but no longer used.

13.4 WITHHOLDING VERSUS WITHDRAWING

A perceived difference between withholding and withdrawing a procedure has influenced some English court hearings. This contrasts with interpretations such as that of the U.S. President's Commission, namely that no ethical distinction exists between initially withholding a therapeutic measure from a patient and instituting that measure but subsequently withdrawing it. The alternative position, spelt out in guidelines from the Hastings Center, is that an initial trial of treatment with the possibility of its cessation is ethically preferable to not commencing it:

> "Having a trial period may make it easier to evaluate a life-sustaining treatment if the effectiveness, benefits or burdens are difficult to assess in advance. It is ethically preferable to try a treatment and to withdraw it if it fails, than not to try it at all" (The Hastings Center 1987: 30).

I suggest that any general response to the issue of "withholding versus withdrawing" runs the risk of missing critical clinical details that affect the decision. For example, a trial of tracheostomy with provision of ventilator support for a patient in respiratory failure as a consequence of advanced emphysema is unlikely to be contemplated if the attendant distress for the patient during subsequent attempts at weaning was judged to outweigh any benefits of that trial. *Withholding* would be indicated rather than initiation with subsequent *withdrawal*. A *legal* as distinct from a moral distinction between withholding and withdrawing was perceived by the Missouri Supreme Court when considering an application for the withdrawal of hydration and nutrition from the PVS patient Nancy Cruzan. The Court distinguished between initial withholding and later withdrawal and held that once a family member consented to provision of treatment to an unconscious relative, he or she could not subsequently negate that consent (Colby 1990).

U.K. court applications for cessation of hydration and nutrition for PVS and near-PVS patients taken in response to tube blockage or dislodgement have raised questions about the extent to which the applicants believed withholding and withdrawing to be ethically equivalent and, as already indicated, necessitate mention of this issue. An example of this sequence was the case of Mr S which came to the

Court of Appeal in 1994, 4 days after medical staff discovered that the gastrostomy tube through which he was being fed had been removed from his body, "probably as a result of his own movement" (*Frenchay Healthcare NHS Trust v S* 1994). Prior to this episode, Mr S had been under heavy sedation and some queries had been raised about the certainty of the PVS diagnosis. A member of the bench prefaced his decision in this case by writing about the "extreme urgency in which it was formulated". Another example, the case of Miss D reached the Family Division of the High Court even more rapidly - 3 days after her gastrostomy tube became detached (Grubb 1997b). It was questioned whether Miss D met all of the requirements for PVS as her condition did not fall wholly within the 1996 Royal College of Physicians (R.C.P.) guidelines. That tube dislodgement had been seen as strengthening the case for cessation of feeding was evident from the report of *The Times* legal correspondent on the hearing. A professor of neurology was quoted to the effect that it had already been planned to seek court permission to cease food and fluids but that "the tube disconnection gave more weight to its case" (Gibb 1997). Whilst reinsertion could be achieved by means of a minor surgical procedure, it was contended that:

> "Not to insert it would be non-interventionist which some people would find easier than active withdrawal of treatment" (ibid).

Evidently withholding could be more readily sanctioned than withdrawing.

13.5 CARE VERSUS CURE

Underlying the specific question of the nature of tube feeding – medical or nursing, which has been at the centre of the argument to adopt withdrawal as a practice following a diagnosis of PVS, is the more general question of the distinction between these two categories. There has been a recurrent presumption that "medical treatment" must have "cure" as its goal rather than "care" in much of the published discussion of PVS and in many court cases. It is then accepted that "care" in the absence of "cure", or at least substantial improvement in a patient's condition, is futile.

Jecker and Self (1991) examined the basis for separation of caring from curing and argued that the origins of nursing lay in the home in undertaking "nurturing tasks" and that an artificial separation of caring from curing had been created by the construction of two stereotypes – "nursing: females: caring" and "medicine: males: curing". Historically, a gender-based separation of the two professions had contributed to a division of labour. They noted that this gender separation had been eroded by the 1990s, however the discussion about grounds for discontinuing hydration and nutrition implies that uncertainty about separation of roles has not caused the role distinction to disappear. Whilst "curing" an individual would be expected to include "caring" as a component, "caring" *per se* does not entail "curing". The split between the two stereotypes breaks down, for example when a physician, in offering palliation to a patient is caring but certainly not curing. Caring, irrespective of whether it occurs in association with curing, implies the establishment of a relationship between patient and carer.

Distinctions between medical and nursing roles, and between caring and curing, have become blurred in recent decades. Most arguments about withdrawal of hydration and nutrition from PVS patients have been framed in the former terms. However, earlier assessments of tube feeding tended to classify it as care. For instance, a 1988 paper from the Stanford University medical ethics committee on the subject of initiating and withdrawing life support acknowledged the distinction felt by many people between cessation of highly technical medical interventions and of the tube administration of hydration and nutrition:

> "These basic measures are regarded more as signs of caring than as treatment" (Ruark and Raffin 1988: 30).

Suggested guidelines for decisions to forgo medical treatment published in the following year from the *Appleton Consensus* recognised an obligation to "continue to offer supportive care" in the course of withholding treatment in observance of the earlier wishes of a patient who had subsequently become incompetent (Stanley 1989). The nature of "supportive care" was not spelt out, nor was its demarcation from "life-sustaining medical treatments". There was said to exist no reason for the use of such treatments on behalf of "reliably diagnosed" PVS patients unless the patient had previously requested them, or the family or caregivers could justify them. The tone of the Stanford and Appleton positions on the physician's responsibilities (a significant issue if withdrawal of support is under consideration) were quite dissimilar. The former held that actual authority over a patient never resided with the physician, whereas the latter credited the physician's clinical wisdom with determining the patient's best interests.

13.6 TUBE FEEDING - NURSING CARE VERSUS MEDICAL TREATMENT

> "What seems to have been accepted without dissent is that artificially provided food and water by nasogastric tube or a gastrostomy is part of medical treatment" (Jennett, 1993a: 106).

> "An overwhelming consensus has developed in recent years that there are no substantial moral or legal distinctions between artificial feeding and other medical treatments" (Cranford, 1995: 464).

> "It is ironic that the only reason that tube feeding has been identified as 'treatment' has been so that it can be withdrawn" (Andrews, 1995).

Two questions promoted by the medical versus nursing issue commonly remain unasked. "Why is the first question, namely, whether a procedure is medical or nursing, being asked?" "In what way is that question relevant to patient management?" Andrews' comment above provides the most succinct response to the first. Placement of any decision-making relating to tube feeding within the responsibility of the physician brings into play the medical prerogative to withhold or suspend any treatment which is judged to be futile. The contention that tube feeding constitutes medical treatment has been central to all of the arguments for its withdrawal if a patient has been diagnosed as in a PVS. A physician is not required to provide *medical treatment* which is regarded as futile even if requested to do so by a patient or a patient's family.

The answer to the second supplementary question, posed above, is presumably that designation as "medical" facilitates withholding. Perhaps the classification of a procedure as being either a medical or a nursing procedure could influence the fee structure applicable to it or the medical insurance benefits payable. Beyond that, the status of procedures which commonly may be undertaken predominantly by nursing staff and, with the increasing demedicalisation of tube feeding and many other procedures, by patients themselves or their families could be regarded as largely irrelevant. The initial placement of a gastrostomy tube is a surgical procedure, its subsequent use and maintenance may continue for prolonged periods without further intervention by a medical practitioner. Insertion of a nasogastric tube might be undertaken (and commonly is) by medical *or* nursing personnel.

Whilst agreement about the medical nature of administering hydration and nutrition via a tube, and about the primacy of medical decisions for its withdrawal, may not be quite as overwhelming as implied in the quotes from Jennett and Cranford above, the emphatic nature of statements such as theirs is undoubted. In reviewing a quarter century of the vegetative state, Jennett stressed the existence of wide international consensus that tube feeding was a medical treatment, whilst Cranford (1990b) cited the "well-reasoned, compelling arguments on why artificial nutrition is a form of medical treatment" as one of the highlights of the U.S. Supreme Court Cruzan decision. These arguments, as advanced by Justice Brennan in support of his dissenting decision, were based on precedents from lower courts, statements from authoritative bodies and the classification status of apparatus and materials in the U.S. health system. His review of lower court cases failed to discover any instance in which feeding by artificial means was differentiated from other forms of life-sustaining treatment (Cruzan v Harmon 1988). Three reports, from the U.S. President's Commission, the American Academy of Neurology (A.A.N.) and the American Medical Association (A.M.A.) were cited. Justice Brennan observed that formulas to be used in tube feeding were regulated as "medical foods" by the Food & Drugs Administration which also regulated feeding tubes as "medical devices". Finally, he cited reports of possible complications of tube feeding and expressed his belief that patients had to be monitored daily by medical personnel.

Substitution of the succinct phrase "artificial feeding" for the longer version "artificial administration of food and water" has almost certainly had a significant influence in shaping attitudes when used in the context of a court application for cessation of tube feeding. Interestingly, it has been observed that the use of "artificial" as a qualification of hydration and nutrition has been more typical of moralists than of nutritionists (Graham 1999). The description of withdrawal as "switching off" of life support, already noted, is likely further to assist in shaping attitudes. Some commentators have sought to influence attitudes even more forcefully, such as an attorney, representing the Jobes family in a court action to withdraw tube feeding from their daughter, who objected to the designation of this form of "artificial support" as "feeding" (Armstrong and Colen 1988).

Rather than complying automatically with the "overwhelming consensus" that tube feeding is unequivocally a medical treatment, I believe it would be reasonable to test the proposition against several criteria. Three criteria which come readily to mind are professional qualification of the operator, the aim of the procedure (care or cure?) and its actual technical details. Considering the qualification of the operator, the A.A.N. has claimed the administration of fluids and nutrition as a medical rather than a nursing procedure and stressed that a gastrostomy requires a physician's judgement to select and monitor it and to undertake its surgical insertion. It is arguable as to whether feeding by means of a gastrostomy tube *remains* a medical procedure after its surgical installation has been completed if, as commonly occurs, its further use is exclusively managed by nursing personnel or by the patient's family under nursing supervision. A case can be made that the only occasions on which medical decision-making can supplant any other is when a gastrostomy tube is initially inserted or when the replacement of a dislodged tube is required. In the latter instance, it is certainly not rare for a nurse or family member to reinsert the tube without recourse to medical expertise. However, tube dislodgement or blockage has, as already noted, provided an opportunity for a medical decision not to continue feeding in some English court cases. The extent to which medical rather than nursing management is required is likely to be even less in the case of a nasogastric tube when the actual initial placement of this is undertaken by a nurse. The trend to demedicalisation of an increasing number of procedures, as patients who require ongoing management of technically complex therapeutic devices revert to being people living in the community and managing their own care, is well illustrated by the manner in which home dialysis will now often be undertaken with minimal medical supervision.

The *aim* of the procedure in question - care or cure – provides a second criterion for separating nursing from medical procedures. The question was taken up by Andrews (1993b) when testifying in the Bland case:

> "I suggested that treatment, by its very nature, was given to treat an abnormality and said that I could not understand what abnormality the food was supposed to be treating - its purpose being to supply normal nutrition to an otherwise healthy body" (ibid: 1600).

As discussed in Chapter 11, disagreement over the aim of feeding in the management of PVS patients has led to its dismissal as futile treatment, an assessment premised on the proposition that it is not achieving recovery of the individual from the neurological disability. The alternative position is that feeding of the PVS patient is intended to achieve no more and no less than the feeding of his or her medical attendant, namely the maintenance of life. Whilst most commentary on the subject has tended to couple "medical" with "treatment" and "nursing" with "care", Lord Goff in his Bland decision uncoupled the two phrases in deciding that, if the provision of hydration and nutrition was not medical treatment, it was part of "medical care" (Grubb 1997a).

When categorising tube feeding on the basis of its burdensome nature because of its technical complexity, it is appropriate to heed Wikler's view that specifying tube feeding as being medical and invasive "makes a fetish out of the details of the method of feeding which would otherwise be regarded as relatively inconsequential" (Wikler 1988). The U.S. President's Commission (1983a) ran no risk of delving into fine detail in studying "life-sustaining treatment". Its application of the term extended from the use of ventilators to "home physical therapy, nursing support for activities of daily living and special feeding procedures" (ibid). Cranford (1984) described the report as being "somewhat ahead of its time". In achieving some balance between the technical details and the intent underlying their specification, Wikler's (1988) extrapolation from the practical implications of cessation of tube feeding to its application as a means of causing death is informative. He suggested that "the road continues past our present resting point". If cessation of tube feeding was justifiable he argued, then similar considerations could be raised to support cessation of any assistance with oral feeding, or even of allowing patients to feed themselves:

> "Though cessation of feeding by mouth seems a big jump from forgoing antibiotics, it is a smaller step from cessation of feeding by tube" (Wikler, 1988: 42).

In reviewing the arguments for the classification of tube feeding as medical treatment, Andrews (1997) summed up three of the propositions which had proved influential in the Bland case and added his personal assessments in parenthesis

> "The argument was heard that tube feeding is treatment – that the food needs a prescription (which it does not) that the tube, nasogastric in the case of Tony Bland, needs professional skills to insert (families had been known to replace them though this is less likely for gastrostomy tubes) and that nutrition has to be supervised by a dietician (preferred but not essential)" (ibid: 595).

An assumption implicit in sustaining the medical nature of tube feeding is that the highest level of technical sophistication will always be provided to the patient, and will be essential for his or her ongoing maintenance. If this is to be judged as "medical" and, consequently withdrawable as part of a medical decision, should the substitution of less sophisticated "nursing' procedures be offered as a substitute? Whilst the use of specialised pumps to propel food through a gastrostomy tube increases the efficiency of this operation, and reduces nursing time involved, the introduction of nutrition through a tube under the influence of gravity was previously the only available method and remains quite effective.

The attitudes of those most profoundly affected by consideration of cessation of tube feeding, namely PVS patients' families, may not necessarily correspond with accounts published from the perspective of physicians and ethicists. Tresch *et al.* (1991a) reported on the results of interviewing family members associated with 33 patients who met criteria for diagnosis as PVS. A sharp distinction emerged between possible management procedures, based on their perceived intrusiveness for the patient. Notwithstanding their expectation that the patient was unlikely to improve, a majority of family members wanted therapy to be maintained. Arguably displaying more discrimination than some commentators on the subject, the majority did not want the patient to be placed on a ventilator but *did* want feeding to continue and "agreed that the tube should not be removed unless another means of feeding was possible" (ibid: 19). This selection of procedures on the basis of their level of intrusiveness, as already noted, generally tends to favour those which entail lower levels of technology over the more "high technology" approaches. Hence, family support was apparent for tube feeding but not for ventilator connection. A survey, by Smith and Wigton (1987), of the views of clinicians and medical students examined respondents' preferences in relation to a number of procedures, including tube feeding, and the underlying reasons for those choices. A majority of respondents opted for use of tube feeding on the basis that it was an example of an ordinary, or obligatory, level of care. A similar conclusion was spelt out in a paper from an Israeli institution subscribing to orthodox Jewish religious principles:

> "Feeding is a basic human necessity, outside the limits of decision-making involved in medical treatment, and therefore should be pursued in the same way that treatment of pressure areas and general hygiene of the body is continued with the dying patient" (Rosin and Sonnenblick 1998: 45).

Considerations of burdensomeness are as applicable to tube feeding as they are to any other procedure, irrespective of its medical or nursing nature. Recurrent episodes of aspiration into the lungs during attempts to feed a patient with metastatic cancer provide an excellent example of a case in which tube feeding was unequivocally burdensome for the patient and best discontinued (Dresser and Boisaubin 1985). Nevertheless, tube feeding appears to be a safe procedure without major complications for most patients. A review of 253 patients receiving tube feeding (the majority by means of a nasogastric tube) at a large medical centre in New Jersey concluded that such feedings were "economical and safely tolerated by most patients" (Cataldi-Betcher *et al.* 1983)

13.7 IS RETENTION OF THE CAPACITY FOR ORAL FEEDING SIGNIFICANT?

I consider that the retention of a capacity to be fed orally by a patient diagnosed as in a PVS is a significant feature of any case in which it occurs if one accepts at face value, and as genuine, the justification typically provided for withdrawal of tube feeding, namely that it represents "medical treatment". If the *motivation* for withdrawal of tube feeding is to adopt a course of action that will reliably end the patient's life, it is disingenuous to couch this in terms of "discontinuing medical treatment" if a specific patient is suitable for substitution of the decidedly "non-medical" procedure of feeding by mouth. It would surely be more honest to state in a patient's notes that it is intended to cease feeding *by any route* because the patient's continued existence is regarded as undesirable. As questions such as that of the medical or nursing nature of "tube feeding" have come to occupy centre stage, the subject of the retention by any patients of the capacity to swallow and, contingent upon this, of the feasibility, efficacy and safety of employing the time-honoured strategy of feeding by mouth has been sidelined. The degree of attention paid to the possibility of oral feeding has varied in inverse proportion to the extent to which the cessation of tube feeding is regarded primarily as a means of ending an existence deemed to be insufferable. A 1994 account of the *substitution* of oral feeding for tube feeding in nursing home patients cautioned that

> "The presence of the tube and its use may create the impression that it is crucial for the maintenance of life" (Leff *et al.* 1994: 132).

Irrespective of the factual basis to this impression in any individual case, its impact in most court proceedings and commentaries on PVS is indisputable.

The question of retention of capacity to swallow by patients in a vegetative state does not lend itself to categorical statements, but it has, nevertheless, been the subject of them. The 1989 position paper on PVS of the A.A.N. stated that:

> "The capacity to chew and swallow in a normal manner is lost because these functions are voluntary, requiring intact cerebral hemispheres" (American Academy of Neurology 1989: 125).

Any nuances intended by the reference to "a normal manner" remain unanswered. Rather more detail, and an answer, were provided by Hansotia (1985) in a review of eight PVS cases. This included an account of a patient considered to "illustrate the characteristic findings in PVS". "Liquid and food placed in her mouth were properly swallowed" (ibid: 1049). Included in the legal proceedings seeking approval for discontinuation of tube feeding of Nancy Cruzan was the comment that "she was able orally to ingest some food" (Robertson 1991). Establishment of a gastrostomy was intended to simplify her feeding. In the series of 110 PVS patients reviewed by Higashi *et al.* (1977), 26% could be fed orally.

Factors likely to be taken into account in determining whether a specific patient is suitable to receive all or part of his or her fluid and nutritive requirements orally include both the likelihood that a reasonable fraction of the nutritional requirements of the patient can be taken orally (as a supplement to gastrostomy feeding), and the extent of risk that aspiration of material into the lungs could occur if the swallowing mechanism is inadequate. An overriding consideration that may lead to a decision in favour of tube feeding despite retention of capacity for swallowing can be the time expended by nursing staff in undertaking oral feeding. The 1995 position paper of the American Dietetic Association on feeding of permanently unconscious patients makes the point that "although patients in a PVS can be hand-fed, most are tube-fed because it is safer and more practical" (Maillet 1995: 231). Whilst refraining from attempts to formulate hard and fast guidelines on the extent to which tube feeding should be provided, the paper advises that "the nutritional concept of 'when in doubt, feed' is essential for the patient in a PVS" (ibid: 234).

The capacity of the specific patient to receive food and fluids orally appears rarely to have influenced a court's consideration of an application for permission to withdraw hydration and nutrition. Following the decision by a Scottish court to sanction such a withdrawal from Janet Johnstone, a patient in a vegetative state whose case was mentioned earlier in this Chapter, one legal commentator drew attention to the lack of any consideration of her capacity to receive food and water by mouth (Kearns 1996). The subject of oral receipt of food and water by PVS patients was discussed, albeit indirectly, in the decision in the case of Anthony Bland. One member of the bench made the point that had Bland retained any capacity to receive materials by mouth, this would not have any implications for the decision approving withdrawal of hydration and nutrition. This endorsement of the cessation of feeding, whether by tube or mouth, was consistent with the point made in the Law Lords' decision that the primary reason for withdrawal was to end Bland's life. Any attempt at weaning onto oral feeding would obviously have had the potential to frustrate that goal. Given the severity of Anthony Bland's PVS, it is most unlikely that any substitution of oral feeding would have been possible. However, the dismissal of oral feeding in that case, transmitted as a precedent to all subsequent cases, could readily apply to other patients who *retained* a capacity for oral feeding. The position adopted by the Law Lords in relation to oral feeding was distinctly at odds with the Conroy case in the U.S. courts a decade earlier. On that occasion, the trial judge said that:

> "The nasogastric feeding tube could be removed, but that nourishment or fluids could not be removed where the patient could take them herself or with the manual assistance of others" (Meyers 1985: 127).

There have been indications that the argument embedded in the Bland decision, namely that withdrawal of hydration and nutrition from PVS patients could be undertaken, irrespective of any capacity to receive these by mouth, has influenced practice in relation to other patients who were not in, or necessarily near to, a PVS. Reports in the English press early in 1999 described police investigations of allegations that patients in some hospitals and nursing homes had been subjected to withdrawal of food and water and sedated (Hornsnell and Foster 1999). In a similar vein, a commentary on a British Medical Association report published in mid 1999 addressed the situation of the generality of patients whose death is not imminent and whose wishes are not known but "for whom it is deemed that their best interests lie in withholding or withdrawing artificial hydration and nutrition" (Luttrell 1999). The report recommended the implementation of extra safeguards for these patients.

13.8 THE CAUSE OF DEATH AFTER WITHDRAWAL OF HYDRATION AND NUTRITION

The issue of the cause of death following withdrawal of hydration and nutrition has been accorded careful treatment in court. The House of Lords, for example, went to considerable pains in providing reasons for its decision in the Bland case. Those responsible for withdrawal have frequently resolved the issue with the simple statement that the brain injury which led to development of PVS was responsible for the patient's death. I doubt that the issue can be so neatly resolved. A common position has been to refer to withdrawal as allowing "an existing pathologic condition to take its natural course" (Taylor 1995). Taylor also exemplified the common approach of bracketing patients in "irreversible coma" with those in the process of dying (other than as a result of withdrawal of hydration and nutrition) in the description of "comatose terminally ill patients". The two concepts, namely that of nature taking its course and of the concurrent presence of a vegetative state and terminal illness, have often travelled together. For instance, in the landmark 1995 case of a 45 year old

Irish woman in a "near-permanent" vegetative state for 23 years which came before the Irish Supreme Court, Justice O'Flaherty considered that "nature should take its course without artificial means of preserving what technically was life" (Irish Correspondent 1995). Chief Justice Hamilton concluded in the same case that as, without nourishment she would die in a short period of time, "she must be regarded as terminally ill" (Wall 1995). (In retrospect, twenty-three years must represent one of the longest periods for which a patient has been regarded as terminally ill).

In relation to the second issue, namely the proximate cause of death following withdrawal, acute dehydration, rather than starvation, has been regularly cited as producing this outcome within days to a few weeks (Cranford 1990a). In the course of replying to criticism of the A.A.N. position paper on PVS, Cranford (1991) added that:

> "If they live beyond four weeks after nutrition and hydration have been stopped, it is possible and likely that someone is feeding or hydrating the patient surreptitiously through the feeding tube" (ibid: 18).

If suspected, this would presumably be grounds for physical removal of a tube rather than merely discontinuing its use.

Consideration of the *cause* of death has often been coupled with the determination of legal *responsibility* for it. An exception to this was contained in the decision of Justice Thomas of the New Zealand High Court in a 1992 case involving a 59 year old man whose brain was considered to be "entirely disengaged" from his body as a result of the Guillain-Barré syndrome (*Auckland Area Health Board v Attorney General* 1993). The patient's respiration was maintained by means of a ventilator and the Court was required to consider an application for a declaration that its withdrawal would not represent culpable homicide. Having drawn attention to the possibility of "clear common sense" differences in culpability between withdrawal of a ventilator from a patient affected by polio and unable to breath, but otherwise fully conscious, and a patient similar to the subject of the application in his decision, the judge concluded:

> "The difficulty is to perceive the rationale which would allow it to be said that the underlying disease was the cause of death when the doctors withdraw the life-support apparatus of one whose condition is irretrievably hopeless but not the cause of death when a doctor withdraws the support from one whose continued life is sustainable" (ibid: 249).

Commenting upon an opinion that a doctor's conduct, if improper, could be regarded as the cause of death but, if proper, would not be so regarded, Justice Thomas concluded:

> "To my mind framing the issue in these terms begs the question: the discontinuance of the ventilator is the cause of death if it is not legally acceptable but not the cause of death if it is!" (ibid: 249).

Andrews (1995) has nominated the medical profession's "desire to avoid seeming to support euthanasia" as being responsible for tortuous arguments to show that doctors are not responsible for the death following withdrawal of feeding from patients with brain damage. In the light of Andrews' interpretation of medical descriptions of withdrawal of hydration and nutrition, it is interesting to note that some advocates of assisted suicide and euthanasia have not hesitated to claim this process as their own. For example, the Dutch euthanasia proponent Pieter Admiraal, in discussion with a group of Minneapolis clinicians on the subject of withholding food from PVS patients, was said to have accused them of doing the same thing as he did while playing games with words (Dolan 1994). Alan Meisel, one of the most authoritative writers on the subject of the "right to die", has criticised the "premise that there is a bright line between passive euthanasia and active euthanasia" (Meisel 1992: 309). He noted that the emotional nature of the term "euthanasia" had been avoided by courts by recourse to descriptions of the practice in such terms as "forgoing life-sustaining treatment" or "terminating life support". A final, novel slant to the question of cause of death following a decision to withdraw hydration and nutrition was provided by Hoffenberg *et al.* (1997) in discussing whether organs should be taken from PVS patients for use in transplantation. One possible approach was to define such patients as dead and then to stop the heart, raising the interesting question of whether the cause of death was the definition or the injection administered to produce cardiac arrest.

13.9 CLINICAL COURSE FOLLOWING WITHDRAWAL OF HYDRATION AND NUTRITION

Some account of the clinical features associated with the withdrawal of hydration and nutrition is reasonable given the euphemistic accounts presented in much of the bioethical literature. The M.S.T.F., in discussing the aftermath of withdrawing food and water, placed the usual time of death at 10 to 14 days after cessation (M.S.T.F. 1994b). It noted that, whereas some patients slip into coma, others continue to maintain sleep-wake cycles until they die. Signs of dehydration were said not to be readily apparent and the characteristic signs of malnutrition did not appear. Cranford (1995) indicated that signs of dehydration may become evident in the last few days of life but asserted that:

> "The patients do not show any of the terrible signs of starvation described by pro-life supporters" (ibid: 464).

Jennett (1992) expressed his belief in similar terms:

> "As for the supposed unpleasant effects of discontinuing food and water, many reports from those with experience testify that with good nursing care death comes quietly and without changes that disturb the carers" (ibid: 1305).

It would seem to be fair comment to observe that both claims were referenced to the same source, as the M.S.T.F. assurance that people in a PVS are incapable of experiencing thirst, namely an article on *The sloganism of starvation* co-authored from the Department of Legal Services, Society for the Right to Die, New York (Ahronheim and Gasner 1990).

Andrews (1993b) has described the death of a specific patient in a PVS when feeding became no longer possible as a consequence of an oesophageal stricture which prevented reinsertion of a nasogastric tube:

> "She took three weeks to die and became more alert, constantly awake and agitated - presumably due to the release of brain stimulating chemicals in response to hypoglycaemia". Andrews continued: "It is one thing to state that she could not have felt any distress because she had a damaged cortex, it is another to be fully convinced (and to convince her carers) that there really was no suffering" (ibid: 1601).

He speculated that heavy sedation may have been worthwhile but eschewed it as being a positive intervention. It might be further speculated that the much shorter time courses often cited for survival in a PVS after withdrawal of hydration and nutrition might owe more than a little to concurrent provision of heavy sedation with consequent respiratory depression.

One aspect of the death of PVS patients following the cessation of food and fluids that was indirectly touched on by both Jennett and Andrews was the impact of participation in this process on carers. An article from a New Zealand nurse dealt specifically with the experience of nurses involved in withdrawal of food and fluids from a PVS patient (Hollows 1995). Most of the nurses were said to have coped by imagining themselves in the patient's situation and deciding that they would not wish to be maintained. The nurses were also said to have felt better once they understood that PVS patients "by definition" were unable to feel anything. Some of the nurses had discussed the procedure with a minister of religion and had been comforted "in his opinion they (presumably PVS patients) were not able to relate to God". (The article did not indicate whether this was also guaranteed by definition.) All of the nurses expressed a wish to have someone professionally trained in counselling and grief management "readily available 24 hours a day". The article compared the assistance provided to the New Zealand nurses with the procedures that had been put in place to accompany the dying of Tony Bland in the U.K. and to support his nursing and medical attendants. These included provision of a psychologist and a help phone line for staff while Bland remained alive followed by debriefing and extended follow up after his death.

13.10 ANALGESIA AND SEDATION DURING WITHDRAWAL OF HYDRATION AND NUTRITION

There is an inherent incongruity in the practice of providing analgesic or sedative agents to PVS patients categorised as non-sentient non-persons incapable of experiencing anything, including pain or thirst. If a patient was regarded as utterly insentient, provision of analgesia would be superfluous: if a diagnosis of PVS has been made with the precision that is claimed to be possible, the responsible clinician has decided that the patient is insentient. In any case, death following withdrawal of hydration has been described by advocates of withdrawal as non-distressing (see above). Presumably, the use of analgesics represents an each-way bet. *If* the patient has been incorrectly diagnosed and retains sentience and *if* death following withdrawal is not completely non-distressing, then all contingencies have been covered. Whilst the case for retention of sensation of external and internal stimuli has been presented in Chapters 5 and 12 respectively, a majority of statements from authoritative medical sources have unequivocally dismissed any possibility of retention of capacity for either sentience or thirst. Nevertheless, Andrews (1993b), in the course of arguing against the withdrawal of food and fluids, considered that very few of his patients in PVS had been so severely brain damaged that they could not experience distress.

It has been suggested that dehydration may itself produce analgesic effects, at least in patients who are terminally ill. An American geriatrician writing of her experience with a group of patients dying from a number of conditions, including cardiac failure and malignancy, noted that those receiving reduced hydration appeared to be less aware of pain than physiologically hydrated patients (Printz 1988). She speculated that this could be a consequence of the accumulation of ketones and/or increased quantities of opioid peptides produced in response to fluid deprivation and starvation. None of her patients had been subject to withdrawal of fluids and food because of PVS.

Spudis' (1991) review of PVS commented on the use of drugs to control possible distress on the part of PVS patients from whom hydration and nutrition had been withdrawn:

> "The most delicate phase of 'easing the withdrawal' concerns the use of sedatives and analgesics" (ibid: 132).

Spudis remarked accurately that this subject had received little attention from the public or from medical philosophers and expressed some disquiet about the "slight difference between a sedating analgesic dose and a dose that inhibits respiration or depresses circulation" (ibid: 132). Lord Goff of Chieveley commented in the Bland case:

> "Furthermore, we are told that the outward symptoms of dying in such a way, which might otherwise cause distress to the nurses who care for him or to members of his family who visit him, can be suppressed by means of sedatives" (*Airedale NHS Trust v Bland* 1993: 871).

Perhaps the administration of mood-altering drugs to carers and family of PVS patients dying after cessation of fluids and food (the potential beneficiaries), rather than to the patients in the interests of those carers, would be a more direct therapeutic option to achieve the same end.

Hoffenberg *et al.* in their 1997 Lancet paper which discussed the possible use of PVS patients as a source of organs for transplantation averred that:

> "A strong case could be made on humane grounds for routine administration of palliative analgesic or psychotropic therapy if these patients were thought to be distressed before or after withdrawal of hydration and nutrition" (ibid: 1321).

A few papers have provided specific details of analgesic/sedative drug therapy for PVS patients. A study by Tresch *et al.* (1991b) undertaken in Milwaukee nursing homes entailed examination of 62 patients nominated by their institutions as being in a PVS. After excluding 11 whom they regarded as misdiagnosed, Tresch *et al.* reported that 14 (or 27%) of the remaining 51 were receiving anti-psychotic drugs. The authors expressed surprise that this practice was so common. A particularly detailed account of the pharmacological accompaniment to withdrawing food and fluids from four "hopelessly vegetative" children was provided from a Miami hospital. Three of these patients received a variety of drugs (including chloral, morphine, midazolam, phentanyl and paracetamol) after cessation of feeding (Alfonso *et al.* 1992). Apparently, the authors of this report did not consider that vegetative states were incompatible with patient distress. In the case of the Irish patient referred to above, a contemporary account in a legal journal included the information that:

> "During her treatment, the ward was given morphine, melleril and valium, and the continuation of these drugs or some of them could ease her passage" (Tomkin and McAuley 1995: 1235).

Attitudes and practices adopted in relation to PVS patients cannot be "quarantined" to this group but will inevitably spill over and impact upon attitudes towards, and management of, others. Any routine approach to a class of disabled patients which does not reach the standards of care applied for patients in general is likely eventually to erode those standards. As the English courts considered a series of well publicised cases which sought the mandatory court approval for withdrawal of hydration and nutrition from patients in, or near to, PVS concern began to be expressed that the clientele for this practice was being quietly extended. An editorial in *The Times* in January, 1999 commented upon a "disturbing trend" for elderly patients in British hospitals to die from dehydration after sedation. The editorial asked:

> "If doctors are expected to refer a case of a patient in a permanent vegetative state to the courts why should they not be expected to do the same for other patients?" (Editorial *The Times* 1999).

13.11 MAKING THE DECISION TO WITHDRAW HYDRATION AND NUTRITION

> "What actually drives death decisions in PVS cases is an objective test based on the convergence of 'best interests' and economic criteria" (Baron 1990).

This moderately cynical assessment of the decision-making process entailed in withdrawal of hydration and nutrition from PVS patients was provided by an American professor of law who declared himself to be a long-time advocate for the right to die. Another perspective, also moderately cynical, on decisions to withdraw food and water from PVS patients was provided by the ethicist Daniel Callahan. He considered, as early as 1983, that denial of nutrition had become the only effective way to make certain that a large number of "biologically tenacious" patients actually die (Callahan 1983). The withdrawal of support to benefit someone other than the patient has been recognised as an influential consideration. Thus, Siegel (1986) has cited prevention of the extraordinary financial burden of long-term care, sparing of the patient's family from the agony of a protracted death and conservation of scarce medical resources as possibilities. Other examples of benefits proposed following a decision to withdraw hydration and nutrition from a PVS patient are a release of health care providers from "the tremendous sense of frustration experienced by all the providers of patient care", the saving of expenditures on patient care and, the availability of treatment to other patients who might not otherwise be able to benefit from it (Brody 1988). In contrast with such pragmatic analyses, Kadish (1992) reflected on how the best interests of an incompetent patient might ideally be determined when cessation of support is under consideration. He dismissed the use of the concept of autonomy in cases in which the patient has not previously indicated a choice and advocated decisions that were "in conformity with the values and commitments that guided the patient's competent life" (ibid: 857).

The trend towards withdrawal of food and water from persons diagnosed as vegetative has progressed to such an extent that many commentators have agreed with the view that it should be *presumed* that PVS patients would not want to be kept alive indefinitely (Angell 1994). As a consequence, it is not uncommon to encounter the proposition that the onus falls on a patient's family to establish that the patient had previously expressed a wish to be kept alive. A statement from the American Thoracic Society asserted that the presumption that a patient in PVS would not wish for continued feeding should prevail unless the patient had previously indicated a wish to have feeding continued (American Thoracic Society 1991). The onus on the family has shifted from a requirement to establish that the patient had wished *not* to be kept alive to establishing that the patient had *wanted* to be kept alive, a complete reversal of the previous U.S. position that clear evidence of a patient's earlier wish *not* to receive food and water was necessary before discontinuation.

The role accorded to patients' previous attitudes in decisions to withdraw any form of treatment has varied from court to court. For example, the Supreme Judicial Court of Massachusetts considering the case of Paul Brophy, diagnosed as being in a PVS after unsuccessful surgery, ruled that tube feeding could be discontinued in a PVS patient if this was consistent with his previously expressed wishes (Steinbrook and Lo 1988). The requirement to take a patient's views into account in the Brophy case stands in contrast to many court decisions taken in the 1990s. For example, an Edinburgh solicitor discussing the decision of the Scottish Court of Sessions approving cessation of providing food and water to Janet Johnstone made the point that this was basically a non-consensual action (Kearns 1996). Unlike Brophy, Mrs Johnstone had not, when competent, given any indication of her wishes in the event that she became unconscious and disabled. The President of the Court of sessions indicated in his decision that there was no weighing to be performed in assessing the patient's best interests. It was argued that, if a patient is in a PVS, her best interests cannot be served by staying alive.

An alternative view about the best interests of someone diagnosed as in a PVS has been presented by Fiona Smith, a Scottish medical practitioner whose family was advised to request discontinuation of her tube feeding when she remained unconscious and diagnosed as in a PVS in Dundee Hospital after a motor vehicle accident in 1995. Having regained consciousness, Dr Smith was reported, in late 1999, to be vocal in her opposition to an Incapacity Bill then before the Scottish Parliament's Justice Committee. She categorised PVS as a "non diagnosis" (Farmer 1999). An article on medical futility shifted even further away from according weight to a patient's previous wishes. In this, Schneiderman *et al.* (1990) attributed the dominance of the concept of patient autonomy in American medicine to a backlash against medical paternalism. In response to that backlash they advocated a reassertion of medical authority, especially in relation to decision-making. The PVS was cited as an example of a condition in which a patient had "no right to be sustained". Discussing decisions to withdraw support, they asserted "physicians should act in concert with other health care professionals, but need not obtain consent from patients or family members" (Ibid: 949). Finally, it is relevant to question the significance of "refusal-like" behaviour when attempts are made to feed severely demented patients who may be candidates for a diagnosis of PVS. If this apparent rejection of feeding by a patient is to be interpreted as indicative of a choice, other aversive responses (such as withdrawal from an unpleasant stimulus) by the same patient cannot consistently be simply dismissed as examples of mindless reflex behaviour occurring in the absence of sentience.

13.12 DIFFERING ROLES FOR FAMILIES IN DECISION-MAKING

> "Such commitment was as persistent as the vegetative state itself" (Tresch *et al.* 1991a).

This observation about the physical and emotional commitment of the families of many PVS patients illustrates one reason why families can lay claim to a significant role in the decision-making process. In making this assessment, Tresch *et al.* were commenting upon the frequency with which family members continued to visit institutionalised patients, often on a daily basis. Even more striking are instances in which families care for a member in a PVS at home (tube feeding and all). The A.A.N., albeit in 1989, asserted, in relation to the significant stake that the family has in decision-making about a PVS patient, that:

> "While the moral and ethical views of health care providers deserve recognition, they are in general secondary to the patient's and family's continuing right to grant or to refuse consent for life-sustaining treatment" (American Academy of Neurology 1989).

This view of the primary importance of the family of a PVS patient contrasts sharply with the position that had been reached in the U.K. in the mid 1990s namely that the family should be consulted and counselled but have no role in decision-making.

A variety of possible reasons exist which might explain the differing status of families on the two sides of the Atlantic. The issue of patient autonomy has certainly been most marked in the U.S. The intense, and profitable, interest shown by the U.S. legal profession in its medical colleagues may encourage families to assert their position more forcefully. Perhaps families argue for entitlements more effectively if these are to be funded from privately purchased health insurance rather than from a government administered health service. A family's decision could be based on a number of quite disparate grounds such as inferences about what the patient would have wished and what is best for him/her, as well as what other family members would want for themselves in a similar situation and what course of action is currently best for them individually or collectively.

English medical paternalism certainly seems to be reasserting itself, perhaps as a backlash against patient autonomy! As the legal correspondent of *The Guardian* commented in reporting on the case of a man who woke up after a 7 year period diagnosed as in a PVS, the health authority responsible for his care had considered cessation of feeding but had abandoned the idea because of his wife's implacable opposition. As pointed out by the legal correspondent "relatives have no right legally to veto doctors' decisions in such cases" (Dyer 1996a). Notwithstanding the many reasons why the family might, intuitively, be assumed to have priority in decision-making the recommendations of a working party of the U.K. R.C.P. emphatically sidelined the family in PVS decision-making for withdrawal of hydration and nutrition:

> "When the medical team is agreed on the course to be taken the relatives should be counselled and their views sought, but (subject to court involvement) the decision is for those professionals who have the care of the patient" (Royal College of Physicians Working Group 1996).

Whilst British guidelines have been progressively sidelining families and offering counselling in lieu of a role in decision-making, considerably more variety is evident in the U.S. Situations in which conflicting views are expressed by family members serve further to complicate the picture. The case of high profile U.S. television presenter Hugh Finn, diagnosed as in a PVS 3 years after a car accident (although claimed by some of the nursing staff and his family to be aware and communicating with them), highlighted the situation of intra-family disagreement. Finn's wife and one of his sisters sought removal of his gastrostomy tube while his parents, his other siblings and some of his wife's family opposed this (Craig 1998). A circuit court judge found in favour of Mrs Finn. This greater opportunity for the family of an American PVS patient to influence decision-making has been reflected in U.S. legal commentary. For instance, Veatch and Spicer (1992) have pointed out that it is not necessarily clear whether disputes over "ineffective care" are scientific or valuative. Whereas a dispute over a scientific issue (eg. What is the probability of an event?) would be resolved in favour of the clinician, dispute over a value issue (eg. Is the outcome, irrespective of its probability, worthwhile?) may not be.

The background to the U.K. trend towards minimisation of the family role in making decisions about a PVS patient has been reviewed by Grubb (1997a). While recognising that there were some dangers in vesting decision-making power in relatives, Grubb argued that there was no "knock down" argument against family decision-making and some good arguments supporting it. The legal standing accorded the family in decision-making on behalf of PVS patients in England was specifically addressed in *Re G.* Faced with an application from the hospital for withdrawal of feeding which was supported by the patient's wife but opposed by his mother, the Family Division of the High Court held that the treating doctor's duty was to act in the patient's best interests. The doctor must take account of the relatives' views but the decision must be the doctor's alone (ibid). Grubb raised the question which (as at 1997, his time of writing) had not arisen of what a doctor would do if *all* of the relatives of a PVS patient objected to withdrawal of hydration and nutrition and predicted that the views of the relatives would have no legal standing.

Whilst assertions that decisions should be left for the doctors and counselling should be provided for the families (instead of a decision-making role) have emanated from medical bodies such as the R.C.P. and the U.K. "Senate of Surgery" (Fletcher 1997), this position has yet to receive unqualified and complete support from the courts. One of the issues addressed in the House of Lords hearing of the case of Tony Bland, and examined by Kennedy and Grubb (1993) in a commentary, concerned the applicability, to the ethical issue of withdrawal of hydration and nutrition, of the proposition that "a doctor meets his duty to the patient if he acts in accordance with a responsible body of medical opinion". This proposition, usually referred to as the "Bolam test" because of the first case in which it formed part of the judgement would, if accepted, establish that the medical attendants were in the best position to decide what was best *for the patient*. Whilst four of the Law Lords affirmed its relevance to the decision to discontinue feeding Tony Bland, the fifth, Lord Mustill, held that its relevance was confined to technical medical considerations such as formulation of a diagnosis or a prognosis. Kennedy and Grubb agreed with Lord Mustill in holding that the Bolam test was not applicable to an ethical decision, noting that there was "no reason in logic why on such a decision the opinions of doctors should be decisive" (ibid: 363). This resembles the distinction drawn by Veatch and Spicer between *scientific* and *value* issues that was noted above. Medical training, in the U.K., the U.S. or anywhere else, affords no special insights into what would be "best" for an individual patient.

A third approach, other than entrusting decision-making authority to family or medical practitioners, could be to nominate a third individual or body, independent of both, to assume this responsibility. Such an approach, which would remove decisions about cessation of feeding from both the patient's family and the treating doctor, was tentatively outlined in a 1997 U.K. green paper issued by the Lord Chancellor. It proposed the establishment of a "Court of Protection" with power to make decisions on behalf of patients unable to do so themselves (Hibbs 1997). An independent doctor or manager appointed by the new Court would have the final say on medical procedures such as sterilisation, electroconvulsive therapy and withdrawal of tube feeding. In response to criticism of the proposal, government sources were reported as insisting that the green paper was "very green" (Cook 1996).

13.13 A POSTSCRIPT ON DECISION-MAKING OUTCOMES

The case of Mrs Janet Johnstone, a patient in a PVS on whose behalf a court declaration was obtained permitting cessation of feeding, has been mentioned on several earlier occasions in this Chapter. An interesting sidelight on the Janet Johnstone case emerges from comparison of newspaper reports of her husband's views at the time of her death and 14 months later. Whilst the medical belief underlying the common advice to families of PVS patients "to allow nature to take its course" (following withdrawal of feeding) and to resume their lives is motivated by an intent to assist them and to relieve the strain imposed by the patient's continued existence, I am not aware of any formal survey of the attitudes of acquiescing families at a later time. Peter Johnstone's comments at the time of his wife's death featured in newspapers throughout the U.K.

> "For me, Janet died a long time ago. I've done my grieving – I didn't need to be there" (Cook 1996).

However, the assessment of a reporter interviewing Mr Johnstone in the following year was that:

> "He didn't need a journalist, he needed a counsellor, a priest and a lot of help".

At one point in the interview, Mr Johnstone said:

- "Look, I'm not the man I used to be, my nature has changed. I used to be a nice quiet gent, and look at me now. I don't mean to be aggressive, but I've got to live with this 24 hours a day".

Mr Johnstone continued:

> "It went to the courts, so it can't be wrong" (Dunkerley 1997).

Even allowing for some journalistic licence, the reporter's assessment that he had never before met anyone who more noticeably said one thing, while his body language and demeanor said the opposite, is notable. If family wishes regarding management of PVS patients are to be accorded weight (as they are in most jurisdictions), collection of some longer term data after withdrawal decisions is clearly indicated.

13.14 RECAPITULATION

Withdrawal of food and water from patients in a PVS has probably been responsible for drawing general community attention to the condition itself to a greater extent than any other factor. This Chapter has considered the issues which have been discussed in arriving at decisions to withdraw support together with some issues not usually discussed, and some of the practical aspects of withdrawal.

Introduction of the case for withdrawing hydration and nutrition from patients in a PVS has almost invariably been based on construction of analogies with withdrawal of other types of medical procedure, most commonly withdrawal of ventilator support. There has been a near universal tendency to lump together *all* treatment measures, ranging from CPR to physiotherapy and then to argue that any one could legitimately be discontinued on the basis of medical judgement. In my assessment, this is a simplistic device and it would be difficult to disagree with Andrews' assessment that the only reason for classifying tube feeding as "medical treatment" is so that its withdrawal from PVS patients can be more readily justified.

Two questions related to the withdrawal of hydration and nutrition which have generated substantial discussion relate to the legal and ethical differences between acts and omissions and to whether there is any significant difference between initially withholding or subsequently withdrawing food and fluids. As regards the first, notwithstanding the peculiarities in English law (acknowledged as such in the Law Lords' decision in the Bland case) that distinguish acts from omissions, the asking of the question appears to me to have overlooked the central point of the *intention* of the agent who acts or omits. On the other hand, whilst a substantial body of writing on medical ethics proclaims the equivalence of withholding and withdrawing, the arguments presented in those English court hearings concerned with non-replacement of an accidentally removed or blocked feeding tube certainly indicate a perception that there exists a stronger case for withholding than for withdrawing.

One question which is liable to be studiously ignored both in commentaries on withholding/withdrawing and in court proceedings concerned with specific patients remains that of the frequency with which patients in a PVS are capable of being effectively fed by mouth. If the case for withdrawal of tube feeding is based on its being an exercise of *medical* discretion concerned with discontinuation of a measure which is deemed to be medical because of the requirement for medical expertise to manage *artificial* hydration and nutrition, then oral feeding would not be proscribed. On the other hand, if as was explicitly stated in the Bland case, the primary intention in cessation of tube feeding was to end the patient's life, then any trial of substitution of oral feeding could frustrate that goal.

The nature of the physiological changes consequent upon cessation of provision of food and fluids is generally dismissed in a one-liner. Inferences about the likely consequences of cessation of tube feeding for patients in a PVS have usually been drawn from clinical experience of terminally ill patients who frequently decline to accept anything by mouth in their last days and are not discomforted by this. Nevertheless, there exist some major reservations about the validity of this analogy. One of the most important considerations, on a day to day basis, when hydration and nutrition is being withheld, becomes the morale of those nursing the patient. Presumably in deference to this, but paradoxically given the unequivocal assertions that patients in a PVS experience nothing, administration of sedatives and analgesics to the patient appears not to have been an uncommon practice.

CHAPTER 14

SOME ECONOMIC CONSIDERATIONS

"Death is a great way to cut down on expenses"
(Woody Allen, quoted by Avorn (1984: 1297) in discussing discrimination in geriatric health policy).

As patients in vegetative and related states are highly dependent on nursing and medical support for their survival, and as that survival can extend over years, it is not surprising that economic considerations have been acknowledged in discussions of the formulation of guidelines for their management. The distinction between the costs generated by an *individual* case and the costs incurred by a health care system in treating a *class* of patients has generally been emphasised during court hearings concerned with the withdrawal of support from any specific patient.

Whilst not specifically addressed in cases such as *Airedale NHS Trust v Bland*, economic aspects have not been far below the surface. However, the economic aspects of the PVS have not often been addressed using data specific for this condition. It is proposed to consider very briefly in the first part of this Chapter some general approaches that have been suggested for deciding on the allocation of health care resources. When these are relevant to PVS, this will be indicated. The remainder of the Chapter will assemble some economic data that has been generated specifically in the course of caring for patients diagnosed as in a PVS.

14.1 ALLOCATION OF HEALTH CARE RESOURCES WITHIN A SOCIAL CONTRACT

One of the most influential approaches to allocation of any category of resources within a community has been that based on the writings of John Rawls. Rawls has advocated the establishment of a "social contract" as an alternative to the application of purely utilitarian procedures for the distribution of resources. The essential feature of his proposal was that a group of rational individuals should agree among themselves upon their concept of justice in resource allocation (Rawls 1999: 130-175). Rawls stipulated that their decision should be formulated in a situation in which none of the participants could know at the time whether he or she would specifically benefit from the decision that was to be made. This stipulation ensured that any decisions would not be subject to the bargaining practices of everyday life.

Having agreed on principles of justice selected within this constraint, the participants would then be permanently bound by them.

Rawls' exposition of his social contract was intended to refer to what he described as "primary goods". These were categorised as "things which rational persons may be presumed to want whatever else they want" (ibid: 158). Whilst Rawls did not originally address decisions about the allocation of health care resources, his proposal has been extended to them on the basis that health is to be regarded as a primary good. A central feature of Rawls' general theory was a requirement for a fair equality of opportunity, as a result of which all participants should have a fair chance to obtain whatever resources are available (ibid: 161). When applied specifically to health care resources, *equality of opportunity to access* has been distinguished from *equality of distribution*. For instance, any system in which everyone received an identical quantum of health care could not be compatible with attempts to target distribution to needs and so to achieve the most effective outcomes. If everyone received an equal share of the available health care resources, the misallocation of those resources would be inevitable. Rawls stressed that inequalities in the distribution of common goods are not necessarily unjust. However, inequalities should be regarded as arbitrary unless they could reasonably be anticipated to lead to everyone's advantage (ibid: 47-72). Of particular relevance to health care resources, although not specifically so framed, he envisaged a principle of *redress* in compliance with which inequalities attributable to uneven natural endowment could be compensated for by diverting additional resources, up to a certain limit, to those deprived by nature (ibid: 165). Considered in the light of redressing disadvantage, one could argue for special consideration of those severely disabled by brain injury in the allocation of health care resources.

Rawls' development of his proposals for social contracting were firmly set in a theoretical context. Their subsequent application to health care issues has inevitably entailed the intrusion of reality. Thus, in proposing the extension of a social contract approach to health care distribution, Daniels (1981) introduced people with illnesses into the formulation of policies. To expect that contracting people can formulate decisions which will affect their own future health status in isolation from what they already anticipate, or suspect, about that is unrealistic.

In adapting Rawls' theory, Daniels (1981) proposed that health care institutions should be incorporated in those required to implement principles of fair equality of opportunity. He stressed that, to the extent that a disease curtails an individual's opportunity to fulfil reasonable life plans, a health care response to it could be formulated in that context. He also pointed out that the introduction of health care issues into social contracting inevitably raised the issues of *what* health care includes and of *whether* it is special. Responding to the first, Daniels noted that health care includes not just the management of disease but also tasks such as the maintenance of health during "non-disease" processes such as pregnancy. Health care also includes cosmetic procedures in relation to which a requirement for equality of opportunity is likely to be strongly contested. In reviewing the heterogeneous nature of health care, Daniels indicated that some types would be acknowledged by most people to be more important than others. This inevitably raises questions about allocating different emphasis to claims for access to different procedures, for example the provision of prolonged care following a diagnosis of PVS. If health care is to be regarded as "special", in comparison with other services provided within a community (with the proviso that some forms are "more special" than others) it may be necessary to approach its allocation in a manner different from that of access to other services.

If a "contractarian" approach were to be applied to allocating a level of resources to people who have been diagnosed as in a PVS, there is little reason to doubt the contention that "reasonable people" would assert that, if they were to be in this condition, they would wish to die by whatever means was permitted. The difficulty that I have with the outcomes of such a "hypothetical contract" is that it is no more than that. Of course no healthy person in his or her right mind would wish to exist in a condition diagnosed as in, or close to, a PVS. However, as discussed in Chapter 10, the available reports from patients who have regained a capacity to communicate with others after having been diagnosed as in a PVS emphatically *do not* express a wish to exit the scene. As was pointed out in that Chapter, what one is *prepared* to tolerate can change drastically in response to what one is *required* to tolerate. The contract that seems reasonable when it is hypothetical would not usually survive the affront posed by reality. One wonders how many of the authoritative contributors on social contracts have actually spent time with others living with the aftermath of severe brain injury.

Daniels (1985) has stressed the importance of distinguishing between needs and preferences when considering health care. On the basis that access to health care offers the prospect of ameliorating curtailment of opportunity imposed by disease, he identified the achievement of normal functioning as its goal. However, he acknowledged the legitimacy of types of health care with less ambitious goals. For instance, when considering access by people with terminal illness or severe mental or physical disability, he concluded that account should be taken of considerations other than justice, most notably of charity. In differentiating between health care needs and preferences, Daniels nominated the basis for, and the strength of entitlement to, health care and the nature of that entitlement as issues.

The question of whether a right to health care exists has been argued in formulating allocation policies. In querying whether community members have a right to receive health care, Buchanan (1984) differentiated imperatives of justice from imperatives of beneficence. Even if, as he has argued, it is not possible to discern a generally acknowledged "right" to health care, it is still possible to argue that there are health care opportunities that everyone in a community "ought" to have. Buchanan concluded that the application of utilitarian principles to provision of a decent basic minimum would be likely to disadvantage the severely disabled. Rather than attempt to derive rights for such patients, he advocated the application of an "enforced beneficence". Daniels (1985), in considering people with very severe, irremediable disability, also wrote of a decent basic minimum to which equitable access should be guaranteed. Precisely *what* is to be included in that minimum is a separate question, but it is inevitable that its content will vary substantially with the circumstances of the community. What represents a decent basic minimum in Manchester may be quite out of the question in Mogadishu. Access to identical health care measures (whether minimum or high technology) will vary enormously with location.

The issues of what constitutes a decent basic minimum and of the grounds for access to it are among the most important in the management of patients diagnosed as in a PVS. A 1983 U.S. report on *Securing access to health care* referred to a decent basic minimum as provision of adequate care without excessive burdens (President's Commission 1983b). This report perceived a social obligation to provide this minimum on the basis of the special nature of health care. Daniels (1985) has written of the decent basic minimum as incorporating those measures likely to be required in order to lessen the impact on the individual's "normal opportunity range" and so "to maintain restore or compensate for normal species-typical functioning" (ibid: 79). If one questions what represents a decent basic minimum for a patient with the most severe disability, such as PVS, it may be argued, as Daniels has done in relation to the "dying elderly" that their opportunities lie in the past and so any notion of fair equality of opportunity is biased against them (ibid: 86). Daniels' bracketing of the terms "dying" and "elderly" recalls the frequent inclusion of "terminal" in descriptions of PVS patients. I believe that, in both instances, the coupling is likely, even if unintentionally so, to be deceptive. The applicable health care considerations if one is "dying' or "terminal" should be recognised as different in nature from those of patients who are medically stable, albeit elderly or in a PVS. However, this often is not the case.

The need for development of a theory of health care distribution has been generally acknowledged. Thus, Fisher and Gormally (2001) have stressed that, in the absence of a well defined decision-making process which takes account of priorities and rationing constraints, health care resources are liable to be allocated in an *ad hoc* manner which will probably be at the mercy of market forces. Similarly, Daniels (1981) has strongly advocated the need to develop a theory of health care distribution. It would be difficult to contrive a more dramatic illustration of the extent to which health care decision-making can run amok in the absence of well defined protocols for allocation than that provided by an episode at the Duke University Medical Centre in 2001. A patient admitted with a blood coagulation deficiency of sudden onset accompanied by gastrointestinal bleeding ran up a $US 5.2 million account before his death 34 days later. Accompanying this, his treatment consumed almost 10% of the annual national U.S. supply of the coagulation factor in which he was deficient (Winslow 2001).

Whilst the majority of commentators appear to have rejected the operation of a free market as the primary method for determining distribution of health care resources, the fairness of this route for distribution of additional resources, over and above those which everyone has equal opportunity to access, may be a different issue. For instance, if a patient or a patient's family opts to forgo expenditure on other items in order to purchase additional health care items, the objection to the operation of market forces may be weaker (with the qualification that the additional health care to be purchased has *not* attracted considerable public subsidy). The diversion of family income and resources to domiciliary care of a member following a severe brain injury, or a diagnosis of PVS, is not uncommon. Some commentators have advocated shifting of the entire burden of funding health care to families who opt to provide ongoing care to a severely disabled member. This position disregards any concepts of a decent basic minimum of care or of any imperative for beneficence.

The complexity inherent in providing resources to the most severely disabled individuals in the community based on "enforced beneficence" as suggested by Buchanan (1984) becomes apparent when its possible adverse impact on those with lesser (albeit severe) degrees of disability is considered. A policy decision to provide support, on grounds of beneficence, to those most severely disabled by brain injury including those diagnosed as in a PVS, may deprive others who, whilst falling short of qualifying for this support, nevertheless score poorly on the criterion of capacity of treatment to restore them to "normality", unless some tapering mechanism was included to bridge the gap between beneficence and capacity for restoration. The majority of new diagnostic and therapeutic technologies developed in the last two decades of the twentieth century have been considerably more expensive than those they have replaced. Economic analyses of health care appear frequently to have been preoccupied with high technology at the expense of less fashionable, traditional health care modalities. This trend has been reinforced by increasing community expectations and demands and by the necessity in many locations to practise (more expensive) defensive medicine in response to increasing risks of litigation. Both factors have placed increased pressure on health care resources and accentuated the need for rationing.

Decision-making is required in allocation of resources at all levels from the construction of a national budget to the provision of care to an individual patient. At the former level, the decision may be between construction of nuclear submarines and introduction of a new preventive medicine program: at the latter, decision may be required as to how much of what *could be* done for a specific patient *will be* done. The second type of decision is increasingly being made in conformity with guidelines which specify patient characteristics required if particular forms of therapy are to be provided. There have been concerted efforts to develop numerical representations of the quality of life that specific patients could experience if provided with specific treatments.

Formulation of fair processes that will permit consistent allocation of health care resources are essential if decisions are not to be made entirely on an *ad hoc* basis or left to market forces. However, it is difficult to envisage how highly subjective inputs on subjects such as perceived quality of life can be accurately incorporated in a quantitative format. Algorithms which aim to indicate who shall and shall not receive a particular treatment may be a useful input to decision-making but not a substitute for it. The most comprehensive attempt to develop a set of formal priorities for access to health care on the basis of community opinion has been that undertaken in the U.S. State of Oregon.

In discussing the application of a classic utilitarian approach to health care allocation in the U.K., Fisher and Gormally (2001) have identified a number of fundamental problems inherent in the Quality-Adjusted Life Years (QALY) approach that underpinned the Oregon initiative. Application of a QALY strategy requires the identification of benefits that can be expected to accrue from different, competing health care procedures followed by the assignment of relative values to them. The number of anticipated years of life, assessed on an actuarial basis, is multiplied by an assessment of its quality (ranging between death =0 and normal =1) to estimate the benefit conferred by a procedure. The relative monetary costs of achieving one QALY for every procedure under consideration could then be compared to arrive at a value-for-money estimation. The application of the QALY concept in Oregon utilised, in the first instance, ascertainment of community perceptions of the relative value of different medical procedures. Fisher and Gormally pointed out that the community feedback produced many anomalous rankings that necessitated a series of "adjustment" stages the input to which was entirely arbitrary. The final listing of value-for-money of all medical procedures was incorporated into Oregon health care policy to direct funding priorities across the full range of medical procedures.

Referring to the process that had been followed in deriving the Oregon scale Fisher and Gormally commented:

> "It is simply incoherent to approach such questions as if there were no evaluative question at all, merely 'brute facts' which are alleged to be observable and measurable independently of evaluation or even as if it were perfectly clear to everyone what are the values involved" (ibid: 59).

It should be apparent that, notwithstanding the analytic elegance of any mathematical procedures that were applied, the output will inevitably owe much to the values of those responsible for allocating priorities. As emphasised in Chapter 10, the evaluation of the quality of the lives of people with disabilities by non-disabled individuals is usually substantially different from that of the subjects themselves.

No more than a moment's reflection should be required to appreciate the possibility of divergence between a community's opinions on the relative merits of different health care allocation options and less prejudiced assessments. To what extent would commentators asserting the validity of the opinions of Oregon residents on resource allocation to people with very severe neurological deficit subscribe to the majority European opinions of the 1930s on anti-semitism, the majority views of 1960s white South Africans on apartheid or the majority views of contemporary U.S. citizens on capital punishment?

The tendency of families who have a member who has been diagnosed as in a PVS to sacrifice other categories of expenditure in order to purchase additional health care has been referred to above. The contribution of families to management of patients with the most severe grades of neurological disability, sometimes in a domiciliary setting, can be remarkable. As with information on survival of patients, it will generally not be available and so will not be incorporated in the total cost of caring for these patients.

Before examining some economic data specific to PVS, it is appropriate to respond to one anomaly that commonly passes undetected in discussion of caring for patients with severe neurological disability accompanied by impairment of consciousness. Reading of the literature on the subject could easily leave the impression that the preservation of health care resources following a decision to withdraw tube feeding from a patient diagnosed as in a PVS equates with the "medical treatment" which is no longer being provided. However, the actual cost of the "medical treatment" that is withdrawn represents no more than a small percentage of the overall cost of caring for the patient. The saving that is achieved is not that of the cost of the tube feeding formula withheld. The saving accrues, almost in its entirety, as a result of the cessation of a requirement for basic care when cessation of feeding is followed by death of the patient.

14.2 ALLOCATION AND REALLOCATION OF RESOURCES TO PATIENTS FOLLOWING A PVS DIAGNOSIS

> "If there is a conflict between the total social good and the good of an individual, public policy is sworn to uphold the public interest" (Lamm 1999: 29).

The resource implications of the PVS have inevitably generated tension between those positions based on public policy and others which take as their starting point the rights of individual patients. Discussing PVS and referring to the Oregon approach of explicitly reducing the allocation of public resources to individuals with certain types of illness Beresford (1997) observed that:

> "This sort of rationing is contentious anywhere, but especially so in a society as wealthy as ours" (ibid: 390).

Nevertheless, he concluded that:

> "It is not difficult to foresee a growing public willingness to skimp on care for the severely brain injured".

He juxtaposed the expenditure on caring for two comatose or vegetative individuals, whose cases had been in the public domain, with examples of glaring deficiencies in the provision of basic public health measures in unrelated areas. The tactic of comparing relative costs of two measures by placing them in an adversarial relationship in order to encourage funding transfer between them is common. Whether there is a defensible method of adjudicating on the relative benefits of the alternative measures to the competing groups of recipients will depend upon the specific circumstances. The assumption implicit in proposals to divert funding from areas considered to lack merit, namely that depriving one will *guarantee* supplementation of the other, can readily be challenged given the institutionalised nature of health care budgets.

The notion that is central to considerations of allocation of health care resources is that of the finite extent of those resources. Implicit in arguments based on scarcity is the presumption that limited resources of a specific type could advantageously be re-applied to alternative uses, more in accord with public policy, if they were to be withdrawn from an existing, unfashionable use. This assumes that it is realistic to reduce different forms of health care services to a common interchangeable scale of monetary value and then to purchase the required quantum of the alternative form of care with the funds generated by abandonment of the pre-existing variety. The extent to which reallocation of resources between two different uses is feasible will depend upon the extent to which the equipment, services or medications required for the substituted alternative will be available for purchase using the funds generated by discontinuation of support for the original application. For example, an additional number of individuals with the required professional background may not be available for hire with the funds freed by discontinuation of employment of others with a different background. Beds may not be readily exchangeable for health educators. Discontinuation of the contribution of *voluntary* untrained or semi-skilled carers, an item never quantified in estimates of the gross domestic product of any state, nor funded from a health care budget, will not provide any additional funding for professionals trained to meet different needs and expecting remuneration commensurate with that training. Transfer of voluntary carers from one area to another is unlikely to be a feasible option in real life if the motivation for their participation derives, as it usually would, from a concern for a specific group of patients. Finally, before applying considerations based on public policy to reallocating budgets between different groups of patients, those charged with formulating that policy should possess a comprehensive and accurate understanding of those groups, a requirement that very few policy makers would meet in the case of patients in a PVS. Avorn (1984) has noted the increasing enthusiasm for using quantitative methods to guide the allocation of health care resources and cautioned that decision-making in relation to the care of individual patients might be reduced to a set of algorithms.

Lamm (1999) cites the indisputable proposition of an earlier author writing on managing scarcity that it is unethical to ignore costs. However, it is simplistic automatically to attribute scarcity of resources entirely to their finite nature without examining the health care budget for evidence of waste. Thus, Avorn (1984) cautioned against uncritically accepting

> "the assumption of scarcity, which is the mainspring for much of the current interest in resource-allocation planning. Granted there is a great deal of waste and inefficiency in the American health-care system… It is only through more intelligent allocation of resources by physicians and more responsible use of resources by patients that we will be able to defend the care of the elderly against the misguided efforts discussed above" (ibid: 1300).

Writing specifically about health care of patients in vegetative states, Sailly (1994) noted an estimate that over 10% of the French social security budget was consumed by expenditure on frivolous, useless or harmful initiatives. He suggested that efforts to apply the wasted 10% to more efficient uses, rather than contesting the 0.12% of these resources devoted to patients diagnosed as in vegetative states, would be more equitable. In another indication of the extent to which health care funds can be wasted, *The Lancet* reported that a study by the U.S. Institute of Medicine estimated that adverse events resulting from diagnostic errors occurred in 2.9 to 3.7% of hospital admissions (Editorial 2000).

Are existing ethical principles appropriate for consideration of the future funding of health care? Lamm (1999) considered that they are not, and in his paper titled *Redrawing the ethics map*, he proposed doing precisely that.

> "Medical ethics needs to be revised if it is to provide meaningful guides to future health policy" (ibid: 28).

In his view the outcome of any conflict between the considerations of individual patients, or groups of patients, and the community majority is clear cut. In contrast with Lamm, Sailly (1994) did not consider that there was a fundamental conflict between economics and the prevailing ethical approach to care of patients in vegetative states. He believed that economic considerations could complement ethical ones and that an economic approach could help to uncover the implicit and explicit choices involved in decision-making. He also stressed the need to recognise the entry of any elements, unmeasurable in monetary units, into an economic analysis of some aspect of health care and cautioned against ignoring these. A similar point was made in the report of a group of U.S. bishops considering issues raised by the management of patients diagnosed as in a vegetative state when they advocated that comparisons of the economic value of various individuals to society should be avoided (United States Bishops' Committee 1992).

Although arguments have frequently been presented in articles on PVS for the curtailment of medical treatment of affected patients on economic grounds, there have been surprisingly few comprehensive studies of the economic aspects of management of patients in vegetative states. More common are accounts of the financial aspects of individual patients, especially those characterised by long survival and/or particularly intensive types of management. The anecdotal nature and dramatic calibre of many of these individual case reports has not constrained their impact on thinking about management of patients in vegetative states generally. It is quite paradoxical that instances of emergence after a prolonged period in a PVS are liable to be dismissed as anecdotal whereas *one-off* cases of extraordinary expenditure apparently elude this categorisation. The archetypal example of this, reported as *The six-million-dollar woman* may reflect "non-neurological" factors such as compensation claims, unlimited availability of health insurance and the prospect of litigation (Paris 1981). As a means of supplementing the limited information on the economics of PVS management, I propose to draw some qualified analogies with the more comprehensive economic information available about patients who have been placed in similar levels of dependency as a result of dementia. In doing this, I shall take into account one prominent feature that the two conditions have in common and several very distinct differences between them. The similarity is that some 25% of PVS cases are said to arise in the course of chronic degenerative conditions, half of which are Alzheimer's disease and the commonest level of support, once consigned to a nursing home, may be sufficiently similar to validate comparisons of cost of care (Ivan 1990). This book is concerned with patients with prolonged unresponsiveness, following one or more *episodic* brain injuries. Patients diagnosed as PVS after suffering from dementia are likely to be in much poorer physical condition than those who have sustained an acute injury and also to have accompanying diseases. Another difference, limiting the application of any analogy, is the progressive nature of Alzheimer's disease in contrast with the relative stability of younger patients who have sustained an acute brain injury. Recent reports of returning awareness among PVS patients contrast with the typically inexorable course of Alzheimer's disease. Thirdly, as "acute episode" unresponsive patients will commonly be younger than demented patients, the identity of a patient's available family members may be parents or spouses rather than children as is the case with demented patients. A further important difference is the liability of PVS patients to develop severe neuromuscular complications with management implications, such as contractures, because of neurological disabilities, other than disturbances of consciousness, not typically shared by dementia patients.

Most physicians, notwithstanding their recognition of those economic aspects of health care issues which affect the community as a whole, continue to believe that their role is to serve the best interests of *their* patients, rather than to seek to remedy the health care system overall by amending the management of individual patients. Responding to a proposal which advocated diversion of resources from some patients to "more productive use within, or even outside the health care system", Youngner (1988) rejected the mixing of concerns about what was best for the individual patient with the question of how society should use its resources:

> "Individual clinicians and institutions should continue to separate concerns about patient welfare from broader social and economic policy issues" (ibid: 2095).

Schiedermayer *et al.* (1989) remarked on the manner in which ethical and economic aspects of treatment decisions were often intimately intertwined. They called for all physicians to "develop the ability to unmask economic issues in medical care" (ibid: 1305). One aspect of the overall management of patients in coma (and potentially liable to pass into a vegetative state), discussed by Shewmon and De Giorgio (1989), concerned the "legal, economic, ethical and social" pressures, under which their medical attendants operated. The thrust of these pressures was increasingly to require prognoses to be formulated earlier in the course of coma.

14.3 ECONOMIC IMPLICATIONS OF VARYING INTENSITY OF CARE OF PVS PATIENTS

The overall cost to a health care budget of caring for patients in a PVS will be the product of the annual cost of caring for a patient and the prevalence of the condition. Any attempt to generate "typical" or "average" economic profiles of the care of PVS patients should be regarded with considerable scepticism not only because of the heterogeneous nature of this population but, especially, because of the variability of the management provided to them. "Averages" are likely to be of little value, and may be positively misleading, in making decisions on behalf of individual patients. The reasons why some patients have received vastly more intensive care (with corresponding inflation of the individual's treatment costs) are varied. However, patients who have required the most intensive (and accordingly expensive) management during their first year are less likely to have survived for extended periods beyond this. Consequently, the inclusion of this group in calculations of the cost of caring for vegetative patients inflates the average expenditure. They are, however, likely to be quite unrepresentative of the description of PVS patients as surviving for a period of years. The occurrence of a subpopulation of patients who incur high levels of intensive care expenditure in the first year, but die whilst in receipt of intensive care or soon after its discontinuation, is a reflection of the absence of sufficiently reliable prognostic indicators of the unconscious patient's future course that are applicable in the early stages after traumatic or ischaemic injury to the brain. The difficulties inherent in accurately identifying patients certain to have an unfavourable outcome, at an early stage of management, have been discussed in Chapter 6.

Apart from the difficulty in predicting more specific outcomes with precision whilst patients remain ventilator-dependent, other reasons for the application of treatment that might commonly be regarded as unduly intensive or unduly prolonged could include the availability of open-ended health care funding for the individual, based on insurance or compensation, and trenchant demands of family members that nothing less will do. Most, if not all, reports of cases falling in this category appear to have emanated from the United States. Cranford (1988) has illustrated the cost variation according to "state, type of institution and support systems", by comparing Minnesota costs of $US 18,000 to $US 25,000 per patient per year with the annual cost of approximately $US 120,000 in a single very well publicised Massachusetts case. The M.S.T.F. on PVS differentiated in its 1994 report between the high initial average cost of medical care (estimated at $US 149,200 for the first 3 months) and the ongoing costs (estimated at between $US 126,000 and $US 180,000 per year) (Multi-Society Task Force 1994b). Its rough approximation of total US costs of caring for PVS patients was an amazing range of $1 billion to $7 billion. However, given the difference of an order of magnitude between Cranford's 1988 figure of average cost in his State of Minnesota and the 1994 figure cited by the M.S.T.F. (of which he was a member), it would seem to be unwise to attach much credence to the M.S.T.F. estimate.

Some reports of groups of patients who, although described as vegetative, received considerably more intensive care for prolonged periods than could reasonably be classed as "typical" could lead to unrealistic figures in calculating total costs to a health care budget. An Israeli article which recounted the course of 49 patients who remained unconscious for periods in excess of 6 months after non-traumatic brain damage concluded that the mean economic cost of each of these patients was that of almost 1000 days of hospital stay in an intensive care facility (Sazbon *et al.* 1993). Another 1993 report, this time of the management of a group of 20 children who had been discharged from U.S. hospitals with a "diagnosis and discharge examination consistent with the vegetative state", revealed that most had continued to receive care that was appreciably more intensive than would be usual during post-acute stages of vegetative states (Fields *et al.* 1993). Thus, 7 of the children had tracheostomies, received oxygen and were provided with cardiorespiratory monitors and 2 received mechanical ventilation. These are not typical features of the management of most PVS patients in the longer term. The annual costs of maintenance of this group of children averaged in excess of $US 90,000.

A report of 23 PVS patients in New York is an example of quite atypical management of a quite atypical group of patients. Individual costs of hospital care (average stay 197 days) ranged from $US 30,000 to $US 427,000 (average $170,000) (Kaufman and Lipton 1992). Of these patients, 10 received ventilator support and an intravenous line in addition to a nasogastric or a gastrostomy tube. All of the patients in this series had gradually become vegetative whilst in hospital, following dementia or other neurologic disorders rather than sustaining an acute brain injury. Nineteen of the 23 patients in the series were aged 65 years or older and 8 were 80 years or older. Without making any judgement on the appropriateness of the level of intensity of treatment provided to a group of patients with such preceding histories, it is likely to have been considerably in excess of that usually required by the much younger PVS patients whose cases have provided the basis for public discussion of the withdrawal of hydration and nutrition. It is unfortunate that such unrepresentative costs should be presented as a guide to expected costs of caring for patients in vegetative states.

Some specific cases have been both expensive and influential. The case of "the six-million-dollar woman", already mentioned, referred to a patient maintained for 18 years as a private or semi-private patient in an acute care hospital (Field and Romanus 1981). Cited by Cranford (1984) were other cases in which costs of $US 280,000 were incurred in the first two years and of $US 224,000 during the first 10 months. Nancy Cruzan, a 32 year old woman whom most of her medical attendants considered by 1990 to have been in a PVS for 7 years was said to be costing "immeasurable anguish to her family and $US 130,000 per year to the state of Missouri" (Angell 1990: 1226). To the extent that consumption of expensive resources has been cited (among other reasons) as a basis for withdrawal of hydration and nutrition from patients who are judged to be in, or close to, a PVS it could be noted that the actual costs of feeding a patient through a nasogastric tube or a gastrostomy are insubstantial compared with the outlays required to provide the types of intensive support measures described above. For instance, in the case of Nancy Cruzan, James Bopp (President of the U.S. National Legal Center for the Medically Dependent and Disabled) observed that the daily cost of her food was $US 7.80 which represented 2.6% of the total cost of her care. Bopp (1990) also quoted a 1987 report from the US Congress Office of Technology Assessment to the effect that some 780,300 people had been receiving tube feeding in hospitals, 54,400 in nursing homes and 14,400 at home in 1980. The savings provided to a health care system as a result of cessation of feeding a PVS patient are not derived from the cost of the nutritional supplies but represent the costs of nursing care. A patient reported by Childs and Mercer (1996a), who first evinced signs of consciousness 15 months after a head injury was estimated to have cost well over $US 1,000,000 by the fifth year after her accident. Finally, an estimate of the costs likely to be incurred in maintaining "full care" for PVS patients in New Zealand was estimated to range from $NZ 3000 to $NZ 12000 per month (Hollows 1995). It is extremely difficult to think of another condition, characterised by the uniformity of recognition and prognosis that has been claimed for PVS, for which such a wide variation in cost occurs within one health care system.

Alternatives to the preceding "high technology" approaches to PVS management may be both more appropriate medically for many patients, and more affordable. For instance, intensive efforts at rehabilitation may be made in the first year with a lessening of expenditure thereafter, either as a result of improvement in condition or reflecting a tapering of rehabilitation. Domiciliary care of patients discharged whilst in a PVS is likely to make considerably smaller demands on health care budgets. A set of guidelines concerned with discontinuation of medical treatment and styled *The Appleton Consensus* by its participants was considered by a large number of discussion groups in 15 countries and comments on it were subsequently collated (Stanley 1992). After identifying the implicit assumption that treatment of PVS patients for more than a short time would deny resources to others, the further proposition was raised that the burden of proof in deciding on whether "life-support" (undefined) was to be continued should be shifted from those arguing for discontinuation to those in favour of retention. The extent to which medical services could be provided to any group of patients was regarded as a decision to be taken at the aggregate level. However, it was argued by some discussants that a "decent basic minimum" of health care (by analogy with standards applied to food and shelter) should be provided to all the citizens in a community. The question of *what* is included in such a minimum is likely to be argued with different responses, presumably varying with the financial resources and living standards of the community concerned. The further question of *who* should decide what is to be included remains to be answered.

The concept of a standard of decent basic minimum care, already considered in general terms above, has been discussed in relation to people who have become highly dependent in the course of dementia. Callahan (1995) guessed that public opinion would accord a high priority to decent nursing and palliative care for demented patients, but a much lower priority to the use of expensive medicine to prolong life. He specifically cited "intermediate-level care" as advocated by an earlier writer, namely "conservative low-technology treatment, and often at home rather than in a hospital" as a middle-way option between aggressive treatment and providing no treatment at all (ibid: 30). Callahan explicitly excluded PVS patients from the middle-way option on the basis that he considered they lacked "selfhood". The concept of "intermediate level" care appears entirely reasonable to me, however the exclusion from it of patients diagnosed as in a PVS appears to be as arbitrary as the notion of "selfhood". An indication of a middle-way treatment option that may be relevant to some PVS patients, is provided by accounts of the care of locked-in patients who have neurological disabilities and risks of complications similar to those of patients in a vegetative state. Of an American group of 18 LiS patients who had survived for at least 5 years and who were reviewed by Katz *et al*. (1992), 11 resided in their own homes, 2 were permanent hospital residents and 5 were in nursing homes. Of the 11 patients living at home, 6 received in excess of 40 hours of hired nursing assistance per week, 2 had from 4 to 15 hours of part-time help per week and three had no outside help. It is likely that the varying levels of care were determined by variations in the medical nature of the associated disabilities as well as in the capacity of family members to provide help. Whilst LiS patients were likely to have a more prolonged life span, they were as disabled physically as PVS patients and similar considerations are likely to be applicable to the two groups.

The monetary costs of caring, in a traditional long care setting, for patients who were severely demented were compared with the costs of a dementia special care unit in a study by Volicer *et al.* (1994). The special care unit differed from its traditional alternative in that patients were homogeneously grouped and cared for by staff trained in the management of Alzheimer's disease. Emphasis was placed on the maintenance of patients' comfort instead of striving for maximum survival. Volicer *et al.* reported that the cost of medical treatments and procedures and medications (over and above costs of residence and nursing) was almost three times greater in the group of patients receiving the traditional rather than the palliative form of management. Comparison between the two groups revealed a higher mortality in that subpopulation of patients in the dementia special care facility with less severe Alzheimer's disease than for comparable patients receiving traditional care. This finding of a better economic outcome from establishment of special care units for Alzheimer's disease resembles the recommendations of Sailly (1994) for PVS patients. Whereas palliation may be indicated from the outset in the case of dementia, it is more likely to become a consideration with the passage of time in PVS as attempts to achieve improvement are tapered off because of lack of response.

14.4 FAMILY IMPLICATIONS

The economic and social impact of vegetative states spreads beyond the patient to affect his or her family to an extent that is equalled by few, and probably surpassed by no other, medical conditions. Conventional medical practice in cases of PVS has often entailed advice to the family, at an early stage after the traumatic or ischaemic episode, to forget the patient or to regard him or her as already dead or as a 'non-person' to be disowned. Unless the affected individual has been the principal wage-earner for the family, the major impact on the family in accepting this advice is likely to be psychological rather than economic (See the postscript to the preceding Chapter). I would expect that unresolved grieving is likely to be a long term complication of abandoning the family member diagnosed as vegetative. "Coming to terms" with loss of the family member by achieving a clear break has been invoked by some medical practitioners not only as a basis for family abandonment but also as a reason for participating in decisions to curtail continued existence of the patient. In purely economic terms, there may be some indirect costs imposed on the community as a consequence of the effects on the social functioning of an affected family after abandonment of the member with brain injury.

The economic burdens upon any family opting to retain and support their disabled member are often considerable. There can be direct effects, in the form of loss of employment income, or less immediately apparent consequences, for example marital breakdown and anti-social and even para-suicidal behaviour on the part of siblings who experience neglect as parents concentrate their total attention on the disabled member. Ambivalence towards the patient may also warp relationships between other family members and skew family decisions in relation to his or her management. Such ambivalence may outlive the family member when a decision to abandon him or her has been implemented. Covinsky *et al.* (1994) reported on the impact on 2600 U.S. families of having a seriously ill family member (including comatose persons) discharged home after the onset of illness. Whilst almost all of the families had hospital insurance, the impact both in caring and financing was often devastating. In almost 20% of cases another family member had to quit work. Most or all of the family savings were lost in 31% of cases. The major source of family income was lost in 29%.

Specific cases often convey the reality of a situation more effectively than aggregated statistics. Andrew Devine, like Tony Bland, was a victim of the 1989 Hillsborough football stadium disaster. He was considered to be in a PVS until 1995, but was then observed to have regained awareness of his surroundings together with the ability to indicate this to observers (Hopkins 1997). In the intervening years, Andrew's father had quit his job as a police inspector to concentrate on helping his wife look after him. The family home was suitably adapted to facilitate caring for him and a daily program of exercises designed to stimulate him was undertaken. In this case, substantial financial support was available from an insurance company, but in many other cases all available family resources have been diverted into assisting the disabled family member. Ultimately, the decision as to whether undertaking domiciliary care of a family member after a diagnosis of PVS was worthwhile will probably depend on the relative values that the family attaches to economic and other, less measurable but more basic, considerations.

The economic burdens likely to be borne by the family of a PVS patient were lumped together with arguments about "invasive medical treatments, futile and thus extraordinary, disproportionate and unduly burdensome" in the decision for withdrawal of nutrition and hydration from Marcia Gray, who had been in a vegetative state for more than a year (United States Bishops' Committee 1992: 622). The likelihood that an acute psychological and a potentially medium and long term economic burden will be imposed on the families of PVS patients has been augmented by arguments that the onus of *continuing* to provide food and water to unconscious patients or of funding their provision should fall on them so reversing the traditional position. Until recently, the onus of proof fell on anyone claiming that the patient's preference was for *discontinuation.* A U.S. physician called for this transfer of the onus of proof to the patient's family, categorising preference for the continued provision of food and fluid to vegetative patients as an "idiosyncratic view" (Angell 1994). Whilst not explicitly spelled out, the tone of this and similar articles inferred that the family should incur financial liability if it held to its "idiosyncratic view" of wishing the affected family member to continue to receive food and water.

Consideration of the impact on his or her family of a very severely disabled person has led some authors to discover a "duty to die" on the part of such patients. Hardwig (1997) has postulated the existence of such a duty founded upon "our technological sophistication coupled with a commitment to our loved ones" (ibid: 34). The "duty" was based on the effects that the patient's continued life may have upon others. In particular, Hardwig nominated the impact on family finances, on family time for other activities and on education and employment opportunities of other family members. According to Hardwig, an exemption from the duty to die could be granted "if my loved ones are truly benefiting from coping with my illness or disability" (ibid: 36), a fairly demanding prerequisite.

14.5 Global Costs of PVS to Health Care Systems

As indicated above, substantial variations occur in the costs of managing individual PVS patients with many of the higher cost estimates being based on prolonged initial periods in intensive care units. Variations between health care systems, and between hospitals, in the duration for which patients are in an intensive care unit will impact markedly on these costs. Even allowing for this, the frequent absence of a common "medium" level of care makes estimates of overall costs to a health care system difficult. Jennett identified this problem in the following terms:

> "In some hospitals, there nowadays seems not much middle ground left between intensive care and relative neglect, even if this is styled by the more positive label of 'self-help'" (Jennett 1976: 595).

While he hoped that improvement in prognostication would soon enable individual patients to be directed into the most appropriate treatment stream, accurate formulation of prognosis at an early stage of treatment is still generally acknowledged to remain a goal, rather than an achievement. Unless the aggregate costs incurred in the intensive care of patients, who are *subsequently* diagnosed as being in a vegetative state are separated off from the (almost invariably) much lower costs when they have been so diagnosed and moved to a technologically less sophisticated setting, any estimate of the expenditure which might be saved by restricting the care available to *diagnosed* PVS patients cannot be formulated. In the continued absence of generally agreed, reliable predictors of subsequent development of a PVS, as distinct from regaining consciousness although remaining severely disabled, it is difficult to envisage how the large component of expenditure incurred *before diagnosis* could be saved.

Quantification of the cost of the intensive component of caring for vegetative patients encounters difficulties similar to those in undertaking this calculation for the terminally ill. Patients in PVS are not terminally ill (despite efforts by some courts in the 1990s to define them as so), but there are similar obstacles to attempts to cost the expenditure on each class of patient (terminally ill and PVS). For instance, an article by a group of bioethicists, physicians and economists noted that the economic data available about terminal care tended

> "to conflate the costs of caring for the terminally ill and the critically ill" (Bayer *et al.* 1983: 1491).

The authors noted also that any attempt to develop cost control strategies applicable to the terminally ill

> "cannot begin by assuming, as if demonstrated, that a large-scale socioeconomic problem exists or that there is a widespread and irresponsible indifference to costs" (ibid: 1493).

The global impact of PVS on any health care system could be estimated from information on its prevalence and the costs incurred in providing a "reasonable" standard of medical care for affected patients, both difficult to estimate. What level is selected as reasonable will depend upon the commentator. It will be somewhere between prolonged maintenance under intensive conditions in an acute care facility and "warehousing" with restricted nutrition and nursing lacking anything recognisable as attempts at rehabilitation therapy. The former could be seen as an immoral diversion of resources to the patient and the latter as an amoral deprivation. A reasonable approach to the care of PVS patients is that adopted in institutions specialised in longer term maintenance of patients and could entail provision of non-intensive therapy with opportunity for the exploitation of any detected potential for improvement. A most comprehensive economic analysis of such a facility exists for Établissements Helio-Marins at Berck (H.M.E.B.), which receives patients from all of France.

14.6 Costs of Caring for PVS Patients in a Specialised Facility

Sailly's study of H.M.E.B. was based on 515 patients who were admitted in coma during the period 1987-1991. Of these patients, 179 subsequently entered a vegetative state and, of those, 24% ultimately regained consciousness. Of the group regaining consciousness, 21% were assessed as being severely handicapped whilst the remaining 3% were classed as either "moderate handicap" or "good recuperation" (Sailly 1994). Considering these groups of patients as a whole, Sailly noted that the average length of stay of all admitted patients was 396 days whilst the average stay for patients who were vegetative at some stage was 558 days. Sailly calculated all costs in 1990 French francs. Grouping all patients in the study as a single group, the average 396 day length of stay was associated with an average cost of 650,000FF. However, when this group of patients was disaggregated into subcategories, some significant cost differences between subgroups became evident.

The younger patients were responsible for much higher expenditure than the older ones. Patients under 20 years of age attracted twice the per capita expenditure of those over 50. Patients who died whilst at H.M.E.B. generated substantially more expenditure than those who survived in accord with the hypothesis that the severity of brain injury is correlated directly with expenditure on intensive care, but inversely with duration of survival. Of the patients who died, those who had experienced trauma incurred considerably higher expenditure than others with cerebral vascular accidents (800,000 FF v 400,000FF). Patients who ultimately remained severely disabled cost twice as much as those who retained a moderate degree of disability or made a good recovery. Patients who were comatose on arrival at H.M.E.B. ultimately cost approximately twice as much as those who were awake at that time.

These results suggest several conclusions. In the first place those patients who were sickest (and so most likely to die) received more attention, at greater cost, than others who had not been so severely affected. Patients who regained consciousness and were able to resume some activities cost less than those who remained moderately handicapped. In the continuing absence of a capacity for reliable early prognostic assessment, the retrospective statistics from H.M.E.B. are unlikely to facilitate the concentration of resources on those most likely to derive the greatest benefit from them. Presumably the much greater unit cost of managing young patients reflects decisions to treat these people more intensively. Similarly, the greater expenditure incurred on those patients who died may reflect the additional intensity of resources directed to them as their condition deteriorated.

In order to achieve an estimate of national costs for management of PVS, Sailly made some assumptions about its prevalence. With a prevalence rate of 2 per 100,000 population and an average daily cost at H.M.E.B. of 1600FF, Sailly calculated that, for the total French population of 57 million, annual costs of caring for patients in a vegetative state would approximate 650,000,000FF, that is 0.12% of the total national health care budget (for 0.0016% of the population). Sailly contrasted the much lower level of concern for PVS patients displayed by key components of the health care establishment, such as the pharmaceutical industry, with that accorded by that establishment to conditions which were of greater concern to the community at large. He commented upon the skewing of costs for comatose and vegetative patients by the much higher costs of their intensive care and he predicted that good domiciliary management of long surviving patients could be better and possibly cheaper.

Information about the absolute costs of caring for patients in a vegetative state is unlikely to be very informative in the absence of additional information. To place the costs of optimal management such as that at H.M.E.B. in context, it would be necessary to compare them with the economic costs of other courses of action. As a first step, the basic costs of living of any non-disabled individual could be subtracted from Sailly's calculations for vegetative patients. Additionally, the costs associated with the alternative of "warehousing" PVS patients could be compared with those of H.M.E.B. management. Unless the community is prepared to follow the course of selecting death as a means of cutting down on expenses, a decision *not* to provide moderate support will introduce new costs of its own. Not only will the occurrence of potentially avoidable complications such as nutritional deficiencies, contractures and decubitus ulcers impose additional management costs, but it is also highly likely that these complications will have a negative impact on the morale of nursing and paramedical staff with a resulting costly staff turnover and burn out. Medical "care" which accepts these deformities as a certain and foreseeable consequence of the inadequate level of support to be provided would also be morally deficient.

As mentioned above, economic comparisons should be drawn not only with what would happen with vegetative and other severely disabled individuals if their support were curtailed, but also with assessing whether resources diverted from PVS patients were likely to be advantageously applied to other groups of patients. Health care personnel are unlikely to be as disposable as chess pieces on a board. If such personnel are motivated by the wish to assist specific groups of patients, it should not be assumed that they can readily be transferred (ignoring their training and inclination) into other areas deemed to be national priorities. The implications of the current fashion of "managed care" for patients in and close to vegetative states are ominous. The underlying impetus in a managed care system, namely that providers have a financial incentive to limit the treatment provided to their patients, will inevitably discriminate against them (Kaveny 1997).

14.7 PREVALENCE OF PVS

Apart from estimating the average costs of care of patients in a vegetative state, the other prerequisite for determining the global cost of PVS to a health care budget is a reliable estimate of the prevalence of the condition. Prevalence, in its turn, is the product of incidence of the condition (that is, of the appearance of new patients) and duration of ongoing survival of affected patients. There are no generally applicable data on the likely life span of PVS patients. Cranford nominated four major factors likely to affect length of survival and suggested that it was not uncommon for patients to survive for five, ten and twenty years. His factors were age (younger patients survive longer), economic circumstances (wealthier patients receive better care), resistance of the body to infections and "changing moral and social views on the appropriateness of stopping treatment, especially medical means of providing hydration and nutrition" (Cranford 1988: 31). As a response to an increasing awareness in the UK in the late 1990s of the possibilities of unexpected emergence from a vegetative state and of its misdiagnosis, a survey to determine the number of people in PVS was initiated (Macdonald 1998). An impediment to this exercise was that the system would be likely to lose track of patients who had been discharged to their homes.

Most prevalence estimates appear to be of a similar order of magnitude. Sailly (1994) cited a prevalence of 2 per 100,000 for France. Estimates of 1200 to 1500 patients in Britain (2-2.5 per 100,000) (Macdonald 1998) are close to the French figures as is an estimate of 2.5 per 100,000 in Japan (Higashi *et al.* 1981). Ivan (1990) has estimated a Canadian figure of 800 (2.8 per 100,000). Cranford's (1988) figure for the U.S. of between 5000 and 10000 patients (1.9-3.8 per 100,000) was presented as an assumption in an article subtitled *getting the facts straight*. The derivation of this estimate was that:

> "The estimate is based on epidemiological studies from Japan showing approximately 2,000 to 3,000 patients in this condition in that country, and an 'extrapolation of that data to the United States, taking into account both a

> doubling of population and our more advanced (and more indiscriminately applied) life-support systems" (ibid: 32).

More recently, Cranford (1995) has cited a prevalence of 10,000-25,000 adults and 4,000-10,000 children in PVS (total of 5.4-13.5 per 100,000) in the U.S., attributing this estimate to the M.S.T.F. The Councils on Scientific Affairs and Ethical and Judicial Affairs of the American Medical Association estimated the US total as 15,000 to 25,000 (5.8-9.6 per 100,000) (American Medical Association Councils 1990). These figures represented a substantial reduction from the estimate of 100,000 (38.5 per 100,000) presented by the A.M.A., appearing in an *Amicus Curiae* capacity in the Cruzan case (Meisel 1995: 636).

Any calculation of likely costs to a health care system of long term maintenance of patients in a vegetative state that is based on the product of unit cost of treatment and life expectancy (as such calculations inevitably will be) is likely to assume as its starting point that these two inputs are independent of each other. This will generally be incorrect. As Shewmon and De Giorgio (1989) inferred from their experience, the patients who ultimately have the poorest outcome (although usually not identifiable in advance) are likely to receive the most intensive (and expensive) treatment but, despite this, to die early and so not to continue to require that expenditure for prolonged periods.

Taking account of the decidedly speculative nature of the calculations on which many of these prevalence estimates appear to have been based and the complete absence of sound information about the levels of medical and nursing care that any national "PVS population" is receiving, no quantification of costs could confidently be regarded as authoritative. Additionally, unless one is proposing to lump all severely disabled patients together, irrespective of whether they completely meet the definition of PVS, the high rate of misdiagnosis of the condition by British neurologists that has been reported by Andrews *et al.* (1996) imposes another major qualification on any estimates of the cost of caring for PVS patients. It would be very surprising if this qualification was applicable only to the UK.

14.8 RECAPITULATION

Some of the economic factors influencing the management of patients in a PVS are shared with most other medical conditions. Irrespective of the health care system under consideration, the level of available resources will be finite, although the actual level will vary widely. As a consequence of this, there is likely always to be conflict between the interests of individual patients and those of the community for which health care is being provided. Again, as a general feature, it is necessary that the interests of the individual patient, which will be a responsibility of his or her medical attendants, should not be overridden as a step towards redirecting the community's resources. Decisions at the systemic level on allocation of resources between institutions, programs etc. will be made by those responsible for oversight at the level of the health care budget. Decisions about the care of the individual patient will obviously have to be formulated within the constraints of the systemic budget but should not be formulated with the objective of promoting systemic goals. Finally, an adequate exposition of the economic basis of any course of clinical management can provide valuable background data for making ethical decisions.

The most useful, and least available, economic information relating specifically to the management of patients in a PVS relates to the unit costs of providing various levels of intensity of care, the duration for which specific types of care are likely to be required and the prevalence of patients requiring care. As discussed in earlier Chapters, information on both the frequency of occurrence of PVS and the likely length of survival of affected patients is quite inadequate. Furthermore, it is clear that the level of care *required* can vary between patients and between times in the case of an individual patient. The level of care *provided* (and funded) to individual patients will vary both with their requirements and with what is available (influenced by factors such as locality, availability of medical insurance or compensation and systemic policies on provision of resources to different types of patient). There have been published reports of individual patients in a PVS whose care was extremely expensive to such a degree as to be clearly unrepresentative of this class of patient as a group. Likewise, the level of intensity (and costs) of care in some published series of patients appear to be unrealistic. Examples of this have included the ongoing use of ventilators and long term intravenous fluid administration to patients diagnosed as entering a PVS in the course of progressive deterioration in the eighth and ninth decades of life.

Any decisions to reallocate resources from one group of patients to another will remain subject to the practicality of securing the monetary value of the services and materials to be withdrawn and the availability of the alternative services and materials to be purchased with the proceeds. The feasibility of achieving this substitution if resources are to be moved from management of patients in PVS to other areas does not appear to have received as much consideration as has the idea of such reallocation.

CHAPTER 15

VEGETATIVE STATES IN COURT

> "One might wonder why an issue which has always been with us has suddenly developed a sense of urgency. The answer – as is often true these days in medicine – is the law" (Editorial *The Daily Telegraph* 1998).

This editorial comment referred to a debate in the British Medical Association (B.M.A.) on the issue of withdrawal and withholding of medical treatment with particular reference to patients in vegetative states. The media and the courts stand out as the two areas outside hospital wards and nursing homes to have been most affected by the issues raised by PVS. Media accounts of PVS have included some of the most sensationalist, but also some of the most accurately informative, accounts of affected patients.

This Chapter will not attempt to review the large number of court cases that have addressed the issue of withdrawal of hydration and nutrition from specific patients in a PVS. Such cases have, numerically, occurred predominantly in the U.S., to a much lesser extent and more recently in the U.K., with which this Chapter will be principally concerned, and in single figure numbers in other jurisdictions. The Chapter has two parts, the first of which will deal, in general terms, with the significance, for clinical management of PVS, of those cases which have come to court and the approaches that have been adopted to permit decision-making. The second part of the Chapter will use the first U.K. case, that of *Airedale NHS Trust v Bland*, to illustrate and consider from a medical perspective issues raised by applications to the courts for withdrawal of support from PVS patients. This case has stimulated a cottage industry of analyses and commentaries and the present examination will be restricted to the implications for subsequent cases of several issues raised in court.

15.1 PVS COURT CASES AS A REPRESENTATIVE SAMPLE OF PVS

The extreme variation in the frequency with which "PVS cases" have been considered by courts within different jurisdictions is likely to reflect the operation of multiple factors that are not readily separable. Court cases may not have eventuated either because withdrawal of hydration and nutrition is regarded in a particular jurisdiction or state as a medical procedure not requiring legal surveillance or, alternatively, because of reticence on the part of the medical profession to implement withdrawal. A pre-existing policy of routinely discontinuing support at an early stage after brain injury when patients are still ventilator-dependent could obviate any requirement for later withdrawal of hydration and nutrition from patients with severe neurological disability, so reducing its prevalence. Issues arising from the funding of long term care could influence approaches to courts as also could a culture in which medical negligence suits were commonplace.

PVS cases which have progressed through the legal system to appellate level have had a substantial impact on attitudes towards patients in a PVS and other patients with unrelated conditions. The prospect of court involvement in decision-making has alarmed the medical profession. For example, one early decision by the Massachusetts Supreme Court elicited the heading *Judges as physicians* in the *New England Journal of Medicine* (Relman 1978). The Court ruled that decisions about termination or institution of life-prolonging measures for terminally ill patients must be made by the courts rather than by physicians, family or ethics committees and the *Journal's* concern touched on the issue of *who* was to make decisions. Subsequent U.S. court decisions were much less assertive on this issue.

Recognition that court decisions about withdrawal of support from patients in a PVS could not be quarantined from clinical decisions relating to patients with similar conditions was explicitly spelt out in the *Amicus Curiae* brief presented by the American Geriatrics Society in the U.S. Supreme Court hearing of the 1990 Cruzan case which dealt with withdrawal of tube feeding.

> "Although Nancy Cruzan is only 32 years old, the ultimate disposition of the issue in this case will have serious implications for the care of the elderly" (Glover *et al.* 1990: 570).

Similar concerns that entrenchment of policies about PVS could impact much more widely prompted another *Amicus Curiae* brief submitted in the Cruzan case by several groups representing handicapped and retarded persons. This brief pointed out that in excess of 800,000 people in the U.S. were in receipt of tube feeding and that almost two thirds of the residents in one State's facilities for persons with developmental disabilities "required full or partial assistance in eating" (Bopp *et al.* 1990).

It is impossible to determine the extent to which those cases involving PVS patients which have reached courts, and, in particular, those that have been referred to superior courts, are representative of the general run of cases of patients in a PVS. In his review of U.S. "right-to-die" cases that entailed the withdrawal of life-sustaining measures, Meisel (1992) proposed that the 50 to 75 appellate court decisions which had been delivered on this subject up to 1992 represented only "the tip of the tip" of the proverbial iceberg. He did not attempt to estimate whether the tip represented an accurate sample of the remainder of the iceberg. Not all of the cases retrieved by Meisel were concerned with patients diagnosed as in PVS; not all entailed the withdrawal of food and water. Meisel contrasted the 50 to 75 appellate court decisions with estimates that some 2900 – 7000 trial court cases in the period 1975 – 1989 had involved withdrawal of treatment. The number of these trial cases which addressed the specific question of withdrawal of nutrition and hydration from PVS patients was not indicated. However, the *Amicus Curiae* brief of the Society for the Right to Die submitted to the Cruzan hearing provided some indication of the frequency with which cases of withdrawal of treatment in general did not come to court. This brief cited an estimate that 10 life support systems were being disconnected each week in Minnesota 5 years previously (Gasner *et al.* 1990). A major limitation of such estimates, however, is the absence of any information concerning the condition of the patients – specifically whether they were terminally ill or stable – and the nature of the "life support" systems. Meisel noted that while trial court litigation did not have the precedential value of appellate court decisions, it nevertheless became incorporated in the behaviour and thinking of health care professionals and patients and their families, in addition to that of lawyers.

Widening the extent of the catchment even further, Meisel (1992) calculated, on the basis of a survey finding that 70% of deaths in U.S. hospitals occur after decisions "to forgo" life-sustaining treatment, that the 2900 – 7000 trial court cases themselves represented only 0.2 to 0.5% of deaths consequent upon such "forgoing". Whilst to *forgo* is commonly taken to be to deny oneself, Meisel's use includes involuntary withdrawal decisions made by others. To assess the relevance of this scaling up for PVS patients would require some indication of the extent to which decisions were taken in response to deterioration in the patient's condition *despite* treatment rather than decisions to cease treatment which could have maintained the patient in a stable condition indefinitely, or only achieved improvement which was regarded as inadequate. It is not possible either to infer how commonly withdrawal of hydration and nutrition from patients in a PVS occurred during this period without referral to *any* court.

In reaching decisions in cases concerned with the withdrawal or withholding of hydration and nutrition from patients in a PVS, courts have adopted a number of approaches. They have generally proceeded either to infer what course of action the patient would have wanted or else to decide what would be "best" for the patient (two approaches which need not necessarily lead to identical answers). Determinations of what the patient *might* have wanted have been based on directives, formulated by the patient in advance or, more frequently, on the advice of surrogates deemed likely to have been familiar with the patient's unexpressed wishes. A variant of this approach, involving the notion of "a brief lucid interval" during which the patient could express a wish before persisting in vegetation, has received short shrift in the U.K. courts as being too fanciful, although it featured in the 1976 New Jersey court decision allowing ventilator withdrawal from Karen Ann Quinlan. On the other hand, court determinations of what would be "best" for the patient usually have taken account of the views of the patient's doctor or family with the decision being based on a combination of familiarity with the patient's previous wishes (if any), as well as on an assessment of contemporary "best interests". The nature of the decision sought by the applicants has ranged from a declaration that a course of action proposed by the patient's doctors would not be illegal to a determination that a specific medical course of action (i.e. withdrawal) was indicated. In some cases, courts have explicitly endorsed the medically recommended withdrawal decision; in others they have only determined that the medical attendants have the legal authority to make that decision.

15.2 THE USE OF ADVANCE DIRECTIVES IN PVS CASES

> "For someone to be asked to decide in advance whether he or she would want dialysis, ventilator or feeding tubes, without knowing what using these procedures would yield is incomprehensible" (Lynn 1991: 102).

The two essential components of any form of advance directive are encompassed in the answers to the questions, "What modification to patient management is to be implemented in following the directive?" and "What set of conditions brings the directive into operation?" The 1993 report of the American Neurological Association on PVS specified three forms of advance directive that could be applicable to affected individuals, namely a living will, an enduring power of attorney and an appointed health care proxy (American Neurological Association Committee on Ethical Affairs 1993). Opinions about the value of advance directives range from support to strong criticism an example of which is Joanne Lynn's assessment above. Notwithstanding the reservation she expressed, information about the likely treatment wishes of patients who are no longer capable of expressing them has been sought both during clinical management and when decisions have been referred to the courts. Whilst Joanne Lynn's criticisms were directed to the practicability of advance directives, the legitimacy of many forms, given their construction, has also been criticised by John Finnis (1994) in a legal analysis of advance declaration statutes. He considered that all "blur and obscure the difference between suicidal intent and other intentions".

There has been considerable geographical variation in the extent to which advance directives have come into use. Whereas legislation sanctioning them had been introduced in most jurisdictions of the United States by the 1990s, they have received much less attention in the U.K. However, by the mid 1990s, both political (the House of Lords Select Committee on Medical Ethics) and medical (B.M.A.) establishments had endorsed their use (Robertson 1995). Addressing the question of the circumstances in which a directive *might not* be followed, a B.M.A. code of practice on advance directives made the point that "a refusal seriously likely to affect other people adversely" may not be legally binding (British Medical Association 1995: 5). Enlarging on possible reasons to account for a directive not binding, the following sentence of the code cited a refusal of basic care measures. Defining basic care was, in its turn, acknowledged to be problematic. At a later stage, the code stated that:

> "Caring for a person whose pain or symptoms are not sufficiently relieved as a result of an advance refusal may impose an intolerable burden on those around them and abandonment of an incapacitated person is unacceptable" (ibid: 15).

By 1999, the B.M.A. ethical guidelines on withdrawal of treatment had come specifically to identify "artificial nutrition and hydration" as medical treatment while acknowledging that this was not a universally accepted position (British Medical Association 1999). The guidelines acknowledged that "neither the nutrition nor the hydration is, in fact, artificial" but that the terminology had become widely used.

While there appears theoretically to be no reason why an advance directive should not specify *either* the provision *or* the withholding of any identified medical procedure, the use of directives has been considered almost exclusively in the latter context.

> "In general, advance directives regarding future treatment decisions are negatively formulated in the sense that they contain a specified refusal of treatment (for instance in the case of irreversible coma/persistent vegetative state (PVS) or severe dementia)" (Berghmans 1998: 32).

In an abandonment of the original philosophical underpinning of individual autonomy and the substitution of one based on a communitarian outlook, some authors have stressed that advance directives entailing refusal of treatment conserve public resources by reducing the need for expensive medical measures. Cantor considered that although general public benefits do not "provide a morally sufficient basis for enforcing advance directives, they do reinforce the argument for upholding a competent person's advance directive" (Cantor 1992: 21). Obviously, a directive requesting the *provision* of a specific medical measure, representing an additional call on resources, would not be so reinforced. It has been suggested that an advance directive can be readily prepared by an individual without any particular knowledge of the medical conditions likely to bring the directive into operation, or of the different forms of treatment to be withheld. For instance, Emanuel *et al.* (1991) claimed, in a trial of the procedure, that a directive could be completed in less than 15 minutes by a group of outpatients and by the Boston general public. Of special relevance to advance directives in anticipation of PVS, Emanuel *et al.* found no substantial difference in that trial between the rate of refusal of "technically advanced interventions and that of artificial hydration and nutrition" (ibid: 894).

Analyses of the issues raised by the withholding of food and water from people in a PVS have usually commenced by considering the right of *competent* individuals to refuse treatment that is necessary for their survival. A competent person, whose capacity for rational judgement has not been affected by clinical depression, should not be compelled to accept medical treatment, even if death is a foreseeable consequence of that refusal. However, the situation becomes more complex when the refusal is that of a person not suffering from a life threatening condition, involves food and water and is patently motivated by an intention to commit suicide. Whilst there may be no legal impediments to a non-institutionalised person opting to end his or her life in this way, circumstances which impose responsibility on others for the welfare of the individual concerned will introduce such constraints. When the actual wording of an advance directive is being considered, Finnis (1994) has drawn attention to a nuance in the use of "terminal" in this type of document. Many American statutes originally defined a terminal condition as one which would soon result in death *whether or not* life-sustaining treatments are employed.

Subsequently, "terminal" has been taken to imply that death would occur *only* if treatment was withheld.

In interpreting advance directives (or, more frequently, in attempting to construct these in their absence on behalf of patients in a PVS) the question of whether withdrawal of hydration and nutrition can be included in them has been controversial. Whereas, originally, such withdrawal was commonly separated from other non-treatment decisions, and its use was related specifically to PVS, both distinctions have been gradually discarded. Sanford Kadish (1992) noted that living-will statutes in the United States typically only applied to persons in "permanent vegetative states, or where death is inevitable and imminent" and the provisions of the living will are instituted after the person becomes terminally ill (ibid: 861). He also pointed out that, at that time of writing, typical living will statutes in many of the 40 odd States which had enacted them excluded the withdrawal of artificial hydration and nutrition. Writing at a similar time in the *American Journal of Law and Medicine*, Cantor (1989) drew attention to the difference between the legal position that no logical distinction existed between removal of a "respirator" and removal of artificial nutrition and the specific exclusion of the latter from living will legislation in many States. State legislation either explicitly excluded nutrition and hydration from procedures which could be withdrawn or else specified the circumstances required to validate withdrawal. The latter included imminent death, irrespective of whether nutrition was provided, and inability of the patient to assimilate nutrition. Subsequently, there has been a trend for statutes to be modified to permit the withdrawal of artificially administered hydration and nutrition. Nevertheless, as of 1993, it was noted during the course of the Bland case in the U.K. that 20 out of 39 American States which had legislated in favour of 'living wills' specifically excluded the termination of life by the withdrawal of food and water (*Airedale NHS Trust v Bland* 1993: 888). Other pre-conditions for withdrawal incorporated in State legislation specified that the continued provision of nutrition would shorten the patient's life or cause severe pain. Some additional background to the factors underlying US practice and legislation was cited in a 1990 review when it recalled the anxiety referred to in the Quinlan case attributable to "the brooding presence of … possible liability" (Weir and Gostin 1990: 1852).

The issue of precisely *what* differentiates treatment from care when interpreting an advance directive has been extensively argued. Notwithstanding concerted attempts to extend the purview of "treatment" so that procedures traditionally regarded as "care" can be rendered subject to medical discretion, I do not believe that the distinction has become a dead issue. It was raised in a U.K. Law Commission report entitled *Mental Incapacity*. In endorsing legislation to support advance directives the Commission argued that "advance refusals" of life-sustaining treatments should

> "not preclude the provision of basic care, defined as the maintenance of bodily cleanliness, relief of sustained and serious pain, and the provision of oral nutrition and hydration" (Doyal 1995: 612).

A 1999 retrospective survey of more than 1000 U.S. patients diagnosed as being in a PVS over a 15 year period indicated that some 44% of these individuals had been fed orally (Strauss *et al.* 1999) raising the question of how difficult or tedious such oral feeding must be for nurses or family before it might be omitted without contradicting the spirit of an advance refusal. The thrust of argument in *Bland* was that tube feeding was medical treatment whereas feeding by mouth was not. It seems fundamental that the scope of any procedure to be withheld should be specified in an advance directive. Commenting upon the case *Re R*, involving a profoundly disabled individual with a very low state of awareness, before the Family Division of the English High Court in 1996, Ian Kennedy (1997) emphasised the inappropriateness of "global" orders stipulating "do not treat" and the necessity for specifying treatment options. On this first occasion when an English court considered the place of "do not resuscitate" orders in medical law, Kennedy stressed that a "do not resuscitate" decision is not equivalent to a decision to forgo *all* life-sustaining treatment. This distinction has also been stressed by others (Shewmon and De Giorgio 1989). Nevertheless, earlier surveys suggest that "do not resuscitate" orders have often been interpreted by hospital staff as precluding a very wide spectrum of medical care ranging from continuing admission to an intensive care unit to withholding all supportive care (Evans and Brody 1985).

Precision in specifying, in an advance directive, *what* is to be provided or withheld will not be of any assistance in implementation unless the *context* in which those measures are to be undertaken and the *prerequisites* to bring them into effect are also specified. The likelihood of *reversibility* of the medical condition bringing the order into effect should also affect its implementation. Preparation of a list of requested interventions may appear to be a tidy way of encapsulating a person's wishes for future management but it could readily miss the more fundamental requirement of recording the person's intent when framing the directive.

Among U.S. court considerations of the application of advance directives for withdrawal of hydration and nutrition from PVS patients, a 1995 decision of the Michigan Supreme Court raised four unresolved issues. How specific must the patient's previous remarks be before these may be interpreted formally as an advance directive? To what extent should a *competent* patient be able to control his or her future care? To what degree can an objective burden/benefit analysis legitimately authorise the withholding or withdrawing of treatment? How are disputes between close members of the patient's family to be resolved? (Dresser 1996). The Missouri Supreme Court, when it required "clear and convincing evidence", or a living will, to establish that the PVS patient Nancy Cruzan would not have wished to receive tube feeding, expressed considerable scepticism about advance directives in general:

> "It is definitionally impossible for a person to make an informed decision – either to consent or to refuse under hypothetical circumstances" (Lo *et al.* 1990: 1229).

The Michigan Supreme Court required evidence that the patient should have previously considered the details of possible future treatment whereas other courts have accepted very general statements often based on others' recollections of conversations with the incompetent individual. With the passage of time, court requirements have shifted from the need to establish that a patient *would not have wanted* the treatment under consideration to permitting withdrawal of the treatment unless it can be established that the patient *would have wanted* it.

W*hat change* in a patient's condition is required to *activate* an advance directive? Lynn has emphasised that standard forms of living wills *should* (Lynn's emphasis) have virtually no impact on the management of PVS patients as these people "do not meet the requirement of dying soon irrespective of treatment" (Lynn 1991: 102). However, the re-interpretation of "terminal" noted above, and the frequency with which discussions of advance directives have used PVS cases as illustrations have realigned the relationship of advance directives to PVS patients. Standard forms of living wills or advance directives commonly specify that the individual not receive nourishment by other means if incapable of self-feeding without specifying a cause for that incapacity. These instructions would be implemented when an individual is dying, or has entered the terminal stage of dementia. However, the way in which directives are generally formulated could permit application to *any* patient diagnosed as vegetative, irrespective of his or her general medical condition. Dresser (1986) has commented, that the commonest flaw in advance directives was patients' inability to anticipate every specific health crisis that could befall them, whilst Emanuel and Emanuel (1993) also identified the necessity for a patient's previously stated preferences to be applied to unanticipated circumstances as a major weakness. However, attempts to overcome the obstacles to implementation of an advance directive in unforseen circumstances by very specific instructions may lead to a preoccupation with technology at the expense of principles.

In practice, the usefulness of advance directives has been limited, not only because many patients have not executed them, but also because existing directives may not have been available or adhered to by clinicians. Most writers who have considered the practicability of advance directives have drawn attention to some substantial obstacles in the way of their implementation. For instance, Emanuel and Emanuel (1993) cited a survey indicating that only 20% of patients completed these; only 31% of directives which had been completed were available when life-sustaining treatment decisions were being made; 23% of those that were available were ignored or overridden. On this basis, very simple arithmetic suggests, that something less than 5% of patients would have their preferences implemented as a result of an advance directive. A number of other patients are likely to have had their previous wishes implemented because these were accurately discerned by their families or doctors. Danis *et al.* (1991) reported that, when advance directives had not been followed, one quarter of the patients were treated more aggressively than they had requested and the remainder were treated less aggressively.

> "Future oriented decisions generally involve hypothetical facts, variable circumstances, and a limited perspective which complicates decision-making. Advance medical directives thus present problems about accurately anticipating a multitude of scenarios involving the dying process of a future incompetent being" (Cantor 1992: 15).

Whilst legislation has not been enacted in the U.K. to validate advance directives and earlier opinions were to the effect that they had no legal status (Higgs 1987), the 1992 Court of Appeal case of *Re T* indicated that an anticipatory refusal of treatment would be legally valid provided that the circumstances in which it was given were appropriate and the intent of the individual was clear (*Re T* 1992). A model advance directive discussed in the *British Medical Journal* in 1995 bracketed serious brain damage together with degenerative brain disease, terminal malignant disease and progressive degenerative disease of nerves or muscle as conditions eligible to bring into effect a directive not to feed other than by mouth (Robertson 1995). The question of how an advance directive specifying not to feed, other than by mouth, is to be regarded in a patient retaining the ability to swallow after diagnosis as PVS seems not to have been seriously addressed.

Despite the lack of any formal legislative backing, living wills requesting withholding of treatment are accorded considerable respect in some U.K. hospitals. For example, a recent contribution to the *British Medical Journal* from a database manager who had experienced a pulmonary embolism and a period of intensive care illustrated this point. Apprehensive about dying intestate, he resorted to writing a will shortly after admission indicating the manner in which he required his *estate* to be distributed. Soon after this, he collapsed and required vigorous resuscitation. Following his recovery, he learnt about "the fuss that (writing a will) caused", namely that it had been assumed to be a "living will" with instructions about withholding resuscitation. The last word of advice to him came from the senior registrar:

> "Let this be a lesson to you. Never mention the word 'will' in a hospital again" (Young 2001).

15.3 SURROGATE DECISION-MAKING

While living wills have many disadvantages, the same may also be said of the alternative in which a patient-nominated or legislatively-specified proxy makes a surrogate decision on behalf of a patient, because such decisions frequently are not in conformity with the wishes of the patient. For example, a study of the wishes of geriatric patients in Chicago comparing them with the decisions of physician-selected proxies from patients' families indicated that the patient would have wanted the proxy to make a decision opposite to that actually made in 24% of cases for tube feeding, 44% for resuscitation and 50% for chemotherapy (Zweibel and Cassel 1989). As only a minority of patients are said to have discussed their likely wishes with prospective proxies, frequent discordance between patient and proxy can be anticipated (Emanuel and Emanuel 1993).

Conflicts of interest between patient and proxy can arise and may be more common than is generally acknowledged. Incompetent patients tend to be both emotional and financial burdens on the family from which proxies are drawn and this may influence decisions (Emanuel and Emanuel 1992). Dresser noted that the U.S. President's Commission on Forgoing Life-Sustaining Treatment favoured the consideration of family interests when determining treatment of an incompetent individual on the grounds that the patient would be likely to have concerns about his or her family's well-being (President's Commission 1983a). However, she asserted that:

> "Family concerns have no permissible influence on the treatment choice, and that considering them only opens the door to the subordination of patients' interests for the convenience of their families" (Dresser 1986: 396).

Balancing this, she acknowledged that it remained questionable whether treatment decisions for incompetent patients can ever be made without considering family interests. A criticism of proxy decision-making even more dismissive than that of Dresser contended:

> "Studies that compare the abilities of persons to predict how their spouses would answer a series of hypothetical questions are more appropriate for game shows" (Miller 1991: 1254).

These assessments of the value of family involvement in decision-making stand in sharp contrast to the views of Joanne Lynn indicated above.

Proxy decision-making may fail if a patient changes his or her mind or if the patient's interests change substantially after discussion occurs. Emanuel and Emanuel (1993) have, rather superficially, dismissed the former as a major concern by comparing the frequency of unstable decisions related to future treatment options with that applying to decisions to marry. Dresser has dealt rather more substantially with this concern and has criticised courts and legislatures for often failing to acknowledge that less weight should be assigned to competent patients' interests in future-oriented decision-making than to those interests relevant to contemporaneous choices (Dresser 1986).

15.4 INTERESTS AS THE BASIS FOR DECISIONS

If advance directive and "best interests" criteria are applied by a court in strict isolation from each other, they may prescribe completely different management decisions for a patient. This is hardly surprising given that *competent* individuals commonly opt for courses of action in everyday life which do not correspond with their best interests. When decisions are to be made on behalf of an incompetent person, the risk is that other interests may intrude into the decision-making process. Dresser (1986) asserts in her article on "hidden values" in the law which affect its dealings with incompetent patients, that certain family and societal interests have surreptitiously entered the legal decision-making process. If so, the standard legal approach of determining what interests the reasonable person in the patient's circumstances could be expected to have might effectively incorporate the concerns of *others* into the decision-making process. An example of this process, which featured in the Cruzan case and with which families of patients with severe brain injury would empathise, is that of protecting the memory of the patient that is retained by the family (Cantor 1992). While not wishing to denigrate the significance for a patient's family of their recollections of him or her, it is indisputable that, to the extent that this factor influences one's assessment of what *the patient* would have wished, one is effectively superimposing the interests of others on that decision. The legal approach could be to pose the question of how a reasonable person in the patient's position would want to be remembered by his or her family.

An American professor of law and ethics, Rebecca Dresser (1986) has called for both courts and legislatures to acknowledge the "separate and potentially conflicting interests" of incompetent patients and their relatives in reaching treatment decisions. She criticised the Quinlan decision on the grounds that:

> "The concerns that the court imputed to Quinlan were instead concerns of her family and of the significant portion of our society that opposes aggressive medical treatment for permanently comatose patients" (ibid: 385).

Whilst family interests are indisputably important, it is equally important that they be identified as such and not presented as patient's interests. The financial implications of maintaining patients in PVS have never been far below the surface. Acknowledgement of this point, followed immediately by a disclaimer that it had not biased the outcome, was a feature of the final decision in the U.K. case of Tony Bland. It may be significant that, in *Bland* and each of the succeeding cases, it was the National Health Service (NHS) Trust responsible for financing care of the patient which approached the court requesting withdrawal of food and water (usually with the support of the patient's family). Dresser nominated financial considerations of caring for PVS patients as a source of conflicting interests and stressed that, in the U.S. judicial system:

> "Courts and legislatures have managed to steer clear of this potential conflict by pretending that resource constraints have no influence on decisions about life-sustaining treatment" (ibid: 403).

The prospect of the routine introduction of financial considerations into clinical decision-making has been explored by Sheldon Berrol (1986b), a specialist in the rehabilitation of patients with head injuries, under the heading *Chilling perspective*. The perspective which chilled Berrol was

> "the recent (*ca* 1986) suggestion within the Department of Health and Human Services, that all new applicants for Medicare be provided copies of living wills" (ibid: 285).

Whilst it may be possible to establish legal procedures that reliably exclude the intrusion of others' interests into decisions that are purported to be made exclusively on the basis of those patients' interests, some commentators have dismissed them as flawed For example, one hospice physician described a living will as:

> "An artificial contrivance similar to tamper-proof packaging for medication, which has been forced upon us temporarily in order to prevent abuses by a legal system that is devoid of compassion or common sense" (Miller 1991: 1255).

Dresser (1994), has shown a comparable degree of scepticism about the adequacy of court proceedings, citing the general tendency of those making decisions on behalf of incompetent individuals to formulate "vague, usually unspoken intuitions on what it would be like to be someone like her" (ibid: 612). In the same article, titled *Missing persons*, Dresser asserted that court-derived answers to the hypothetical question of what an incompetent patient might choose if she were competent are likely to be "indeterminate enough to permit almost any treatment option preferred by a patient's family, guardian or physician" (ibid: 616).

15.5 LEGAL CONSIDERATION OF LIFE-SUPPORT SYSTEMS

In his comprehensive review of U.S. court cases relating to the withdrawal of life-sustaining measures, Alan Meisel (1995) draws attention to the imprecise and non-specific meaning of the term "life-support system", commenting that its use in determining what treatment can be forgone is "unfortunate, unhelpful and potentially misleading". Whilst entirely concurring with Meisel's criticism of the vagueness of the term and its uselessness, I am unable to accept his inference that the variety of nursing and medical modalities that have been grouped, for purposes of discontinuation, under a common semantic umbrella should be treated as equivalent to each other. If, as I suspect is likely, community acceptance of decisions to discontinue treatment is accorded in proportion to its perceived "high-tech" nature, any representation of tube feeding as dependent on complex technology as, for example, in coupling the verb "switching off" to "life-support system" will, predictably, influence community attitudes to its discontinuation. In drawing attention to the varying levels of intensity of the range of procedures that are increasingly described under the rubric of "life support system", I am *not* advocating that the level of intensity or of "extraordinariness" *per se* should be reintroduced as the basis for deciding whether a procedure can be withdrawn. What I *do* wish to emphasise is the frequent correlation between the intensity of a procedure and its "burdensomeness" *for the patient*. I believe that the grounds for not utilising "higher technology" procedures such as total parenteral nutrition or long term ventilation should rest on their *intrusiveness* for the specific patient under consideration and *not* on their technical elegance or expense.

The U.S. President's Commission report (1983a) provides ample precedent for an all inclusive categorisation of "life-sustaining treatment":

> "Although the term includes respirators, kidney machines, and all the paraphernalia of modern medicine, it also includes home physical therapy, nursing support for activities of daily living, and special feeding procedures, provided that one of the effects of the treatment is to prolong a patient's life".

To place it in context, the report was issued 7 years after the Quinlan case, which approved disconnection of a patient in a PVS from a ventilator, and in the same year as the first cases to approve the withdrawal of hydration and nutrition from such patients. If the President's Commission report is to be read consistently and literally, as it must be to equate "special feeding procedures" with "all the paraphernalia", one could anticipate successful applications to withdraw "home physical therapy" and/or "nursing support for activities for daily living" from PVS patients on the grounds that they are burdensome and futile. Such a course of action would assuredly lead ultimately to the patient's death, albeit over a longer time scale and with even more emotional impact upon the nursing staff than occurs at present with withdrawal of the provision of food and water. I am not aware that applications for withdrawal of either of these "life-sustaining treatment" modalities has yet come before a U.S. court.

Applications to U.S. courts exclusively for ventilator disconnection from PVS patients, as documented by Meisel, ceased at the time of commencement of applications for approval of withdrawing hydration and nutrition. Applications for ventilator disconnection from patients with other conditions did not cease at the same time. The first instance of a successful application to a court for withdrawal of hydration and nutrition from a vegetative state patient was concerned *not* with cessation of *enteral* feeding but with discontinuation of administration of sustenance *parenterally,* using an intravenous catheter. This is a much more technologically specialised, demanding and potentially hazardous exercise than (enteral) tube feeding into the gut. If the general acceptability in the community at large of discontinuation of any medical procedure is proportional to its invasiveness, then the withdrawal of intravenous nutrition and hydration is an ideal intermediate between removal of a ventilator and that of a feeding tube. Shewmon and De Giorgio (1989) have commented that, prior to the acceptance of withdrawal of hydration and nutrition, ventilator disconnection before spontaneous respiration was regained from comatose patients considered likely to have a poor outlook represented the only effective way of reducing the prevalence of PVS.

15.6 PVS IN CONTINENTAL EUROPEAN COURTS

Citations in the English language medical literature relating to PVS rely heavily on reports from English language sources. Although this is a common feature of most medical literature, the lack of citation of non-English language articles on PVS may reflect the existence of fewer publications on this subject in other languages. It should also engender some caution in extrapolating from the voluminous U.S. literature on management practices to other nations. PVS cases certainly have had a lower profile in European courts then in the U.S. or U.K. The extent of the difference in the numbers of PVS court cases between European jurisdictions (other than the U.K.) and the U.S. has been brought out by Grubb *et al.* in a 1998 review *Reporting on the persistent vegetative state in Europe*. There had been approximately 20 court cases in England concerned with the withdrawal of hydration and nutrition by the time of this report. However, the report noted that such cases had been considered "on very few occasions" by courts in the Netherlands, Germany, Scotland and Ireland. On those infrequent occasions, withdrawal was held to be lawful. The issue of withdrawal had not arisen in a French court at the time of the report.

In seeking to explain the substantial differences between European nations in attitudes to PVS, Grubb *et al.* cited the impact of differing roles for the legal system in regulating medicine. In the U.K., the doctor-patient relationship is closely regulated by law, whereas a medical code of ethics, independent of the legal system, operates in France. Another possible explanation could be the absence of a written constitution in the U.K. contrasting with the existence of such constitutions in other European countries "as applicable to patients in PVS as they are to all citizens". A third possibility proposed by Grubb *et al.* to explain international differences related to the promulgation in some European countries of codes of medical ethics drawn up by national organisations responsible for regulating the practice of medicine.

A comparative survey of medical practitioners' attitudes towards treatment-limiting decisions may explain the wide variation between countries in the frequency of appearance of PVS court cases. Rather than lumping all treatment-limiting decisions together as has invariably been done by English courts and medical authorities, the survey of Grubb *et al.* sought information on attitudes towards treatment limitation in two different situations. Their questions related to the appropriateness of not treating "acute infections and other life-threatening conditions" and the "withdrawal of artificial hydration and nutrition" from patients in a PVS. An aim of the researchers was to determine the extent to which doctors in different European countries considered decisions concerned with the non-treatment of infections to be different in kind from decisions to withdraw artificial hydration and nutrition. At one extreme, doctors in the Netherlands and the U.K. considered the non-treatment of acute infections or other life-threatening conditions and the withdrawing of artificially administered hydration and nutrition to be similarly appropriate (namely 84% v 70% and 90% v 73% in the two countries respectively). At the other extreme, doctors in Germany, France and Ireland regarded withdrawal of artificially administered hydration and nutrition as much less appropriate than not treating acute infections (namely 16% v 58%, 14% v 78% and 53% v 100% respectively). Evidently, practitioners in the latter three countries do not automatically regard decisions to withdraw hydration and nutrition from PVS patients as equivalent to decisions not to treat acute infections.

15.7 THE U.K. TEST CASE: AIREDALE NHS TRUST v BLAND

The case of Anthony Bland was the first instance in which the withdrawal of hydration and nutrition from a patient in a PVS was tested in an English court. The case progressed through three courts and produced decisions from nine judges. It established precedents which have been followed in English courts and taken into account in other jurisdictions. I intend to examine several specific aspects of the "Bland" case which have been frequently invoked in subsequent cases involving PVS patients and to consider their influence (*Airedale NHS Trust v Bland* 1993).

Anthony Bland sustained a crushed chest in a spectator stampede at the Hillsborough football ground in April, 1989. As a consequence of cessation of respiration, he suffered very extensive hypoxic brain damage, failed to regain consciousness and was subsequently diagnosed as being in a PVS. His doctor contacted the coroner in August, 1989 to enquire about the legality of withdrawing feeding through a nasogastric tube and withholding antibiotics in the event of infection. The coroner suggested that legal advice should be obtained and, on the basis of this, the Airedale NHS Trust which was responsible for the care of Anthony

Bland issued an originating summons in September, 1992 which came before the Family Division of the High Court in November of that year. This sought a declaration as to the lawfulness of discontinuing:

> "All life-sustaining treatment and medical support measures designed to keep Anthony Bland alive in his existing persistent vegetative state including the termination of ventilation, nutrition and hydration by artificial means and that they could lawfully discontinue and thereafter need not furnish medical treatment to him except for the sole purpose of enabling him to end his life and die peacefully with the greatest dignity and the least pain, suffering and distress" (ibid: 824).

The judge in the Family Division granted the declaration and the Official Solicitor, appearing on behalf of Bland, appealed to the Court of Appeal. When this affirmed the judge's decision, the Official Solicitor appealed to the House of Lords on the basis that the proposed course of action was both a breach of the doctor's duty to care for his patient, indefinitely if need be, and a criminal act. This appeal was dismissed in February, 1993.

The three aspects of the Bland case to be considered are the medical features which strengthened its "test case" status, the nature of tube feeding and the relevance to the court decisions of Bland's doctors' intentions in withholding tube feeding. Whilst the appearance of cases with such novel features that they are destined to become test cases may occur in an entirely fortuitous and unpredictable manner, some cases exemplify so well the points on which a decision is required for the first time that it becomes difficult not to suspect that they were selected specifically for that purpose. The case of Anthony Bland illustrated the issues raised by PVS much more effectively than any of the cases that entered the English courts in the following 4 years. No expert witness dissented from the diagnosis of his being in a PVS. He was considered also to be an extreme case. For example, Keith Andrews, arguably with more experience of PVS than any other English clinician, having had some 50 affected patients in his care to the time of the hearing, expressed the opinion that Bland was the most severe case of a vegetative state that he had seen (ibid: 828). The other expert witnesses included Bryan Jennett and Peter Behan, a professor of neurology, who had been instructed by the Official Solicitor to examine the patient.

15.8 MEDICAL ADVANCES AS A SOURCE OF NEW ETHICAL PROBLEMS

Technical novelty is the ideal meat for any test case which is to be heavily based on input from a non-legal discipline. Some of the judges in the Bland case considered that its novelty required matching novelty on their part. It is clear from the wording of their decisions, that relatively recent advances in intensive care permitting survival beyond the acute stage of patients, some of whom subsequently became vegetative, had been totally conflated with major advances in the maintenance of patients who *had become* vegetative. Thus, Lord Hoffman in his Court of Appeal decision concluded that until relatively recently:

> "A person who had irreversibly lost consciousness would quickly have died: from lack of nutrition or from one of the many complications which have afflicted Anthony Bland's body over the past three years and which medical technology has been able to hold at bay" (ibid: 850).

Lord Browne-Wilkinson's confusion was adequately evidenced in his allusion to the modern technological developments which had underpinned the maintenance of individuals certified as brain dead, while acknowledging that Bland was not dead, but then expressing his belief that:

> "Modern technological developments such as tube feeding enabled him to be sustained in a state of 'living death'" (ibid: 878).

Unless one is prepared to extend the ambit of "modern" back into the first half of the twentieth century, any proposition that development of such feeding is the recent advance which has occasioned clinical situations such as that of Bland, necessitating an attendant new ethic, has a singularly unconvincing ring to it. The court decisions had no relevance to withholding the "high technology" intensive care procedures which had enabled Bland to survive the acute stage after brain injury, but were exclusively concerned with withdrawal of decidedly "routine" non-intensive support measures.

Some paradoxical features of Anthony Bland's medical management emerged during the court proceedings. Expert testimony before the Family Division of the High Court about the management of vegetative patients revealed that it had become accepted as good practice both in the U.K. and elsewhere to agree, in consultation with patients' families, to withhold antibiotics and cardiopulmonary resuscitation in the event of complications that would justify the use of these measures in patients not in a PVS (ibid: 827). This is not a contentious position. Yet, Anthony Bland had received vigorous antibiotic therapy for repeated bacterial infections during the three years elapsing after his doctor first raised the question of withdrawing food and water with the coroner in 1989, 4 months after the accident in which he was injured. It remains inexplicable that, despite the existence of an agreed position shared by family and doctors, namely that his death was the desired outcome, the legally incontestable and commonly selected option of *not* treating infections had been passed over for several years. In the absence of vigorous antibiotic therapy, he is most unlikely to have survived long enough for the court hearings and, if so, there would not have been a test case.

Keith Andrews testified that Tony Bland's high susceptibility to recurrent life-threatening infections presaged a relatively short life expectancy (presumably even *with* continuing vigorous use of antibiotics) (ibid: 828). Perhaps because of its apparent naivety, the question as to *why* no decision to withhold vigorous antibiotic therapy had been made during the years elapsing before the case finally entered court does not appear to have been posed during the court proceedings. The failure of Tony Bland's doctors to withhold antibiotics was subsequently perceived to be an obvious issue by a House of Lords Select Committee which considered the Bland case and its implications and queried why inappropriate treatment with antibiotics had been provided to Tony Bland, given that recovery from the successive infections occasioning their use could add nothing to his well-being. In the absence of this continuing treatment, the Select Committee recognised that the case was unlikely to have come to court (House of Lords Select Committee 1994).

Two comments in the Court of Appeal hearings suggested a reason why failure of Bland's medical attendants to withhold antibiotics during the extended period before his case first came to court did not attract judicial attention. Sir Thomas Bingham suggested that discontinuation of antibiotics might result in the patient dying "perhaps less peacefully than on withdrawal of artificial feeding" (*Airedale NHS Trust v Bland* 1993: 841). Similarly, after mentioning antibiotic use, Lord Justice Hoffman opined that:

> "Withdrawal of nourishment is the most gentle and controlled way in which to allow him to die" (ibid: 856).

The experience, on which these inferences were based was not indicated. A letter in the *British Medical Journal* during the hearing of Bland case, written from a position of opposition to euthanasia, enlarged on antibiotic withholding.

> "Should he develop an overwhelming pneumonia it would be an entirely legitimate medical decision if antibiotics were not given. He might then die. If so he would die from pneumonia and the persistent vegetative state; if the proposed plan is followed, he will inevitably die of intentional starvation and the persistent vegetative state" (Fergusson 1992).

Andrews (1992b) commented in the same issue of the *Journal* in the following terms:

> "When voluntary euthanasia is accepted as a legal method of medical care, starvation is highly unlikely to be an accepted way of assisting the death of the patient. Why then should we choose this method for involuntary euthanasia?" (ibid).

A discordant note in relation to the management of Tony Bland was struck by M.A. Tudor (1993b), a rehabilitation specialist from the Royal Hospital and Home, Putney (subsequently the Royal Hospital for Neuro-disability). She noted that little attempt appeared to have been made to improve his quality of life as all published photographs had shown him in bed affected by contractures and with a nasogastric tube. In response to her letter to the *British Medical Journal*, the geriatrician responsible for the care of Tony Bland accused Tudor of being ignorant, patronising and insulting. He referred to "a vigorous and intensive rehabilitation programme" similar to "those carried out in many units around the country as well as Putney" (Howe 1993). In the following month, the *Journal* carried a letter from Keith Andrews which responded, *inter alia* that Tony Bland could not have received the type of rehabilitation programme carried out at Putney in a general unit with little or no experience of the PVS. More significantly, Andrews questioned what standard courts would accept as "rehabilitation" before a decision is made in future cases that lack of response validates withdrawal of feeding (Andrews 1993d). Insofar as accounts of subsequent court cases are accessible, this fundamental question has yet to be specifically addressed.

15.9 TUBE V MOUTH: MEDICAL V NON-MEDICAL PROCEDURES

The significance of establishing a distinction between tube feeding (medical) and feeding by mouth (nursing) in the Bland case is that subsequent pronouncements on the subject from legal and medical authorities have claimed that, in the U.K., *medical* procedures may be withdrawn at the discretion of a doctor if considered to be futile. The Bland case was notable for the rigidity of presentation of the proposition that, provided a treatment or procedure was adjudged to be "medical", its application or withdrawal should be considered uniformly alongside all other "medical" procedures. In the intensity of its expression, this categorisation now exceeds the abandoned traditional distinction between ordinary and extraordinary measures which was not mentioned in any of the judgements. Implicit in the ordinary-extraordinary distinction (albeit usually not acknowledged in criticism of it) was the concept that either term was to be applied in a *relative*, contextual sense. Nevertheless whilst the medical-non-medical distinction can become completely dependent upon circumstances, the absolute nature of the distinction, as it has been interpreted by English courts when applied to patients in a PVS, makes no provision for this in its application. The absurdity of this was brought out (one presumes inadvertently) by the claim of James Munby Q.C., appearing for the Official Solicitor on behalf of Anthony Bland, that any "medical measure" ranging from tube feeding to dialysis or organ transplantation would be *equally* required by Bland if specifically indicated by his condition. Sir Thomas Bingham, very reasonably found this suggestion:

> "So repugnant to one's sense of how one individual should behave towards another that I would reject it as possibly representing the law" (*Airedale NHS Trust v Bland* 1993: 841).

Similarly, the dismayed response of Lord Justice Butler-Sloss to Munby's contention that, in the event of

> "a cardiac arrest or a similar failure, it would be the duty of the doctors to perform a heart bypass operation or a kidney transplant" (ibid: 848)

(allowing for imperfections in the technical medical detail) seems perfectly reasonable to me. By the device of bracketing renal transplantation and tube feeding in the same category of "medical treatment", Munby and the Official Solicitor instructing him made a major contribution to ensuring that any court would judge the latter to be as inappropriate as the former and accordingly reject it. In racing parlance, the Official Solicitor, in adopting this vitalist position, could be described as "running dead".

The contention of Butler-Sloss LJ that the duty of doctors towards a patient in a PVS does not extend to prolonging the patient's life at all costs appears unexceptionable (ibid: 849). However, the lumping together of tube feeding and renal transplantation within the single category of "medical treatment" has effectively substituted "any cost" for "all costs". While Sir Thomas Bingham MR acknowledged the gross variation possible between different medical procedures in the extent of physical invasion of a patient's person, and privacy, he refrained from any attempt to decide what might or might not be *reasonable* in the light of the benefits conferred by the procedure in question for the specified patient. His attention was directed exclusively to the question of whether *criminal liability* depended upon the relative invasiveness of the different procedures which it was proposed to withhold (ibid: 841). His negative finding presumably implies that unconsented touching and unconsented amputation of a limb would incur a similar degree of criminal liability.

Slippage occurred in the argument that tube feeding, by virtue of its artificiality, must be regarded as medical treatment when Butler-Sloss LJ proceeded to widen the catchment considerably by referring to "medical care" to avoid "the uncomfortable attempt to draw a line" between spoon feeding and tube feeding of a helpless patient (ibid: 844). The medical-non-medical distinction was further eroded by Lord Browne-Wilkinson in deciding that the removal of Tony Bland's nasogastric tube was not an act, as:

> "The tube itself, without the food being supplied through it, does nothing" (ibid: 881).

This appears to come perilously close to the position of those arguing that the *provision* of food through a tube is not a "medical" procedure.

15.10 WHATEVER HAPPENED TO INTENT?

> As to the element of intention, or *mens rea*, in any judgement there can be no real doubt that it is present in this case: the whole purpose of stopping artificial feeding is to bring about the death of Anthony Bland. (Lord Browne-Wilkinson) (ibid: 844).

The submission of the Official Solicitor in the hearing of the Bland case before the Court of Appeal was summarised by Bingham MR as including two propositions. The first was that the proposal to withdraw hydration and nutrition was intended to cause death. The second was that therefore it was necessarily criminal. There does not appear to have been dissent from any of the judges in the three courts through which the Bland case passed that the intention of the withdrawal of hydration and nutrition was to cause the patient's death. However, in each of the decisions which addressed the question, it was concluded that no *actus reus* existed. Butler-Sloss LJ concluded that Bland's doctors were not under a duty of care to continue feeding and, consequently, no unlawful act or omission would arise (ibid: 848). Lord Lowry not only discounted the existence of any "guilty act" because it was not in Bland's interests to be supported but decided that his doctors would be acting unlawfully if they *continued* his support (ibid: 877). Lord Browne-Wilkinson, as noted in the preceding section considered that the nasogastric tube "does nothing". Therefore, he reasoned that, even if *removal* of the tube was regarded as a positive act (contrary to his view), it would not constitute the *actus reus* of murder (ibid: 881). Lord Goff indicated that, as withdrawal of support from Bland would not represent a breach of a duty of care owed to the patient, the act (or omission) was not illegal (ibid: 868).

In an interesting placement of the proposed withdrawal in a wider legal context, he spelled out his interpretation of the difference between withdrawal and active killing:

> "Whereas the law considers that discontinuance of life support may be consistent with the doctor's duty to care for his patient, it does not, *for reasons of policy*, consider that it forms any part of his duty to give his patient a lethal injection to put him out of his agony" (my emphasis) (ibid: 868).

15.11 THE BLAND CASE AS A PRECEDENT

The decisions delivered in *Airedale NHS Trust v Bland* clearly indicated that their Lordships were acutely aware that this case would be invoked as a precedent. Lord Browne-Wilkinson emphasised that his judgement related only to the case under consideration and did not seek to lay down a new regimen (ibid: 880) and also that he expressed no view on the appropriate decision in any future case in which a patient might retain some level of consciousness (ibid: 884). Lord Mustill warned that the pressures of such an extreme case might distort the law leading to false conclusions in more finely balanced cases (ibid: 885). It would, he considered, be too optimistic to expect that future cases could be resolved on the basis of the Bland case (ibid: 887). Whilst the *Bland* precedent has been adopted, the disclaimers about its applicability to other patients with dissimilar features have been largely ignored. As the patient's need for ventilation was neither expressly indicated, nor implied, in the court proceedings, one can only speculate on the reasons for the inclusion of provision for its discontinuation in the schedule. One possible reason might be to strengthen the inclusion of food and water under the medical rubric of "life support".

The future implications of the 'Bland' case, not only for patients in a PVS but also for those with other conditions, may be of concern even if one considers the decision to have been reasonable. Thus, one bioethicist considering it and the second case to come before an English court, namely *Frenchay Healthcare NHS Trust v S*, acknowledged that:

> "A good case could be made both for discontinuing Tony Bland's tube feeding and for not reinserting S's tube".

Nevertheless, he warned that:

> "The problem with these cases is not so much their outcomes as the reasoning behind the decisions, what this reveals about trends in law and practice, and what this kind of thinking is likely to allow in the near future" (Fisher 1994).

Aside from the question of why individual cases of PVS have come before the courts, the question of the extent to which those cases which have proceeded through the system, and attracted considerable publicity, have been representative of the majority of PVS cases remains uncertain.

15.12 PUBLICATION AND PATIENT CONFIDENTIALITY

Obstacles to reconstructing the early legacy of the Bland case in the following four years have included non-reporting of cases, court orders suppressing publication of patient details and the tendency for cases to remain unreported (and under-reported) once the initial excitement generated by the first test case has subsided. Publication of patient-identifying information has been a contentious issue when they have emerged from a vegetative state or are to have food and water withdrawn following a court hearing. The *British Medical Journal* expressed reservations about publishing a paper describing a series of cases of misdiagnosis of PVS because the patients' direct consent to publication was unobtainable and because media publicity of some identified cases could permit their matching with clinical details in the *Journal* (Smith 1996). The degree of identification of patients who were the subject of court cases has ranged from extensive reporting of all details in mass media, in addition to medical and legal journals, through suppression of the identity, not only of the patient and family, but of the hospital, and even of *all* involved parties, including the health authority.

The basis for suppression of all identifying information was specifically canvassed in the cases *Re G* and *Re C*. In *Re G*, the patient's wife and mother, together with the hospital in which he was a patient, sought to have a hearing in chambers to obtain a declaration that provision of hydration and nutrition could be discontinued. The family's reason for seeking a hearing in chambers was to spare them distressing publicity. The Official Solicitor, appearing on behalf of Mr G, opposed this request and sought a hearing in open court with safeguards to preserve the anonymity of all concerned. The judge undertook a balancing exercise in which the interests of the patient, the family and the hospital were offset against the public interest. Taking account of the court's responsibility to provide reassurance to the public, he considered that the case was "very much in the public domain" and that there was a very clear balance in favour of the public interest. The substantive hearing took place in open court with restriction on publication of any identifying details, extending even to the names of the instructing solicitors (Grubb 1995a).

Media interest in Mr C continued after withdrawal of hydration and nutrition, and his death, notwithstanding previous restriction on publication. The Official Solicitor applied for guidance as to the continuing validity of an order preventing publication of any identifying details. The ruling recognised that there could be an adverse impact upon the doctors and nurses involved and their care of the patient if it were known that their anonymity might be breached after the patient's death. Their decisions, it was held, "should be untrammelled by the fear of publicity", establishing an interesting precedent for professionals making decisions on controversial issues. In finding that the order on confidentiality should survive Mr C's death, the judge noted that a public interest in freedom to report details had not been argued in that case and that "public interest" was not synonymous with "public curiosity" (Grubb 1997c).

15.13 INCIDENCE OF PVS COURT CASES AFTER AIREDALE NHS TRUST V BLAND

Twelve months elapsed before the second English court case to seek withdrawal of hydration and nutrition came to court. Grubb (1994) speculated that this may have resulted from a failure of doctors and families to agree on a court application. He also speculated that doctors may have been unwilling to approach a court in these circumstances "even if the wishes of the relatives are not strictly relevant to a determination of the patient's best interests" (ibid: 207). Nine additional declarations permitting withdrawal of hydration and nutrition had been made by the High Court by November, 1996 and it was reported in February 1997 that a further six applications had been made (Macdonald 1997a). A member of the B.M.A.'s Ethics Committee commented at that time:

> "Hopefully it is a statistical blip"

but added that the number of applications had been

> "much lower than some predictions. At one stage we were being told there was going to be a mass clear-out of long term wards, with the cases running into the hundreds, which has not happened" (ibid).

A spokesperson for the same Committee, quoted in November, 1996, referred to the issue of whether applications for withdrawal were being confined to PVS patients:

> "When we looked at vegetative patients, we thought that was a discrete condition and it (i.e. PVS) wouldn't have applications for other cases" (Dyer 1996c).

Broadening of the scope of court orders will be considered below.

15.14 ENTRENCHMENT OF PVS AS A SINGLE ENTITY

Notwithstanding the pathological heterogeneity of affected patients, the lack of reliable diagnostic investigations and the potential for clinical imprecision in recognising unconsciousness (or failing to recognise consciousness), courts in the U.S. and the U.K. have established PVS as a well demarcated medical condition. Many of its predominantly negative clinical features are shared by patients with severe neurological damage who fail to meet diagnostic requirements for PVS. Even the most cursory consideration of the cases coming into the English courts after *Bland* confirms the original prediction of Jennett and Plum of the existence of a spectrum of conditions, despite categorisation of all as "PVS" cases.

Whilst some of the patients whose cases came before the English courts after *Bland* manifested indications of awareness inconsistent with the criteria previously nominated as necessary for a PVS diagnosis, translocation from the ward to the courtroom has conferred considerably more precision on PVS and its diagnosis than was previously available. For example, in *Bland* the Master of the Rolls asserted unambiguously that:

> "The absence of cerebral function is not a matter of surmise: it can be scientifically demonstrated. The space which the brain should occupy is full of watery fluid" (*Airedale NHS Trust v Bland*: 834)

With respect, the autopsy report on Anthony Bland hardly supported the Master's claim (see Chapter 2). Lord Hoffman pointed out that:

> "No one has ever recovered any vestige of consciousness after being in a persistent vegetative state for more than a year" (ibid: 853).

Apart from the clear inaccuracy of this contention and its incompatibility with published reports such as those cited in Chapter 9, the correspondence columns of the *British Medical Journal* in the same year described Andrew Devine, another PVS victim of the Hillsborough stadium disaster who had done precisely that (Tudor 1993b).

The contention from *Bland* that PVS is a clinically discrete condition which a patient is either *in* or *not in* was contradicted by some of the following cases which came to court. For instance, in *Frenchay Healthcare NHS Trust v S*, the evidence was "not as emphatic and not as unanimous" as it had been in *Bland* (ibid: 408). S was described by a neurology professor as appearing to suffer pain. Another discordant feature was the inability of the attending clinicians to reduce his high dose of sedatives. The confounding effect of this on reliable adjudication on his conscious state appears to have escaped notice. Another two of the cases following *Bland* were stated in court not to meet the Royal College of Physicians criteria for diagnosis of PVS. Mrs H was described as being able to track objects with her eyes (Dyer 1997b). Miss D, according to the legal correspondent of the *Guardian*, retained the capacity for a number of responses, including visual tracking. Three reports provided by medical expert witnesses stated that this 29-year-old former university student was in a PVS but also, paradoxically, advised that, according to the existing guidelines, she was not (Dyer 1997a). One of the expert witnesses, Bryan Jennett, expressed "quite a lot of uneasiness", apparently not about the possibility of misdiagnosis, but about nonconformity of the guidelines with the clinicians' assessment (ibid).

A New Zealand case several years after *Bland*, which was strongly influenced, by it, illustrated the extension of its conclusions to less emphatic situations. The patient in *Re G* was considered not to be in PVS but to be so close to it as to have a quality of life no different from a person in that condition. The court agreed to consent to withdrawal on the patient's behalf and to base this decision primarily on consideration of "best interests" (*Re G* 1997). A commentary on *Re* G noted that this case did not fit within "the extreme factual situation" applying to *Bland* (namely, the New Zealand patient was not considered to be in PVS whereas Tony Bland was) and advocated widening of withdrawal decisions based on "a more-or-less objective conception of a life worth living" (Peart and Gillett 1998). This commentary involved less rather than more objectivity in its assertions that G retained no *meaningful* way of communication and had no prospect of *meaningful* recovery or of *meaningful* improvement, did not have a *meaningful* life nor a life which was *meaningfully* able to be thought of as a life. In another example of basing a decision on an extension of *Bland* the Irish High Court decided in *In the matter of a ward of court* that a patient who appeared to be able to distinguish between her nurses and strangers, although "not fully PVS" was near enough (*In the Matter of a Ward of Court* 1995: 416). The extension to other patients, not meeting the diagnostic requirements, of management decisions based specifically on PVS has been increasingly accepted. By 1999 B.M.A. guidance on the subject of treatment withdrawal asserted that there was no reason to differentiate between decisions for PVS patients and others (British Medical Association 1999).

15.15 WHOSE INTERESTS?

> "Thus, perhaps inevitably in the absence of an advance statement from the person concerned, the interests being served are at best speculative and at worst actually the interests of others" (McLean 1999: 492).

In the absence of any formal recognition of advance directives, English court cases involving the withdrawal of hydration and nutrition from PVS patients have relied heavily on two propositions. These are that the "best interests" of such individuals can be adequately decided by others and that compliance with those interests will not be achieved by continuation of support. The concept of "best interests" has been criticised by a number of English legal commentators, including some who were entirely in agreement with the court decisions to end the life of Tony Bland and other patients in a similar condition. Their criticism, as exemplified above by that of McLean, was directed, not to the decision but to the logic underlying it. Ian Kennedy (1998) in analysing the case of Re C, dismissed "best interests" as an empty notion that was "not good enough for a court to decide on".

English courts have identified a number of parties, including the patient, his or her family and the medical and nursing attendants as possibly having an interest in the fate of PVS patients coming before them. As the invariable plaintiff in English cases, the relevant NHS Trust has also had an interest. For example, Tony Bland was said to require the attention of two nurses for 4-5 hours every day (*Airedale NHS Trust v Bland*: 828), which would represent a significant expenditure for the Airedale NHS Trust. Lord Hoffman observed that the Trust wished to have the case considered on grounds of "unlimited resources" (ibid: 857). Nevertheless, as indicated in the course of Lord Mustill's decision, the question of whether the resources provided to Tony Bland could be put to better use was "never squarely put although hinted at from time to time" (ibid: 893). The magnitude of resource commitment to a patient by an authority seeking to have support withdrawn would vary from case to case, being lower in patients such as Mr S who were cared for at home. What may be less evident is that the interests of others who have no association with a specific case may be adversely affected by the precedent that it creates. A particularly graphic account of an immediate impact of the Bland decision upon others has been provided by one of the medical staff of the institution which subsequently became the Royal Hospital for Neuro-disability. On the night that their Lordships handed down their judgement in *Bland*, relatives of patients in the brain injury unit at the Royal Hospital and Home, Putney were reported to be

> "angry, frightened and distressed, being fearful that their loved ones would be affected by the ruling. They vented their feelings on the nurses, and I know that many of these caring people went home saddened" (Tudor 1993b).

The House of Lords had in effect asserted that Anthony Bland had no further interest in being kept alive and that his doctors were under no duty, and were not entitled, to keep him alive. As it was also concluded, not only that Bland need not continue to receive hydration and nutrition, but also that his medical attendants were *obliged* to discontinue this form of support, it is not difficult to envisage the basis for the concerns of other patients' families if they wished for its continuation.

The potential for a conflict of interest between the family and the patient has been noted above in discussing the general issue of surrogate decision-making. The question of whether Anthony Bland may have had an (indirect) interest in advancing the interests of his family by preventing the erosion of their happy memories of him was raised, but dismissed, in Lord Mustill's judgement:

> "It seems to be stretching the concept of personal rights beyond breaking point to say that Anthony Bland has an interest in ending these sources of others' distress" (*Airedale NHS Trust v Bland* 1993: 894).

Whilst there was family unanimity in *Bland*, which contributed to its suitability as a test case, this was not so in the second case (*Frenchay Healthcare NHS Trust v S* 1994: 407) when the patient's father was said to have agreed to reinsertion of the feeding tube and its continued use whereas his mother was not in favour of this. In the fourth case (*Re G*), the patient's wife thought that continued provision of food and water was not in his best interests whereas his mother wished his feeding to continue (Grubb 1995a).

The interests of the medical and nursing staff caring for G were recognised in the argument that they might be reticent about becoming involved in supervising withdrawal of hydration and nutrition from *future* patients if their identity was disclosed in the course of the hearing. Another way in which staff interests might require consideration was pointed out by Lord Goff in his *Bland* judgement. He observed that:

> "The outward symptoms of dying in such a way (i.e. following withholding of food and water) which might otherwise cause distress to the nurses who care for him or to members of his family who visit him, can be suppressed by means of sedatives" (*Airedale NHS Trust v Bland* 1993: 871).

The context indicated that, whereas the distress belonged to the staff and family, the sedatives were to be administered to the patient. A striking example of the administration of pharmaceutical agents to one subject exclusively in the interests of others was provided by a recent recommendation for routine administration of a general anaesthetic and muscle relaxants to brain dead subjects during surgical removal of organs for transplantation. The basis for this recommendation was to prevent the potentially distressing experience, for operating theatre staff, of witnessing movements by organ donors in the course of surgery (Young and Matta 2000). Whilst a patient, once diagnosed as brain dead, lacks interests, others in a PVS are regarded as having diminished interests at best. The interests of the fetus carried by a woman in a PVS have been held to trump those of the mother as she would have effectively been deprived of "the sort of interests which normally underpin treatment decisions" (Peart *et al.* 2000).

Discussion in court has concentrated on the question of *who* should decide just *what* the interests of PVS patients are rather than that of whether actions most favourable to the PVS patient's interests can be discerned by others on his or her behalf. Legal arguments aside, Meilaender (1997) has drawn attention to the difference that arises when *others* make decisions for incapacitated patients. His principal point was that an important distinction exists between refusing treatment for oneself and refusing it for another. Patients' choices about their own treatment will involve judgements about quality of life. The assumption that others can make that choice on behalf of patients recalls Andrews' comments specifically discussing PVS patients: "Quality of life is something I have, not something you tell me I have" (Laurance 1996b).

Two methods, proposed in *Bland*, for deciding what would be *best* for the patient, as distinct from what he or she previously wished, have been either to visualise what the patient *might* request if granted a transient interval of awareness or to allocate to someone else, usually doctors or judges, the "right" of deciding precisely what is in the patient's best interests. As regards the first approach, Hoffman CJ suggested that if Anthony Bland were to be "momentarily restored to consciousness with full knowledge that he would shortly revert to his PVS", his doctors would be required to respect his wishes if he asked for withdrawal of hydration and nutrition (*Airedale NHS Trust v Bland* 1993: 852). Similarly, in the Irish case *In the Matter of a Ward of Court* which drew extensively on the Bland case, the initial trial judge proposed the formulation of a view on what the ward's wishes *would* have been had she been granted a momentary lucid and articulate period (*In the Matter of a Ward of Court*: 418). Quite apart from the absolutely fictional nature of this approach, the opinions expressed in court in the two cases about *precisely what* the patient would have wished (invariably death) were substantially at odds with reports of the attitudes of other people who have emerged from vegetative states (Chapter 9).

In considering *who* would be the appropriate person to make a decision for the patient Sir Stephen Brown, in the first *Bland* hearing, cited the 1957 case of *Bolam v Friern Hospital Management Committee* as a guide to the acceptability of the patient's doctors making a decision to withdraw hydration and nutrition (ibid: 829). This earlier decision had held that if a doctor's treatment of his or her patient was in accord with a large and responsible body of medical opinion, then it was legally acceptable. The *Bolam* precedent has been severely criticised by legal commentators including those who agreed with the final Bland decision. For example, Kennedy and Grubb (1993), while broadly endorsing the decision of the Law Lords, referred to Lord Mustill's dissent from the other four Law Lords in suggesting that the Bolam precedent should apply only to "the ascertainment of the medical raw material, such as diagnosis, prognosis and appraisal of the patient's cognitive functions" (ibid: 365). They suggested that the inclusion of a reference to the *Bolam* decision in the House of Lords *Bland* decision was intended primarily to bolster a conclusion already reached on other grounds rather than being intended as the decisive argument. In the course of his decision, Lord Mustill also acknowledged that judges had no more expertise than doctors when deciding on a patient's best interests (*Airedale NHS Trust v Bland*: 896). He had previously expressed his opinion on the lack of competence or entitlement of *anyone* to make decisions on behalf of others in terms of the distinction between the right to choose *one's own* death and the right to choose someone else's (ibid: 885).

15.16 TIME FOR CONSIDERATION

At several stages during judicial consideration of the request for a declaration that discontinuing the provision of food and water to Tony Bland would not be illegal, the point was stressed that, at least in the short term, any future requests for discontinuation of support for patients in a PVS should be considered in court. Recommendations that court hearings be required to approve future withdrawals of hydration and nutrition immediately set the provision of these services aside from every other type of medical treatment, notwithstanding the accompanying contention that tube feeding is *no different* from any other type of treatment. Decisions to discontinue the provision of medical treatment, including ventilation, renal dialysis and antibiotic therapy among others, to incompetent patients are made routinely on a large scale in medical practice without any requirement for court consideration. Nevertheless, in considering the case of Tony Bland and advising on court hearings for similar cases, the Family Division of the High Court, the Court of Appeal and the House of Lords all effectively placed tube feeding of PVS patients, and its cessation, in a category of its own.

The course to be followed in applying to a court for a declaration that tube feeding of a patient in a PVS may be discontinued was first outlined in 1996 in a Practice Note from the Official Solicitor (Practice Note 1996). Subsequently, with the appearance of cases manifesting a widening spectrum of features, and the change in terminology recommended by the Royal College of Physicians, that Practice Note was superseded. The revised version, issued in 2001, substituted "permanent" for "persistent" and required that the diagnosis of a permanent vegetative state not be made until the patient had been in a continuing vegetative state for 12 months following head injury or 6 months following other causes of brain damage. Presumably in response to earlier cases in which patients did not meet all criteria specified for diagnosis, the revised Practice Note emphasised that:

> "Diagnostic guidelines are not statutory provisions and a precise label may not be of importance" (Practice Note 2001).

The Court's concern should be whether there was any evidence of awareness or any possibility of change.

While each subsequent PVS patient had a day in court, as recommended in *Bland*, this was all that several had. Three cases of withdrawal of tube feeding out of the first 10 after *Bland* came to court as matters of urgency. These were *Frenchay Healthcare NHS Trust v S* (1994), *Swindon and Marlborough NHS Trust v S* (1995) and *Re D* (1997). In each case, the element of urgency was imparted by the accidental interruption of tube feeding. In the first case this resulted from dislodgement of the tube and, in the other two, from its blockage.

As already noted, the 12 month interval elapsing between *Bland* and *Frenchay v S* suggested to Grubb the possibility that this delay may have reflected a lack of consensus between the families of patients diagnosed as vegetative and their treating doctors. The hearing of *Frenchay NHS Trust v S* was treated as a matter of great urgency on the basis that the decision whether or not to resume feeding could not be deferred. In this case, the feeding tube was observed to be dislodged on January 10 and the case was in court on January 14. When the Official Solicitor requested an extension of time in order that a further neurological examination of S could be undertaken, this was disallowed. It was observed that the application could not be presented in the same "leisurely" way as a case where there was no pressure on time and a second opinion from an independent neurologist was not sought. In commenting on this case, Grubb queried whether the court had established, during its expedited hearing, that S was actually in a PVS. Having noted the remark of Sir Thomas Bingham that:

> "The evidence in this case is not as emphatic and not as unanimous as that in Bland's case", Grubb agreed and furthermore observed that although "S was sedated, he appeared to have some volitional behaviour, he seemed to feel distress and suffer pain" (Grubb 1994: 207).

These characteristics are not consistent with those of a PVS patient as envisaged either in the original description or in subsequent guidelines. As the follow up to *Bland*, *Frenchay v S* can hardly be said to have buttressed the decision of the first case or to have established a consistent procedural approach. The Bingham judgement averred that *Frenchay v S* did not involve an emergency situation in which application to the court was not necessary but proceeded to explain the dispensation from provision of two independent medical opinions as a reflection of its urgency. The reticence of the Frenchay Healthcare Authority to initiate temporary intravenous fluid administration pending a court decision contrasted with its subsequent use of this measure following dislodgement of a feeding tube from another of its patients, Catherine Roberts (Chapter 9).

In the case of *Swindon and Marlborough NHS Trust v S*, the next case after *Frenchay v S* which came to court later in 1994, the feeding tube of Mrs S, a 48 year old woman who had been unresponsive for 2 years following unsuccessful neurosurgery to remove a tumor, became blocked. Although only notified of the blockage late on a Friday afternoon, the Official Solicitor arranged an independent examination of Mrs S, who was being cared for at home, and a court hearing occurred on the Saturday afternoon, approving discontinuation of feeding (Grubb 1995b).

The case of Miss D was the tenth case concerned with withdrawal of hydration and nutrition from a patient in a PVS when it came to court in March, 1997 on the third day after dislodgement of a gastrostomy tube (Grubb 1997b). A feature of this case was that, preceding her loss of consciousness, Miss D was said to have been depressed when she expressed serious dissatisfaction with her quality of life. A history of depression should have encouraged her carers to interpret negative wishes with caution. The tendency of the non-disabled to discount depression in individuals with disabilities, discussed in Chapter 10, merits recall. These three cases are not in accord with the frequently advanced proposition of a lack of any significant ethical difference between *withdrawing* and *withholding*. It is difficult otherwise to comprehend the basis for great urgency in any of these cases. Accidental interruption of tube feeding converted the question facing the patient's medical attendants in each case from one of *withdrawing* to one of *withholding* and this was apparently regarded as more persuasive.

15.17 LEGAL EUPHEMISMS

> "Emollient expressions such as 'letting nature take its course' and 'easing the passing' may have their uses, but they are out of place here, for they conceal both the ethical and the legal issues" (*Airedale NHS Trust v Bland* 1993: 884).

The semantic fluidity evident in the vocabulary selected in articles and statements on PVS, including that entailed in the actual naming of the condition, has been influential in shaping the perceptions of medical personnel and the general public about affected individuals. The vocabulary employed in judicial decisions reveals some underlying perceptions. For instance, expressions such as "grotesquely alive" and as "not living a life at all" used by Lord Hoffman in the Court of Appeal (ibid: 854) were emotive in the extreme. Yet, ironically, in the course of delivering *his* judgement, Hoffman complained about the use of emotive language by the barrister retained by the Official Solicitor to represent the patient's interests. Interestingly Lord Hoffman acknowledged the assistance that he had received from reading the manuscript of Dworkin's book *Life's dominion* whilst preparing his judgement (ibid: 855). Dworkin's pejorative derivation of the noun corresponding to vegetative to categorise the PVS patient as "a manicured vegetable" has been remarked already in Chapter 1 (Dworkin 1993: 180). In delivering judgement on the application to withdraw support from Tony Bland in the Family Division of the High Court, Sir Stephen Brown set out his perception of the events after withdrawal in the following terms "the lack of sustenance would bring an end to the physical functioning of the body of Anthony Bland and he would in terms 'die'" (*Airedale NHS Trust v Bland* 1993: 825) (Sir Stephen's emphasis). He referred also to the retention by Tony Bland of "only the shell of his body" (ibid: 832).

The Bland case has not had a monopoly on colourful prose. A court hearing in 2000 was told of two patients who had been diagnosed as in a permanent vegetative state and were in "a twilight zone of suspended animation where death commences though some form of life continues" (Gibb 2000). The Irish Supreme Court in *In The Matter of a Ward of Court* (1995) surpassed the House of Lords in its "emollient" expressions. Chief Justice Hamilton observed of the patient, who had been fed by tube for 23 years, that without the benefit of this support she "would die within a short time and so must be regarded as being terminally ill" (ibid: 405). If applied logically and consistently, this reasoning would bode ill for patients receiving insulin for diabetes, home dialysis for renal failure or cyclosporin to prevent immune rejection of a transplanted heart, as without these supportive measures all certainly would die within a short time. The B.M.A. in its guidance on *Withholding and Withdrawing Life-Prolonging Medical Treatment* noted the inevitable inclusion of such individuals within definitions of terminal illness, which had been suitably adjusted to include patients in a PVS, and recommended the adoption of a number of "procedural safeguards" to avoid over-inclusivity (British Medical Association: 2001). The House of Lords Select Committee established in the wake of *Bland* restored some precision and honesty to the language with its definition of terminal illness, namely

> "An illness which is inevitably progressive, the effects of which cannot be reversed by treatment (although treatment may be successful in relieving symptoms temporarily) and which will inevitably result in death within a few months at most" (Select Committee House of Lords 1994).

Application of this definition would exclude PVS on the basis of its non-compliance with the first and last conditions.

The Irish Supreme Court in *In the Matter of a Ward of Court* attached considerable importance to the issue of whether any medical or nursing procedure was "natural" or otherwise. Thus, Lynch J considered that the patient should be allowed "to slip away naturally" by withdrawal of "abnormal artificial means". Apart from introducing the subjective and decidedly imprecise classification of 'normal' and 'abnormal', preoccupation in legal decision-making with "natural" and "normal" as identifiable classes with distinct, identifiable implications is highly questionable. Whilst the preceding examples of the creative use of language in courts have been drawn from cases in England and Ireland, any anthology of U.S. PVS court language would include some superb examples capable of holding their own in any company. The 1987 New Jersey hearing which authorised withdrawal of food and water from Nancy Jobes was told that some nurses believed that she responded appropriately to them. The appearance of what nurses described as "tears" was discounted by Dr Daniel Carlin with a turn of phrase which would have done George Orwell proud, namely "an unemotional collection of secretions in the corner of Mrs Jobes' eyes" (*In the Matter of Jobes*: 440).

15.18 WHAT WAS THE QUESTION ADDRESSED BY THE COURTS IN AIREDALE NHS TRUST V BLAND?

The "crafting" of the "correct question" has been identified as an important component of the decision in the *Bland* case (Savell 2001). In devising that question, Lord Browne-Willkinson decided that it should be whether it was in Bland's best interests "to continue the invasive medical care involved in artificial feeding". He emphasised that this was not the same as:

> "Is it in Anthony Bland's best interests that he should die?" (*Airedale NHS Trust v Bland* 1993: 883).

Had the "correct question" not been discovered, it is questionable whether their Lordships could have reached the same decision. Savell (2001), in reviewing the case 8 years later drew attention to a "filtering process" in the sense that a different description of the case would have been possible at a number of junctures. For example, opportunities for alternatives included the nature of tube feeding, whether it was beneficial or futile, whether its cessation was an act or an omission and whether its continuation was a necessity or an assault.

Commentaries on the subject of withdrawal of hydration and nutrition from patients in vegetative states have frequently concluded that the House of Lords decided that this procedure was legal. However, more specific commentary on this case has suggested that the decision would be more accurately summarised as one which ruled that the doctors responsible for the care of Anthony Bland had followed a proper process in deciding on what would be best for him. Consequently, their actions were held not to be illegal. Thus Lord Browne-Wilkinson considered that the question before the court was

> "not whether the court thinks it is in the best interests of Anthony Bland to continue to receive intrusive medical care but whether the responsible doctor has reached a reasonable and bona fide belief that it is not" (*Airedale NHS Trust v Bland* 1993: 883).

As mentioned above, several of their Lordships cited the earlier case of *Bolam v Friern Hospital Management Committee* (1957) to the effect that a belief could be reasonable if it accorded with the views of "a responsible body of medical opinion". The B.M.A. document cited on this issue of reasonableness was a discussion paper, not a definitive statement. A subsequent English court decision (*Bolitho v City and Hackney Health Authority* 1997) and an earlier Australian one (*Rogers v Whittaker* 1992) emphatically departed from a professional standard as the exclusive basis for assessing the reasonableness of medical decisions. Savell (2001) commented that the English court found that a practice could be unreasonable even though supported by a body of medical opinion whilst the Australian case abandoned a professional standard as the sole criterion for assessing the standard of medical care.

The U.K. High Court, the Court of Appeal and the House of Lords, all of which considered the Bland case, are required to rule on the *legality* as distinct from the *morality* of the course of action before it. Thus, Lord Browne-Wilkinson, recalling the issue of intent raised by Lord Goff, queried how withdrawal of hydration and nutrition from Anthony Bland could be legal whereas the administration of a lethal injection to him (to achieve precisely the same end result) would not be:

> "I find it difficult to find a moral answer to that question. But it is undoubtedly the law" (*Airedale NHS Trust v Bland* 1993: 880).

Rather more to the point, in his judgement, Lord Mustill categorised the law as "morally and intellectually misshapen".

Exemption of Anthony Bland's doctors from any guilt for his death following cessation of tube feeding was considered by Lord Mustill to depend "upon a very special application of the doctrine of causation" (ibid: 892). He envisaged the judgements that had been reached by the High Court and Court of Appeal as putting the ordinary law of causation into reverse. Rather than deciding whether the act (in this case, the cessation of feeding) was itself unlawful and then examining its causative relationship to Bland's death, Lord Mustill identified a variant in which application of "a special rule of causation" determined the nature of the act. Expressed more bluntly, an Australian legal commentary on their Lordships' reasoning in *Bland* concluded that to argue, as was done in this case, that the *real* cause of Anthony's death was the Hillsborough disaster and not the action of the doctors "is the logic of Alice in Wonderland, as is the purported 'distinction' between omission and commission" (Gerber 1994). Examined from a non-legal position, the most surprising aspect of both the court hearings and the ultimate decisions in *Airedale NHS Trust v Bland* appears to me to be the conscious diversion of successive benches towards the *mechanics* of proposed actions at the expense of the *intent* of those actions as the basis for their criminality or otherwise.

Perhaps the divergence between the law (on which decisions were based) and other considerations was most aptly summed up by Lord Browne-Wilkinson:

> "It is important, particularly in the area of criminal law which governs conduct that society's notions of what is law and what is right should correspond" (*Airedale NHS Trust v Bland* 1993: 881).

His lordship refrained from suggesting which position should be adjusted to achieve that correspondence. Subsequently, a legal commentary observed when commenting on "law-led ethics" that "legal precedent is no substitute for ethical argument" (Keown 2000).

15.19 RECAPITULATION

The cases of some patients in a PVS have entered courts when the medical attendants, and/or other members of the patient's family have sought approval to withhold or withdraw nutrition and hydration from the patient. Court cases relating to such patients have been heard with an extremely uneven distribution, almost all having occurred in the U.S. apart from some two dozen in England. The extent to which cases that have gone to court are representative of other cases that have not done so is unknown. Nevertheless, it is clear that the decisions reached in courts have exerted a substantial influence on attitudes to, and management of, others in a PVS as well as patients severely disabled with other medical conditions.

Courts have adopted several approaches in determining the outcome of applications for withdrawal of tube feeding from patients in a PVS. Advance directives have featured in decisions by U.S. courts. Limitations to their usefulness have included their non-availability when required and imprecision in specifying the medical conditions envisaged as bringing them into operation. Possible changes in a patient's wishes after a directive was prepared and the potential for adverse effects on medical and nursing staff complying with a directive to withdraw support may also complicate its implementation. Conflicts between the interests of the patient and those of his or her nominated proxy may also arise.

An alternative approach of seeking to decide on a course of action that is in the *best interests* of a patient generally requires a court to undertake a highly conjectural exercise which has been recognised as such by legal commentators and some jurists. In some instances, the course of action indicated by a *best interests* approach may be diametrically opposed to that requested in an advance directive.

Courts have increasingly moved to accepting withdrawal as the "default" position in the absence of evidence of a patient's contrary wishes. Inclusion of the withdrawal of tube feeding as equivalent to the withdrawal of life support modalities which are technically much more complex and invasive has been contested although U.S. and U.K. courts have generally lumped any form of procedure described as "life support" into a common category. This does not appear to be a position with which medical practitioners in all countries concur.

The case of *Airedale NHS Trust v Bland* which was the first to enter an English court has exerted a strong influence on subsequent cases in England and some other jurisdictions. The Bland case was notable for the extreme vitalist position adopted by the barrister presenting the case against withdrawal of feeding and his presentation evoked some strong negative responses from the bench. It was also notable for the paradox that Bland's medical attendants had elected not to withhold antibiotic treatment in response to any of the severe infections to which he had been subject *before* the case came to court. Such withholding, which would have been ethically and legally incontestable, is likely to have removed any need for an application to withdraw feeding.

Whilst the decision in *Bland* was delivered with the qualification, by some of the judges, that it may not have been identical in "less extreme" cases of PVS, the precedent of *Bland* appears to have been invoked without qualifications in subsequent English court cases. This trend has been especially noticeable in some cases in which conflicting evidence was presented about the diagnosis. I would question the extent to which successive benches hearing this case have established with certainty that the medical facts about PVS, as they understood them, were soundly established.

CHAPTER 16

CONTINUING UNRESPONSIVENESS IN THE FUTURE

The preceding fifteen Chapters have considered the basis for the prevailing understanding of vegetative states following brain injury and, especially, the manner in which the extensive literature on the subject has led to the attitudes towards affected individuals that are prevalent in both the health care and wider communities. In writing them, I have attempted to draw attention to those aspects of the literature which I regard as unreasonably neglected and insufficiently emphasised although central to any comprehensive account of these conditions. In my assessment, much of current teaching about vegetative states is insecurely based on assumptions.

Whilst much of my appraisal of evidence about vegetative states to this point has necessarily been negative, I intend now to introduce some positive suggestions of ways in which the understanding and management of patients diagnosed as being in vegetative states might be improved. It is unlikely that any single measure will produce dramatic improvement in the management of patients who remain unresponsive for prolonged periods after brain injury. Rather, it is reasonable to hope that gains can be made as a result of the cumulative impact of a number of approaches, some of which may seem, in isolation, to be more relevant in some health care systems than in others. Many of them may already be in use or under trial in one form or another.

16.1 A MORE OBJECTIVE NOMENCLATURE IS REQUIRED

The acronym "*PVS*" has acquired a life of its own. Whereas the term in its original form in which "*P*" denoted "*persistent*" may have facilitated communication among clinicians and assisted with concentration of collective attention on a group of patients who had previously been poorly characterised, its continued retention has become an obstacle to better patient management. I believe the concept of "*PVS*" to be seriously flawed both methodologically and sociologically. Methodologically, the attachment of the term "*PVS*" (irrespective of the imputed meaning of "*P*") or of the phrase "*the vegetative state*" to a group of clinical features represents the use of arbitrarily defined cut-off points to impose an all-or-nothing category on a continuous distribution. The likely existence of such a continuum of conditions was acknowledged in the original paper of Jennett and Plum but, together with other reasonable qualifications expressed at that time, it has become a casualty of a predilection for tidiness of expression at the expense of accuracy. Incidentally, the success of "*PVS*" as a term provides an excellent example of the dominance of acronyms in technical vocabularies in the latter part of the twentieth century.

Sociologically, as discussed in Chapter One, the power of a simplistic description to convey a forceful picture of the person to whom it is applied has been overwhelming. This, and the impression of scientific precision conveyed by the term, have been highly persuasive when introduced into a legal context. Impressions and attitudes invariably shape assessments and judgements. There has been a high frequency of transformation of the description "vegetative" into the form of the noun "vegetable", or, in a Australian context, "vegie".

To conclude that the "PVS" terminology is unsatisfactory is not claimed to be either novel or original. Many of those who have written on the subject have called for a change but the prevailing conclusion has been that this would not be possible. In the collective opinion of the International Working Party on the Vegetative State, the word "vegetative" generated a nihilistic attitude to any form of treatment but:

> "Nevertheless it was considered that the term is so ingrained in medical and legal terminology that it would be difficult to introduce new terminology at this stage" (International Working Party 1996: 5).

16.2 POSSIBILITIES FOR PREVENTION OF PVS SHOULD BE EXPLORED

As with any medical condition, strategies directed towards its prevention should logically constitute a first management option. Three possibilities for the prevention of PVS are apparent. In the first place, any success achieved with programs that aim to reduce the occurrence of traumatic brain injury or to avoid conditions predisposing to cerebral vascular accidents and cerebral hypoxia could reasonably be expected to reduce the incidence of cases of vegetative states. Secondly, to the extent that the appearance of cases of people in a PVS has resulted, as often asserted, from improvements in the early management of head injury permitting the survival of patients who would otherwise have died it would seem reasonable to predict that the ongoing continuation of that improvement in intensive care practice should be accompanied, not only by the saving of life in the short term, but by improved outcomes among survivors. To predict this in the case of the intensive care of patients with brain injury is to do no more than to highlight the *continuing* improvement in medical practice that is part and parcel of the advocacy of clinical medical research. Similarly, likely improvements in the early management of cerebral vascular accidents should have the effect, not only of saving lives, but also of lessening levels of residual disability among survivors.

A third possible approach to reducing the occurrence of cases of PVS could be to predict the outcome in individual cases of brain injury at an early stage and to withdraw ventilator support from those patients whom, it was judged, were going to have an "*unfavourable*" outcome. Discontinuation of ventilator support of patients not breathing spontaneously has been an available option, to be exercised in the case of patients not benefiting from the technology, since it was refined in the middle of the twentieth century. If any particular therapeutic measure is not likely to benefit a patient, it has always been legitimate, as a general principle, for a medical practitioner to withhold or withdraw that measure. Contrary to some popular impressions, it was not necessary, on medical grounds, for the concept of brain death to be discovered and defined in order for decisions to be made to withdraw ventilator support from patients with a devastating degree of brain damage. (Apprehension about litigation may have been an inhibitory influence in some situations, notwithstanding sound medical indications). One is not obliged to continue treatment which is unlikely to be of benefit to a patient. Withdrawal would be discussed with patient and/or family and, in the event of their disagreement with the proposition would often not be implemented. However, as discussed in earlier Chapters, the medical decision appears likely increasingly to prevail in the U.K. when there is disagreement.

The technique which has been most frequently applied to achieving early discrimination between "favourable" and "unfavourable" outcomes in patients with severe brain injury has entailed the measurement of somatosensory evoked potentials (SEP). The possible qualification to application of SEP testing for this purpose that has been identified in reports of use of the technique, but dismissed by some SEP protagonists as not sufficiently inhibitory to prevent its use, is that a small percentage of patients who were predicted by SEP to have an "unfavourable" outcome could actually have had a "favourable" one if support had been continued. However, the other issue on which I suggest (in Chapter 6) that the use of SEP measurement as a means of identifying patients with a likely "unfavourable" outcome comes to grief is that of the poor discriminative capacity of the technique. Thus the rubric of "unfavourable outcome" as identified acutely by SEP fails to discriminate between patients with three discrete types of outcome. One subpopulation of patients with an adverse SEP result will die, irrespective of what acute treatment is provided. A second, and the smallest, subpopulation will continue to be regarded as in a vegetative state at 6 months. The third subpopulation of those with unfavourable SEP results at the acute stage will be observed to regain consciousness and recover, albeit to an extent insufficient to permit independent living. At the present time, SEP technology appears unable to discriminate between these three groups at the acute stage following brain injury when patients remain ventilator dependent and withdrawal of this support is likely to lead to death.

If the available SEP technology were to improve to the extent of permitting reliable differentiation between the three types of outcome classed as "*unfavourable*", I would anticipate that most of the community, whether able bodied or disabled, would accept the practice of early ventilator disconnection from those patients whom SEP indicated would die irrespective of the treatment that was provided. On the other hand, I suspect that a majority of the disabled community, and their families and friends, would find early withdrawal of ventilator support from the third subpopulation of patients, namely those for whom SEP results predicted an inability to resume independent living, totally unacceptable. This interpretation runs counter to that of many non-disabled commentators who consider that no one with a high level of dependency would wish to continue to live and advocate accordingly that none should have that opportunity. Kadish (1992) has drawn an interesting distinction between one's approach to this question depending upon the identity of the disabled subject. In discussing Dworkin's finding that respondents expressed a preference for death if they were to be faced with senile dementia, Kadish re-phrased the question so that it related to a decision *on behalf of another individual*. He reported that a number of respondents indicated that:

> "They themselves would prefer to die rather than to hang on to a life so limited. They are not so ready, however, to inflict the same fate on another person on the basis of their own preference" (ibid: 873).

Responses to the proposition that ventilator support be discontinued at an early stage from those individuals indicated by SEP to be destined to be in a vegetative state at 6 months (assuming that this level of discrimination became technically feasible) would presumably be mixed and would be likely to reflect the extent of understanding of vegetative states in the general community. This leads on to a third positive suggestion.

16.3 POLICY FORMULATION SHOULD BE RESPONSIVE TO ADEQUATELY INFORMED COMMUNITY INPUT

As the management decisions which have been made in instances of high profile cases of PVS have affected the medical management of other individuals with entirely different medical conditions, and will inevitably continue to affect others throughout the community, it is entirely reasonable for the wider community to have the opportunity to influence development of public policy about the manner in which patients with continuing unresponsiveness should be treated. I believe that there should be adequate presentation of all that is known (and, equally important, acknowledgement of what is *not* known) about people diagnosed as vegetative, followed by extended discussion, before policy is formulated. This certainly has not occurred to date in any location. That decisions resting on analysis of technical medical detail require input of medical expertise is incontestable. The same cannot be said, however, of decisions about the personhood status of specified categories of patients and the management courses explicitly selected on the basis of those personhood decisions.

Some writing on vegetative states has accepted the existence of "persons" as a subpopulation of "human beings". The defining attributes of "persons" correspond with the capacities which are defined as lacking in vegetative states. Personhood cannot be diagnosed by a biopsy or a scan. Medical personnel are as entitled as philosophers, ethicists, lawyers and those within other fields of expertise to express their opinions on the subject and to specify sets of criteria giving entitlement to "personhood". On the basis that all *experts* become *lay people* once outside the confines of their special expertise, anyone with a value system is likely to possess views as to what a person is. On *this* subject, we are all, at the same time, experts and lay people. The assessment formed by the family of a young man in a prolonged unresponsive state may be based on a more profound perspective of his personhood status than that of any published authority on the subject.

Some of the positions asserted by sections of the medical community, in relation to the diagnosis of PVS, could not be seen by the non-medical community and by medical practitioners in other specialties as other than unsupportable self-delusion. The 1989 declaration of the American Academy of Neurology quoted in Chapter 3 to the effect that:

> "Only a neurological organization can make a definite statement on the neurological facts as the Academy does"

comes readily to mind as a striking example of this. This approach of talking down to anyone not in the peer group and justifying a statement exclusively on the authority of those presenting it recalls the 1957 article on scientific outlook by the chemist Michael Polyani:

> "In the days when an idea could be silenced by showing that it was contrary to religion, theology was the greatest single source of fallacies. Today, when any human thought can be discredited by branding it as unscientific, the power exercised previously by theology has passed over to science; hence, science has become the greatest single source of error" (ibid: 480).

What I believe is required in initiating any wider community debate about the possible nature of ongoing unresponsiveness and the way in which affected individuals are to be regarded is some acknowledgement from medical sources of the manner in which assumptions relating to the subject have frequently been traded as proven facts. There is no logical reason why the repeated assertion of an assumption, increasingly shorn of its original qualifications, should validate its metamorphosis into an unchallenged fact, but this is precisely what has happened with many claims relating to patients diagnosed as in a PVS as exemplified in earlier Chapters. It is necessary to acknowledge that many questions about these patients that are unanswered may remain unanswerable and that value judgements may have to be applied to answers that are probabilistic at best.

16.4 NEURO-REHABILITATION SHOULD BE INSTITUTED EARLIER AFTER BRAIN INJURY

It would intuitively appear more likely that outcomes after brain injury could be improved with a consequent lessening of the period spent by some patients in an unresponsive state if cognitive rehabilitation programs, which included family members whenever possible, could be initiated at the earliest practicable stage, perhaps as soon as the immediate threat to life has abated in an intensive care unit. Against this, it has been argued that the utmost rest with minimisation of sensory input to the patient is the preferable course. The mounting of randomised control trials of these two approaches to resolve the question of which is superior has not proved to be practicable, nor is it likely to become so. Given the possible range of neurological differences between successive patients after brain injury, randomisation would soon be likely to conflict with the medical practitioner's clinical judgement as to which course was likely to be optimal for a specific patient. Furthermore, it would probably create an ethically unsustainable situation in the relationship of ward staff to families if some patients were to receive much more intensive attention than others.

The general acceptance of the association between a prolonged period in coma and an unfavourable outcome provides a case for early, rather than minimal, intervention. The association could be interpreted solely as an indication that both length of the period in coma and ultimate outcome are dependent upon severity of the original brain injury. However, it is equally legitimate to infer that lengthening of the duration of coma *itself* adversely affects the ultimate outcome. The latter interpretation throws the onus of proof firmly on those opposed to attempts at expediting arousal.

Speculating on the basis of recent findings in neuroscience research which have drawn attention to previously unsuspected plasticity in the nervous system, detected dividing neurones in the brains of adult patients and isolated multipotential stem cells from the brains of mature animals, one might anticipate the existence of a considerably greater potential for recovery by the injured brain than was envisaged in the past. This would strongly support the adoption of more vigorous rehabilitation efforts, provided adverse unwanted effects of this were considered to be unlikely. The possibility of producing habituation as a result of excessive sensory stimulation was raised in Chapter 4, but if this was avoided, any risks of early attempts at rehabilitation would appear to be outweighed by possible benefits.

16.5 DIVERSE MEDICAL AND PARAMEDICAL SKILLS ARE REQUIRED IN THE MANAGEMENT OF PATIENTS WHO REMAIN UNRESPONSIVE AFTER BRAIN INJURY

As discussed in Chapter 11 when dealing with positive aspects of the management of patients in a PVS, the outlook of neurologists and neurosurgeons frequently appears to be at variance with that of rehabilitation specialists. Whilst the former have a crucial role, together with intensivists, in the early detection and rectification of any remediable conditions and in preventing aggravation of the initial injury, their contribution once a vegetative state has developed is, according to Richard Beresford as noted in Chapter 8, limited to getting the diagnosis right. However, it is not difficult to detect a *proprietorial* attitude towards vegetative states, which extends to the patients affected by them, in the writings of some neurological specialists. Similarly, one sometimes senses the existence of an adversarial relationship between neurosurgeons and rehabilitation specialists. Consider, for example, the dismissive attitude of Ronald Cranford, recorded in Chapter 8, towards the specialised communication system used by Andrews *et al.* (1996). Management of patients diagnosed as vegetative should be undertaken by a multidisciplinary team. Responses to programs of structured sensory input are likely to be very gradual and to require repeated assessment by members of such a team with the requisite skills.

16.6 RESOURCES SHOULD BE PROVIDED FOR SPECIALISED FACILITIES WHICH ARE LIKELY TO HAVE A HIGHER REHABILITATION SUCCESS RATE

Many of the reports of patients emerging from a vegetative state that were discussed in Chapter 9 came from clinics or institutions with a specific interest and expertise in working with these patients. In the absence of any comprehensive sets of data on prevalence, let alone longer term outcomes, of patients in vegetative states, it is not possible to be adamant about the value of specialised referral centres which concentrate their efforts on this group of patients. It would, however, be surprising if they did not achieve better results than any likely to occur in those younger patients with longer term unresponsiveness after brain injury who have been consigned to nursing homes for the elderly. Specialised facilities such as those at Putney in the U.K. and Berck-sur-Mer in France are likely to offer the best chance of *detection* of any improvement and probably also of *initiating* or *accelerating* that improvement by meticulous attention to those aspects of a patient's condition likely to obscure or impede it. As with almost all aspects of vegetative states, it is not possible to eliminate confounding factors when assessing outcomes. In the case of specialised neuro-rehabilitation facilities, it may well be that the profile of their admissions reflects the persistence and commitment of the patient's family rather than representing an unselected sample of patients with a common problem. Witness the single-mindedness of the relatives of patients, regarded as vegetative, who have persisted with the patients while their vegetative state has not done so. When considering specialised facilities intended specifically for those who have been diagnosed as vegetative, it is worth noting that selection processes have commonly operated *against* these patients to exclude them from more conventional rehabilitation programs. These, like many medical facilities, often make strenuous efforts to pick the likely winners.

Potential disadvantages of specialised facilities include their cost of operation which will significantly exceed that of any basic "care and maintenance" regime. As suggested in Chapter 14, it is likely that the greatest expense may be incurred by younger patients and by those with the most severe complications (and so least likely to survive for an extended period). It is also likely that costs will be greatest in the early stages and can be expected to taper as less ambitious goals replace those initially in place for patients who show little or no improvement and the transition to long term care occurs. Another substantial disadvantage of specialised central referral facilities is the potential deleterious effect either of separation of the patient from his or her family or, alternatively, of family relocation when home and institution are geographically separated. An alternative to specialised institutional placement, if that is not available, and a possible sequel to it when it is, can be domiciliary care together with adequate support of the family carers.

16.7 PATIENTS DO BETTER WHEN FED

The issue of nutrition in relation to patients with severe brain injury has most commonly come to prominence in the context of its withdrawal, accompanied by that of hydration, when both are being administered by nasogastric tube or percutaneous endoscopic gastrostomy tube. However, as indicated in Chapter 11 when discussing positive management, the increased level of catabolism that occurs in patients with brain injury will predictably generate a substantial increase in their nutritional requirements. That this need is commonly *not* adequately met is graphically illustrated by the underweight and frequently emaciated condition of patients in a vegetative state. Reference was made, in Chapter 6, to the frequent occurrence, in patients with anorexia nervosa, of cerebral atrophic changes resembling those reported on CT scans of vegetative patients. It was suggested there that the subnutritional status of many vegetative patients might aggravate the atrophic changes initiated by the brain injury itself. It has been adequately demonstrated that subnutritional status impairs neuronal multiplication in young humans and experimental animals. Consequently, it is likely also to retard the neuronal multiplication which recent studies imply could be a practical proposition during repair following injury to the *adult* human brain. There appear to be good grounds for advocating the implementation of strategies to augment the nutritional status of patients.

Withdrawal of nutrition and hydration from patients considered to be in, or near to, a PVS has been sanctioned by courts of several jurisdictions, as summarised in Chapter 15. Whilst these cases have usually been framed in terms of the withdrawal representing the course of action that the specific patient would have wanted, or of being in the best interests of the patient, the U.K. hearings in *Airedale NHS Trust v Bland* resulted in explicit statements of a more direct intent. As stated by the Official Solicitor's barrister appearing on behalf of Bland and recognised by the Law Lords in the course of decisions approving withdrawal, this course was being taken with the intention of ending Bland's life. One of the judgements specifically drew attention to the distorted situation that intentionally ending his life by withdrawal of hydration and nutrition was legal in the U.K. whereas achieving the same end by means of a lethal injection would be illegal. This recruitment of the legal strategy of withdrawal of hydration and nutrition to support the concept of the right to die and thence of legalised euthanasia appears likely to be a temporary conjunction. Thus, once legislation authorising euthanasia has been passed, as in the Netherlands, it is most unlikely that any solution that is as slow and as potentially disconcerting for the nursing staff as withdrawal of hydration and nutrition from their patient will continue to be practised. The comments attributed to the prominent Dutch euthanasia practitioner Dr Admiraal condemning withdrawal as an unacceptable technique, which were included in Chapter 13, say as much.

Leaving aside the recruitment of withdrawal of hydration and nutrition as one, legally applicable, method of ending life, I accept that *any* therapeutic measure, including the provision of feeding by means of a tube, may legitimately be withdrawn if it has become ineffective and/or burdensome for the patient. I would have no objection to the withdrawal of feeding which for any reason (for example, failure of absorption from the gut) was ineffective for maintenance of nutritional status, which was burdensome in requiring a disproportionate effort to achieve it or which was being gratuitously administered to a dying patient.

16.8 RESEARCH WITH PATIENTS IN VEGETATIVE STATES IS NEEDED TO IMPROVE MANAGEMENT

Any specialised facility intended for the care and attempted rehabilitation of patients in a vegetative state is likely to be learning from observation of its patients and their responses to various protocols on an ongoing basis. In this sense, such facilities are likely to be undertaking continuous research in parallel with providing treatment. Nevertheless, I envisage at least three areas in which formal approaches to research into continuing unconsciousness after brain injury is strongly indicated.

The first research topic concerns the application of functional imaging technology to separate the spectrum of conditions encompassed by the present terminology into subgroups with differing prognoses who are likely to benefit from different management approaches. Present indications are that the use of functional magnetic resonance imaging may be the most worthwhile approach to differentiating groups of patients with different functional deficits and differing prognoses. It is of interest, in passing, to note that positron emission tomography, the application of which to PVS patients was first reported in 1987 and which has often been claimed in reviews, rather than in primary articles, to have considerable diagnostic power, has been the subject of very few recent reports enhancing its value in diagnosis.

The second area which, I believe, would be likely to benefit from intensive research is that of the improvement of technology designed to facilitate communication with patients judged to be unresponsive by conventional criteria. It may be that the experimental development of this technology remains disproportionately in advance of the training of adequate numbers of medical and paramedical personnel in its use.

Finally, there appears to be a limited place, in highly specialised centres, for examination of deep brain stimulation following the introduction of electrodes. As indicated in Chapter 11, this remains an approach with more to offer as a basic research tool with which to gain information about disordered brain function in general than as a therapeutic measure for the individual patient. Conceivably, electrical stimulation may provide some new insights into the pathophysiology of the injured brain. The response to such stimulation may also assist in the identification of subpopulations of unresponsive patients who have different prognoses. Given its highly invasive nature, this area of research raises ethical issues which are considerably more substantial than either of the preceding two. The uncertainty over the likelihood of benefit to the individual patient who is the research subject, as distinct from longer term benefits to a *class* of patients further compounds those issues. The necessity to obtain proxy consent on behalf of patients incompetent to provide or withdraw consent directly augments the ethical complexity. To accept that patients scheduled for withdrawal of support because they were no longer persons could, for the same reason, be supported for *use* in experimentation would be unconscionable.

16.9 IN CONCLUSION

Whereas the concept of a vegetative state may have been regarded, when introduced, as a modest proposal to facilitate communication between practitioners and so to encourage the accumulation of data, it has increasingly served to entrench opinions as fact and to inhibit attempts to improve rehabilitation strategies. Notwithstanding the substantial gaps that exist in understanding consciousness and the unresponsiveness that defines PVS, pronouncements installing it as an archetypal condition determining attitudes towards patients with a variety of other conditions have become commonplace. It is time for reappraisal of the subject of vegetative states.

REFERENCES

Adams, J.H., D.I. Graham. and B. Jennett. "The neuropathology of the vegetative state after an acute brain insult." *Brain* 123.7 (2000): 1327-1338.

Affidavit of Carol J. Gill. In the United States District Court for the District of Oregon. 30 November 1994.

Agardh, C.D., I. Rosen. and E. Ryding. "Persistent vegetative state with high cerebral blood flow following profound hypoglycemia." *Annals of Neurology* 14.4 (1983): 482-486.

Ahronheim, J.C. and M.R. Gasner. "The sloganism of starvation." *The Lancet* 335.8684 (1990): 278-279.

Airedale NHS Trust v Bland (1993) AC789; (1993) 2 WLR 315; 1 All ER 821. Citations are to the All England Reports.

Alfonso, I., W.A. Lanting., D. Duenas., *et al*. "Discontinuation of artificial hydration and nutrition in hopelessly vegetative children." *Annals of Neurology* 32.3 (1992): 454-455

Alkire, M.T., R.J. Haier., S.J. Barker., *et al*. "Cerebral metabolism during propofol anaesthesia in humans studied with positron emission tomography." *Anesthesiology* 82.2 (1995): 393-403.

Alkire, M.T., R.J. Haier., N.K. Shah., *et al*. "Positron emission tomography study of regional cerebral metabolism in humans during isoflurane anaesthesia." *Anesthesiology* 86.3 (1997): 549-557.

American Academy of Neurology Executive Board. "Position of the American Academy of Neurology on certain aspects of the care and management of the persistent vegetative state patient." *Neurology* 39.1 (1989): 125-126.

American Academy of Neurology. Quality Standards Committee. "Practice parameters: assessment and management of patients in the persistent vegetative state." *Neurology* 45.5 (1995): 1015-1018.

American Congress of Rehabilitation Medicine. "Recommendations for use of uniform nomenclature pertinent to patients with severe alterations in consciousness." *Archives of Physical Medicine and Rehabilitation* 76.2 (1995): 205-209.

American Medical Association Council on Ethical and Judicial Affairs *Current Opinions*. Section 2.18. Chicago: American Medical Association, 1986.

American Medical Association Council on Scientific Affairs and Council on Ethical and Judicial Affairs. "Persistent vegetative state and the decision to withdraw or withhold life support." *Journal of the American Medical Association* 263.3 (1990): 426-430.

American Medical Association. *Amicus Curiae* brief, Pp 11/12, Cruzan v Director, 497 U.S. 261 (1990).

American Medical Association. Council on Ethical and Judicial Affairs. "The use of anencephalic neonates as organ donors." *Journal of the American Medical Association* 273.20 (1995): 1614-1618.

American Medical Association, Council on Ethical and Judicial Affairs. "Medical futility in end-of-life care." *Journal of the American Medical Association* 281.10 (1999): 937-941.

American Neurological Association Committee on Ethical Affairs. "Persistent vegetative state: Report of the A.N.A. Committee on Ethical Affairs." *Annals of Neurology* 33.4 (1993): 386-391.

American Physiological Society. *Handbook of Physiology. Vol. 1 Control of Food and Water Intake*. Edited by C.F. Code. Washington, D.C 1963.

American Thoracic Society Bioethics Task Force. "Withholding and withdrawing life-sustaining therapy." *Annals of Internal Medicine* 115.6 (1991): 478-485.

Andersson, B., and W. Wyrwicka. "The elicitation of a drinking motor conditioned reaction by electrical stimulation of the hypothalamic 'drinking area' in the goat." *Acta Physiologica Scandinavia* 41.2-3 (1957): 194-198.

Andrade, J. "Learning during anaesthesia: A review." *British Journal of Psychology* 86.4 (1995): 479-506.

Andrews, K. "Managing the persistent vegetative state." *British Medical Journal* 305.6852 (1992a): 486-487.

Andrews, K. "Letting vegetative patients die." *British Medical Journal* 305.6867 (1992b): 1506.

Andrews, K. "Recovery of patients after four months or more in the persistent vegetative state." *British Medical Journal* 306.6892 (1993a): 1597-1600.

Andrews, K. "Patients in the persistent vegetative state: problems in their long term management." *British Medical Journal* 306.6892 (1993b): 1600-1602.

Andrews, K. "Should PVS patients be treated?" *Neuropsychological Rehabilitation* 3.2 (1993c): 109-119.

Andrews, K. "Managing patients in a persistent vegetative state." *British Medical Journal* 307.6908 (1993d): 870.

Andrews, K. "Tortuous arguments evade the issue." *British Medical Journal* 311.7017 (1995): 1437.

Andrews, K. "International Working Party on the management of the vegetative state: Summary report." *Brain Injury* 10.11 (1996): 796-806.

Andrews, K. "Vegetative state - background and ethics." *Journal of the Royal Society of Medicine* 90.11 (1997): 593-596.

Andrews, K., L. Murphy., R. Munday., *et al.* "Misdiagnosis of the vegetative state: retrospective study in a rehabilitation unit." *British Medical Journal* 313.7048 (1996): 13-16.

Angell, M. "Prisoners of technology. The case of Nancy Cruzan." *New England Journal of Medicine* 322.17 (1990): 1226-1228.

Angell, M. "The case of Helga Wanglie. A new kind of 'Right to Die' case." *New England Journal of Medicine* 325.7 (1991): 511-512.

Angell, M. "After Quinlan: The dilemma of the persistent vegetative state." *New England Journal of Medicine* 330.21 (1994): 1524–1525.

Anon. "Managing the persistent vegetative state." *British Medical Journal* 305.6858 (1992): 886.

Anon. "'I was right to let my girl live after horror smash." *The Standard Recorder* (Basildon) 11 January 1996.

Anon. "Tighter rules on when to allow coma victims die." *The Weekly Telegraph* (London) 21 February 1996.

Anon. "Dilemma for judge in right to die case." *The Daily Express* (London) 21 March 1997.

Anon. "Church bars euthanasia but not all forms of assisted death." *The Daily Telegraph* (London) 30 July 1998.

Anon. "Coma victim's mother attacks testing plan." *The Independent* (London) 9 April 1996.

Appassamy, M. "Doctors said he'd never wake up. They were wrong." *The Daily Express* (London) 27 March 1997.

Armstrong, P.W. and B.D. Colen. "From Quinlan to Jobes: the courts and the PVS patient." *Hastings Center Report* 18.1 (1988): 37-40.

Artmann, H., H. Grau., M. Adelmann., *et al.* "Reversible and non-reversible enlargement of cerebrospinal fluid spaces in anorexia nervosa." *Neuroradiology* 27.4 (1985): 304-312.

Arts, W.F.M., H.R. van Dongen., J.V. Hof van Duin., *et al.* "Unexpected improvement after prolonged posttraumatic vegetative state." *Journal of Neurology, Neurosurgery, and Psychiatry* 48.12 (1985): 1300-1303.

Asai, A., M. Maekawa., I. Akiguchi., *et al.* "Survey of Japanese physicians' attitudes towards the care of adult patients in persistent vegetative state." *Journal of Medical Ethics* 25.4 (1999): 302-308.

Ashwal, S., J.F. Bale., D.L. Coulter., *et al.* "The persistent vegetative state in children: Report of the child neurology society ethics committee." *Annals of Neurology* 32.4 (1992): 570-576.

Ashwal, S. and R. Cranford. "The brain of Karen Ann Quinlan. Authors' reply." *New England Journal of Medicine* 331.20 (1994): 1381.

Ashwal, S., R.K. Eyman. and T.L. Call. "Life expectancy of children in a persistent vegetative state." *Pediatric Neurology* 10.1 (1994): 27-33.

Astrup, J. "Energy-requiring cell functions in the ischemic brain." *Journal of Neurosurgery* 56.4 (1982): 482-497.

Attia, J. and D.J. Cook. "Prognosis in anoxic and traumatic coma." *Critical Care Clinics* 14.3 (1998): 497-511.

Auckland Area Health Board v Attorney-General. (1993) 1NZLR 235.

Austin, G. "So whose life is it anyway?" *The Daily Express* (London) 9 January 1996.

Avila, D. "The brain of Karen Ann Quinlan." *New England Journal of Medicine* 331.20 (1994): 1382.

Avorn, J. "Benefit and cost analysis in geriatric care: Turning age discrimination into health policy." *New England Journal of Medicine* 310.20 (1984): 1294-1301.

Bach, J.R. and V. Barnett. "Ethical considerations in the management of individuals with severe neuromuscular disorders." *American Journal of Physical Medicine and Rehabilitation* 73.2 (1994): 134-140.

Baillie, P., and S.D. Morrison. "The nature of the suppression of food intake by lateral hypothalamic lesions in rats." *Journal of Physiology* 165.2 (1963): 227-245.

Bakran, A. "Organ donation and permanent vegetative state." *The Lancet* 351.9097 (1998): 211-212.

Banja, J.D. "Does the Americans with Disabilities Act protect persons in the persistent vegetative state?" *Journal of Head Trauma Rehabilitation* 8.4 (1993): 108-111.

Baron, C. "On taking substituted judgement seriously." *Hastings Center Report* 20.5 (1990): 7-8.

Bauby, J-D. *The diving-bell and the butterfly*. London: Fourth Estate, 1997.

Bauer, G., F. Gerstenbrand. and E. Rumpl. "Varieties of the locked-in syndrome." *Journal of Neurology* 221.1 (1979): 77-91.

Bayer, R., D. Callahan., J. Fletcher., *et al.* "The care of the terminally ill: Morality and economics." *New England Journal of Medicine* 309.24 (1983): 1490-1494.

Beca, J., P.N. Cox., M.J. Taylor., *et al.* "Somatosensory evoked potentials for prediction of outcome in acute severe brain injury." *Journal of Pediatrics* 126.1 (1995): 44-49.

Beecher, H.K. "A definition of irreversible coma. Report of the Ad Hoc Committee of the Harvard Medical School to examine the definition of brain death." *Journal of the American Medical Association* 205.6 (1968): 337-340.

Bennett, H.L., H.S. Davis. and J.A. Giannini. "Non-verbal response to intraoperative conversation." *British Journal of Anaesthesia* 57.2 (1985): 174-179.

Bennett, M.R. *The idea of consciousness*. Amsterdam: Harwood, 1997.

Beresford, H.R. "The persistent vegetative state: a view across the legal divide." *Annals of the New York Academy of Sciences* 835 (1997): 386-394.

Berger, S. "EU rule will allow medical research on handicapped." *The Daily Telegraph* (London) April 7 1997.

Berghmans, R.L.P. "Advance directives for non-therapeutic dementia research: some ethical and policy considerations." *Journal of Medical Ethics* 24.1 (1998): 32-37.

Bernat, J.L. "How much of the brain must die in brain death?" *Journal of Clinical Ethics* 3.1 (1992a): 21-26.

Bernat, J.L. "The boundaries of the persistent vegetative state." *Journal of Clinical Ethics* 3.3 (1992b): 176-80.

Bernat, J.L. "A defense of the whole-brain concept of death." *Hastings Center Report* 28.2 (1998): 14-23.

Bernat, J.L. "Refinements in the definition and criterion of death." In *The definition of death*, edited by S.J. Youngner, R.M. Arnold and R. Schapiro, 83-92. Baltimore: Johns Hopkins University Press, 1999.

Bernat, J.L. "Questions remaining about the minimally conscious state." *Neurology* 58.3 (2002): 337-338.

Berrol, S. "Evolution and the persistent vegetative state." *Journal of Head Trauma Rehabilitation* 1.1 (1986a): 7-13.

Berrol, S. "Considerations for management of the persistent vegetative state." *Archives of Physical Medicine and Rehabilitation* 67.5 (1986b): 283-285.

Billings, J.A. "Comfort measures for the terminally ill. Is dehydration painful?" *Journal of the American Geriatrics Society* 33.11 (1985): 808-810.

Blacklock, J.B., E.H. Oldfield., G. DiChiro., *et al.* "Effect of barbiturate coma on glucose utilization in normal brain versus gliomas. Positron emission studies." *Journal of Neurosurgery* 67.1 (1987): 71-75.

Block, R.I., M.M. Ghoneim., S.T. Sum Ping., *et al.* "Human learning during general anaesthesia and surgery." *British Journal of Anaesthesia* 66.2 (1991): 170-178.

Bodenhamer, E., J. Achterberg-Lawlis., G. Kevorkian., *et al.* "Staff and patient perceptions of the psychosocial concerns of spinal cord injured persons." *American Journal of Physical Medicine* 62.4 (1983): 182-193.

Bolam v Friern Hospital Management Committee 1 WLR 582, 1957.

Bolitho v City and Hackney Health Authority 3 WLR 1151, 1997.

Bopp, J. "Choosing death for Nancy Cruzan." *Hastings Center Report* 20.1 (1990): 42-44.

Bopp, J., T.J. Marzen., M.M. Nimz., *et al.* "Abridged brief as *Amici Curiae* of the Association for Retarded Citizens of the United States *et al.*" *Journal of the American Geriatrics Society* 38.5 (1990): 580-587.

Borthwick, C.J. "The permanent vegetative state: Ethical crux, medical fiction?" *Issues in Law and Medicine* 12.2 (1996): 167-183.

Borthwick, C. "A small claim for speciesism." *Monash Bioethics Review* 17.2 (1998): 30-34.

Bowcott, O. "Fan's recovery 'unique'. Soccer victim's emergence from vegetative state began in 1994." *The Guardian* (London) 27 March 1997.

Boyle, M.E. and R.D. Greer. "Operant procedures and the comatose patient." *Journal of Applied Behavior Analysis* 16.1 (1983): 3-12.

Braakman, R., W.B. Jennett. and J.M. Minderhoud. "Prognosis of the posttraumatic vegetative state." *Acta Neurochirurgica* (Wein) 95.1 (1988): 49-52.

Braithwaite, S. and D.C. Thomasma. "New guidelines on foregoing life-sustaining treatment in incompetent patients: An anti-cruelty policy." *Annals of Internal Medicine* 104.5 (1988): 711-715.

Brennan, Z. "Coma blunder ends in horror." *The Sunday Times* (London) 21 February 1999.

Brett, A.S. and L.B. McCullough. "When patients request specific interventions. Defining the limits of the physician's obligation." *New England Journal of Medicine* 315.21 (1986): 1347-1351.

Bricolo, A., S. Turazzi. and G. Feriotti. "Prolonged posttraumatic unconsciousness. Therapeutic assets and liabilities." *Journal of Neurosurgery* 52.5 (1980): 625-634.

Brierley, J.B., J.H. Adams., D.I. Graham., *et al.* "Neocortical death after cardiac arrest." *The Lancet* 2.7724 (1971): 560-565.

British Medical Association. Medical Ethics Committee. *Discussion paper on treatment of patients in persistent vegetative state*. London: British Medical Association, 1992.

British Medical Association. Medical Ethics Committee. *B.M.A. guidelines on treatment decisions of patients in a persistent vegetative state*. London: British Medical Association, 1994.

British Medical Association *Advance statements about medical treatment*. London: BMJ Publishing Group, 1995.

British Medical Association. "*Withholding and withdrawing life-prolonging medical treatment. Guidance for decision making*." London: BMJ Books, 1999.

British Medical Association. "*Withholding and withdrawing life-prolonging medical treatment*" 2nd Edition. London: BMJ Books, 2001.

Brodersen, P. and E.O. Jorgensen. "Cerebral blood flow and oxygen uptake, and cerebrospinal fluid biochemistry in severe coma." *Journal of Neurology, Neurosurgery, and Psychiatry* 37.4 (1974): 384-391.

Brody, B.A. "Ethical questions raised by the persistent vegetative patient." *Hastings Center Report* 18.1 (1988): 33-36.

Brown, J. "The persistent vegetative state: Time for caution?" *Postgraduate Medical Journal* 66.779 (1990): 697-698.

Bruhn, P. "Disturbances of vigilance in subcortical epilepsy." *Acta Neurologica Scandinavia* 46 (1970): 442-454.

Brule, J.F., F. Danze. and D. Vallee. "État végétatif: problèmes thérapeutiques." *Revue Francais Dommage Corporel* 14 (1988): 191-195.

Buchanan, A.E. "The right to a decent minimum of healthcare." *Philosophy and Public Affairs* 13 (1984): 55-78.

Burge, F.I. "Dehydration symptoms of palliative care cancer patients." *Journal of Pain and Symptom Management* 8.10 (1993): 454-464.

Burke, W.J. "Persistent vegetative state." *Neurology* 40.2 (1990): 384.

Busalacchi, P. "How can they?" *Hastings Center Report* 20.5 (1990): 6-7.

Byrne, P.A. and R.G. Nilges. "The brain stem in brain death: A critical review." *Issues in Law and Medicine* 9.1 (1993): 3-21.

Byrne, P.A., E.J. Kurt., D.D. Campbell., *et al.* "Quinlan re-examined." *Linacre Quarterly* 64.2 (1997): 58-65.

Callahan, D. "On feeding the dying." *Hastings Center Report* 13.5 (1983): 22.

Callahan, D. "Terminating life-sustaining treatment of the demented." *Hastings Center Report* 25.6 (1995): 25-31.

Calvert, R.J. "Ethics of life support and resuscitation." *New England Journal of Medicine* 318.26 (1988): 1756.

Cameron, P., D.G. Titus., J. Kostin., *et al.* "The life satisfaction of nonnormal persons." *Journal of Consulting and Clinical Psychology* 41.2 (1973): 207-214.

Campbell, A.G.M. "Children in a persistent vegetative state." *British Medical Journal* 289.6451 (1984): 1022-1023.

Cantor, N.L. "The permanently unconscious patient, non-feeding and euthanasia." *American Journal of Law and Medicine* 15.4 (1989): 381-437.

Cantor, N.L. "Prospective autonomy: on the limits of shaping one's postcompetence medical fate." *Journal of Contemporary Health Law and Policy* 8.1 (1992): 13-48.

Carlsson, C., M. Hagerdal., A.E. Kaasik., *et al.* "The effects of diazepam on cerebral blood flow and oxygen consumption in rats and its synergistic interaction with nitrous oxide." *Anesthesiology* 45.3 (1976): 319-325.

Carroll, L. *Through the Looking Glass*. London: The Folio Society, 1962 (1872).

Cassel, E.J. "The nature of suffering and the goals of medicine." *New England Journal of Medicine* 306.11 (1982): 639-645.

Cassell, E.J. "Clinical incoherence about persons: The problem of the persistent vegetative state." *Annals of Internal Medicine* 125.2 (1996): 146-147.

Cataldi-Betcher, E.L., M.H. Seltzer., B.A. Slocum., *et al.* "Complications occurring during enteral nutrition support: A prospective study." *Journal of Parenteral and Enteral Nutrition* 7.6 (1983): 546-552.

Celesia, G.G. "Persistent vegetative state." *Annals of Neurology* 33.4 (1993): 391.

Chen, R., C.F. Bolton. and G.B. Young. "Prediction of outcome in patients with anoxic coma: A clinical and electrophysiologic study." *Critical Care Medicine* 24.4 (1996): 672-678.

Childs, N.L. and W.N. Mercer. "Late improvement in consciousness after post-traumatic vegetative state." *New England Journal of Medicine* 334.1 (1996a): 24-25.

Childs, N.L. and W.N. Mercer. "Misdiagnosis certainly occurs." *British Medical Journal* 313.7062 (1996b): 944.

Childs, N.L., W.N. Mercer. and H.W. Childs. "Accuracy of diagnosis of persistent vegetative state." *Neurology* 43.8 (1993): 1465-1467.

Chortkoff, B.S., C.T. Gonsowski., H.L. Bennett., *et al.* "Subanesthetic concentrations of desflurane and propofol suppress recall of emotionally charged information." *Anaesthesia and Analgesia* 81.4 (1995): 728-736.

Chugani, H.T., M.E. Phelps. and J.C. Mazziotta. "Positron emision tomography study of human brain functional development." *Annals of Neurology* 22.4 (1987): 487-497.

Clancy, R. "Coma wife's family supports fight by doctors to let her die." *The Daily Telegraph* (London) 29 August 1995.

Cohen, J. "My ordeal in limbo." *The Daily Mail* (London) 12 February 1996.

Colby, W.H. "Missouri stands alone." *Hastings Center Report* 20.5 (1990): 5-6.

Colover, J. "Persistent vegetative state." *The Lancet* 350.9087 (1997): 1324.

Conley, S.B, J.T. Brocklebank., I.T. Taylor., *et al.* "Recurrent hypernatremia: A proposed mechanism in a patient with absence of thirst and abnormal excretion of water." *Journal of Pediatrics* 89.6 (1976): 898-903.

Cook, F. "Family's right-to-die battle is over at last." *The Mail on Sunday* (London) 2 June 1996.

Cork, R.C., J.F. Heaton., C.E. Campbell., *et al.* "Is there implicit memory after propofol sedation?" *British Journal of Anaesthesia* 76.4 (1996): 492-498.

Cornwell, J. "Back from the dead." *The Sunday Times (London)* 2 June 1996.

Covinsky, K.E., L. Goldman., F. Cook., *et al.* "The impact of serious illness on patients' families." *Journal of the American Medical Association* 272.23 (1994): 1839-1844.

Cowey, A. "Current awareness: spotlight on consciousness." *Developmental Medicine and Child Neurology* 39.1 (1997): 54-62.

Craig, O. "Hugh Finn is in a coma. His wife wants his feeding tubes removed: his parents refuse, insisting that he is aware of everything." *The Sunday Telegraph* (London) 27 September 1998.

Crane, P.D., L.D. Braun., E.M. Cornford., *et al.* "Dose dependent reduction of glucose utilization by pentobarbital in rat brain." *Stroke* 9.1 (1978): 12-18.

Cranford, R.E. "Termination of treatment in the persistent vegetative state." *Seminars in Neurology* 4.1 (1984): 36-44.

Cranford, R.E. "The persistent vegetative state: the medical reality (Getting the facts straight)" *Hastings Center Report* 18.1 (1988): 27-32.

Cranford, R.E. "Persistent vegetative state." *Neurology* 40.2 (1990a): 385-386.

Cranford, R.E. "A hostage to technology." *Hastings Center Report* 20.5 (1990b): 9-10.

Cranford, R.E. "Neurologic syndromes and prolonged survival: When can artificial nutrition and hydration be forgone?" *Law, Medicine and Health Care* 19.1-2 (1991): 13-22.

Cranford, R.E. "Withdrawing artificial feeding from children with brain damage." *British Medical Journal* 311.7003 (1995): 464-465.

Cranford, R. "Misdiagnosing the persistent vegetative state. An apparently high rate of misdiagnosis demands critical review and action." *British Medical Journal* 313.7048 (1996): 5-6.

Cranford, R.E. "Policy should be balanced with concern for the family." *British Medical Journal* 318.7200 (1999): 1754-1755.

Cranford, R.E. and D.R. Smith. "Consciousness: The most critical moral (constitutional) standard for human personhood." *American Journal of Law and Medicine* 13.2-3 (1987): 233-248.

Cranford, R.E. and H.L. Smith. "Some critical distinctions between brain death and persistent vegetative state." *Ethics in Science and Medicine*, 6.4 (1979): 199-209.

Cravioto, H., J. Silberman. and I. Feigin. "A clinical and pathologic study of akinetic mutism." *Neurology* 10.1 (1960): 10-21.

Crick, F. "Function of the thalamic reticular complex: The searchlight hypothesis." *Proceedings of the National Academy of Science USA.* 81.7 (1984): 4586-4590.

Crisci, C. "Persistent vegetative state." *Neurology* 40.2 (1990): 384-385.

Cruzan v Harmon, 760 S.W. 2d, 408, 1988

Daly, B.J. "Withdrawal of food and fluid." *AACN Clinical Issues in Critical Care Nursing* 1.1 (1990): 187-197.

Daniels, A. "In a coma, hearing talk of death." *The Daily Telegraph* (London) 13 February 1996.

Daniels, N. "Health care needs and distributive justice." *Philosophy and Public Affairs* 10 (1981): 146-179.

Daniels, N. "*Just health care*." Cambridge: Cambridge University Press, 1985.

Danis, M.M., L.I. Southerland., J.M. Garrett., *et al.* "A prospective study of advance directives for life-sustaining care." *New England Journal of Medicine* 324.13 (1991): 882-888.

Danze, F., J.F. Brule. and K. Haddad. "Chronic vegetative state after severe head injury: Clinical study, electrophysiological investigations and CT scan in 15 cases." *Advances in Neurotraumatology* 12. Supplement (1989): 477-499.

Datlof, S., P.D. Coleman., G.B. Forbes., *et al.* "Ventricular dilation on CAT scans of patients with anorexia nervosa." *American Journal of Psychiatry* 143.1 (1986): 96-98.

Davis, D.W., R.A. Hawkins., A.M. Mans., *et al.* "Regional cerebral glucose utilization during althesin anesthesia." *Anesthesiology* 61.4 (1984): 362-368.

De Bruxelles, S. "Coma student given no hope refused to die." *The Times* (London) 11 June 1998.

De Giorgio, C.M. and M.F. Lew. "Consciousness, coma, and the vegetative state: Physical basis and definitional character." *Issues in Law and Medicine,* 6.4 (1991): 361-371.

de Lima, J., A.R. Lloyd-Thomas., R.F. Howard., *et al.* "Infant and neonatal pain: anaesthetists' perceptions and prescribing patterns." *British Medical Journal* 313.7060 (1996): 787

De Renzo, E. "Surrogate decision making for severely cognitively impaired research subjects: The continuing debate." *Cambridge Quarterly of Healthcare Ethics* 3.3 (1994): 539-548.

Deliac, P., E. Richer., J. Berthomieu., *et al.* "Évolution électrophysiologique sous stimulation thalamique des états vegétatifs persistants post-traumatiques." *Neurochirurgie* 39.5 (1993): 293-303.

Dennett, D.C. *Consciousness explained.* Boston: Little, Brown and Co., 1991.

Devinsky, O. "Neurological aspects of the conscious and unconscious mind." *Annals of the New York Academy of Sciences* 835 (1997): 321-329.

DeVolder, A.G., A.M. Goffinet., A. Bol., *et al.* "Brain glucose metabolism in postanoxic syndrome. Positron emission tomographic study." *Archives of Neurology* 47.2 (1990): 197-204.

DeYoung, S. and R.B. Grass. "Coma Recovery Program." *Rehabilitation Nursing* 12.3 (1987): 121-124.

Dimond, S.J. "Tactual and auditory vigilance in split-brain man." *Journal of Neurology, Neurosurgery, and Psychiatry* 42.1 (1979): 70-74.

Dixon, N.F. and S.H.A. Henley. "Unconscious perception. Possible implications of data from academic research for clinical practice." *Journal of Nervous and Mental Disease* 179.5 (1991): 243-252.

Dolan, J.M. "Should we withhold food from patients in a persistent vegetative state?" *Journal of Head Trauma Rehabilitation* 9.4 (1994): 62-69.

Dougherty, J.H., D.G. Rawlinson., D.E. Levy., *et al.* "Hypoxic-ischemic brain injury and the vegetative state: Clinical and neuropathologic correlation." *Neurology* 31.8 (1981): 991-997.

Doyal, L. "Advance directives. Like a will, everybody should have one." *British Medical Journal* 310.6980 (1995): 612-613.

Doyal, L. and L. Doyal. "Why active euthanasia and physician assisted suicide should be legalized." *British Medical Journal* 323.7321 (2001): 1079-1082.

Dresser, R. "Life, death, and incompetent patients: Conceptual infirmities and hidden values in the law." *Arizona Law Review* 28.3 (1986): 373-405.

Dresser, R. "Missing persons: Legal perceptions of incompetent patients." *Rutgers Law Review* 46.2 (1994): 609-719.

Dresser, R. "Dworkin on dementia. Elegant theory, questionable policy." *Hastings Center Report* 25.6 (1995): 32-38.

Dresser, R. "Still troubled. In *re Martin*." *Hastings Center Report* 26.4 (1996): 21-22.

Dresser, R.S. and E.V. Boisaubin. "Ethics, law, and nutritional support." *Archives of Internal Medicine* 145.1 (1985): 122-128.

Dunkerley, C. "First person." *Scotland on Sunday* (Edinburgh) 17 August 1997.

Dworkin, R. *Life's dominion. An argument about abortion and euthanasia.* London: Harper Collins, 1993.

Dyer, C. "BMA examines the persistent vegetative state." *British Medical Journal* 305.6858 (1992): 853-854.

Dyer, C. "'Vegetative' patient wakes up after seven years. Recovery raises doubts over prognosis of 'right to die' cases." *The Guardian* (London) 16 March 1996a.

Dyer, C. "BMA will review guidelines on PVS." *British Medical Journal* 312.7033 (1996b): 725-726.

Dyer, C. "High Court to rule on whether woman in near-vegetative state can be left to starve. Is a flicker of life enough?" *The Guardian* (London) 16 November 1996c.

Dyer, C. "Home news. Family backs hospital's plea on patient in coma. Doctors ask court to cut life support." *The Guardian* (London) 21 March 1997a.

Dyer, C. "Court to let 'living death' woman die." *The Guardian* (London) 17 July 1997b.

Editorial. "Life and death: the line gets finer." *The Independent* (London) 19 March 1996.

Editorial. "How persistent is PVS?." *The Daily Telegraph* (London) 27 March 1997.

Editorial "Fine line between life and death." *The Daily Telegraph* (London) 7 July 1998.

Editorial. "Relative trust. Disturbing allegations of 'backdoor' euthanasia" *The Times* (London) 6 January 1999.

Editorial "When primum non nocere fails." *The Lancet* 355.9220 (2000): 2007.

Ehrensing, R.H. and G.F. Michell. "Similar antagonism of morphine analgesia by MIF-1 and naloxone in *Carassius auratus*." *Pharmacology, Biochemistry and Behaviour* 17.4 (1982): 759-761.

Ellman, I.M. "Can others exercise an incapacitated patient's right to die?" *Hastings Center Report* 20.1 (1990): 47-50.

Emanuel, E.J., and L.L. Emanuel. "Proxy decision making for incompetent patients." *Journal of the American Medical Association* 267.15 (1992): 2067-2071.

Emanuel, L.L., M.J. Barry., and J.D. Stoeckle. "Advance directives for medical care - a case for greater use." *New England Journal of Medicine* 324.13 (1991): 889-895.

Emanuel, L.L. and E.J. Emanuel. "Decisions at the end of life. Guided by communities of patients." *Hastings Center Report* 23.5 (1993): 6-14.

Emanuel, L.L., E.J. Emanuel., J.D. Stoeckle., *et al.* "Advance directives. Stability of patients' treatment choices." *Archives of Internal Medicine* 154.2 (1994): 209-217.

Engelhardt, K. "Organ donation and permanent vegetative state." *The Lancet* 351.9097 (1998): 211.

Enzmann, D.R. and B. Lane. "Cranial computed tomography findings in anorexia nervosa." *Journal of Computer Assisted Tomography* 1.4 (1977): 410-414.

Evans, A.L. and B.A. Brody. "The do-not-resuscitate order in teaching hospitals." *Journal of the American Medical Association* 253.15 (1985): 2236-2239.

Evans, D.W. "Organ donation and permanent vegetative state." *The Lancet* 351.9097 (1998): 212.

Fackler, J.C. and M.C. Rogers. "Is brain death really cessation of all intracranial function?" *Journal of Pediatrics* 110.1 (1987): 84-86.

Falk, R.H. "Physical and intellectual recovery following prolonged hypoxic coma." *Postgraduate Medical Journal* 66.775 (1990): 384-386.

Farmer, H. "Miraculous coma mum fights new euthanasia legislation." *The Universe* (London) 21 November 1999.

Fenwick, A.J. "Applying best interests to persistent vegetative state - a principled distortion?" *Journal of Medical Ethics* 24.2 (1998): 86-92.

Ferguson, P.R. "Causing death or allowing to die? Developments in the law." *Journal of Medical Ethics* 23.6 (1997): 368-372.

Fergusson, A. "Letting vegetative patients die." *British Medical Journal* 305.6867 (1992): 1506.

Ferriman, A. "Mind over matter." *The Guardian* (London) 19 November 1996.

Ferriman, A. "Flicker of hope from brain damage victim astonishes doctors." *The Independent* (London) 27 March 1997.

Field, R.E. and R.J. Romanus. "A decerebrate patient: Eighteen years of care." *Connecticut Medicine* 45.11 (1981): 717-719.

Fields, A.I., D.H. Coble., M.M. Pollack., *et al.* "Outcomes of children in a persistent vegetative state." *Critical Care Medicine* 21.12 (1993): 1890-1894.

Finnis, J. 'Living will' legislation. In *Euthanasia, clinical practice and the law*, edited by L. Gormally, 167-176. London: Linacre Centre, 1994.

Fisher, A. "Old law and new ethics: Bland's case and not feeding the comatose." *Law and Justice* 117.1 (1993a): 4-18.
Fisher, A. *Law and Justice* "Letter to the Editor." 118 (1993b): 147-148.
Fisher, A. "Consciousness: the new test of life." *The Catholic Herald* (London) 4 March 1994.
Fisher, A. and L. Gormally. *Healthcare Allocation: an ethical framework for public policy*. London: The Linacre Centre, 2001.
Fitzsimons, J.T. "Thirst." *Physiological Reviews* 52.2 (1972): 468-561.
Fletcher, D. "Tougher rules on when to let coma victims die." *The Daily Telegraph* (London) 13 February 1996.
Fletcher, D. "Surgeons told when to let a patient die." *The Daily Telegraph* (London) 10 December 1997.
Flohr, H. "Sensations and brain processes." *Behavioural Brain Research* 71.1-2 (1995): 157-161.
Foley, J.M. "The experience of being demented." In *Dementia and aging: ethics, values and policy choices*, edited by R. Binstock, S. Post and P. Whitehouse, 30-43. Baltimore: Johns Hopkins University Press, 1992.
Fox, P.T. and M.E. Raichle. "Focal physiological uncoupling of cerebral blood flow and oxidative metabolism during somatosensory stimulation in human subjects." *Proceedings of the National Academy of Science, USA* 83.4 (1986): 1140-1144.
Fraser, L. "The coma victim saved by a buzzer." *The Mail on Sunday* (London) 6 April 1997.
Freeman, E.A. "Coma arousal therapy." *Clinical Rehabilitation* 5.3 (1991): 241-249.
Freeman, E.A. "The clinical assessment of coma." *Neuropsychological Rehabilitation* 3.2 (1993): 139-147.
Freeman, E. "The coma exit chart: Assessing the patient in prolonged coma and the vegetative state." *Brain Injury* 10.8 (1996): 615-624.
Freeman, E.A. "Community-based rehabilitation of the person with a severe brain injury." *Brain Injury* 11.2 (1997a): 143-153.
Freeman, E.A. "Protocols for the vegetative state." *Brain Injury* 11.11 (1997b): 837-849.
Freeman, E.A. Personal Communication. 2002.
French, J.D. "Brain lesions associated with prolonged unconsciousness." *A.M.A. Archives of Neurology and Psychiatry* 68.6 (1952): 727-740.
Frenchay Healthcare NHS Trust v S 2 All ER 403, 1994.
Fuller, P.R. "Operant conditioning of a vegetative human organism." *American Journal of Psychology* 62.4 (1949): 587-590.
Gallup, G.G. "Chimpanzees: self-recognition." *Science*, 167.3914 (1970): 86-87.
Gamble, E.R., P.J. McDonald. and P.R. Lichstein. "Knowledge, attitudes, and behavior of elderly persons regarding living wills." *Archives of Internal Medicine* 151.2 (1991): 277-280.
Gasner, M.R., F. Rouse., and R. Wasserman. "Abridged brief as *Amicus Curiae* of the Society for the Right to Die, inc., in support of the request of the parents of Nancy Beth Cruzan for a Supreme Court hearing." *Journal of the American Geriatrics Society* 38.5 (1990): 577-579.
Gerber, P. "Withdrawing treatment from patients in a persistent vegetative state." *Medical Journal of Australia* 161.11-12 (1994): 715-717.
Giacino, J.T. "Disorders of consciousness: Differential diagnosis and neuropathologic features." *Seminars in Neurology* 17.2 (1997): 105-111.
Giacino, J.T. and N.D. Zasler. "Outcome after severe traumatic brain injury: Coma, the vegetative state, and the minimally responsive state." *Journal of Head Trauma Rehabilitation* 10.1 (1995): 40-56.
Giacino, J.T., N.D. Zasler., J. Whyte., *et al.* "Recommendations for the use of uniform nomenclature pertinent to patients with severe alterations in consciousness." *Archives of Physical Medicine and Rehabilitation* 76.2 (1995): 205-209.
Giacino, J.T., N.D. Zasler., D.I. Katz., *et al.* "Development of practice guidelines for assessment and management of the vegetative and minimally conscious states." *Journal of Head Trauma Rehabilitation* 12.4 (1997): 79-89.
Gibb, F. "Judge will decide if woman can be left to die." *The Times* (London) 21 March 1997.
Gibb, F. "Rights act does not bar mercy killing." *The Times* (London) 26 October 2000.
Gilbert, W.S. Libretto of *The Mikado or The Town of Titipu* 1885.
Gill, C.J. "Suicide intervention for people with disabilities: A lesson in inequality." *Issues in Law and Medicine* 8.1 (1992): 37-53.
Gillett, G.R. "Why let people die?" *Journal of Medical Ethics* 12.2 (1986): 83-86.
Gillies, J.D. and S.S. Seshia. "Vegetative state following coma in childhood: Evolution and outcome." *Developmental Medicine and Child Neurology* 22.5 (1980): 642-648.
Gledhill, R. "Conference to back 'death with dignity'." *The Times* (London) 7 August 1998.

Glover, J.J., A. Mastroianni., K.R Anderson., et al. "Abridged brief as *Amicus Curiae* of the American Geriatrics Society in support of the petitioner, Nancy Beth Cruzan, by her parents and co-guardians Lester L. and Joyce Cruzan." *Journal of the American Geriatrics Society* 38.5 (1990): 570-576.
Goff, R. "A matter of life and death." Medical Law Review 3.1 (1995): 1-21.
Goodwin, J.S. "Mercy killing: mercy for whom?" *Journal of the American Medical Association* 265.3 (1991): 326.
Gormally, L. "Definitions of personhood: Implications for the care of PVS patients." *Ethics and Medicine* 9.3 (1993): 44-48.
Graham, D.I., D. McLellan., J.H. Adams., *et al.* "The neuropathology of the vegetative state and severe disability after non-missile head injury." *Acta Neurochirurgica* 32 Supplement (1983): 65-67.
Graham, P.G.P. "Artificial hydration and nutrition. It is time to take a stand." *Homiletic and Pastoral Review* 99.5 (1999): 8-19.
Greaves, G. "Andrew is wakening from his coma but we were right to let our son die." *The Daily Express* (London) 28 March 1997.
Greenwald, A.G. "Unconscious cognition reclaimed." *American Psychologist* 47.6 (1992): 766-779.
Griffiths, D. and J.G. Jones. "Awareness and memory in anaesthetized patients." *British Journal of Anaesthesia* 65.5 (1990): 603-606.
Grigg, M.M., M.A. Kelly., G.G. Celesia., *et al.* "Electroencephalographic activity after brain death." *Archives of Neurology* 44.9 (1987): 948-954.
Grubb, A. "Incompetent patient in PVS: reinsertion of a feeding tube." *Medical Law Review* 2.2 (1994): 206-208.
Grubb, A. "Incompetent patient in PVS; views of relatives and 'best interests'." *Medical Law Review* 3.1 (1995a): 80-84.
Grubb, A. "Incompetent patient in PVS: cared for at home." *Swindon and Marlborough N.H.S. Trust v S. Medical Law Review* 3.1 (1995b): 84-86.
Grubb, A. "The persistent vegetative state: A duty (not) to treat and conscientious objection." *European Journal of Health Law* 4.2 (1997a): 157-178.
Grubb, A. "Incompetent patient (PVS): Withdrawal of feeding and compliance with RCP guidelines." *Medical Law Review* 5.2 (1997b): 225-227.
Grubb, A. "PVS patient: disclosure after death." *Medical Law Review* 5.1 (1997c): 108-110.
Grubb, A., P. Walsh, and N. Lambe. "Reporting on the persistent vegetative state in Europe." *Medical Law Review* 6.2 (1998): 161-219.
Guerit, J-M., D. Verongstraete., M. de Tourtchaninoff., *et al.* "ERPs obtained with the auditory oddball paradigm in coma and altered states of consciousness: clinical relationships, prognostic value and origin of components." *Clinical Neurophysiology* 110.7 (1999): 1260-1269.
Gulbrandsen, G.B. and K. Kristiansen. "Response habituation in unconscious patients." *Neuropsychologia* 10.3 (1972): 313-320.
Haider, M., P. Spong. and D.B. Lindsley. "Attention, Vigilance, and Cortical Evoked-Potentials in Humans." *Science* 145.3628 (1964): 180-182.
Haig, A.J. "The persistent vegetative state." *New England Journal of Medicine* 331.20 (1994): 1380.
Hall, J.K. "Should nurses implement 'death by dehydration'-decisions? Caring for corpses or killing patients?" *Nursing Management* 25 October (1994): 81-89.
Hall, S. "Judge's decision on tragic dental patient. Coma man's right to die." *Derby Evening Telegraph* (Derby) 18 November 1995.
Hallows, N. "Suspension spotlights end-of-life issues." *BMA News Review* April 14 1999.
Hansotia, P.L. "Persistent vegetative state. Review and report of electrodiagnostic studies in eight cases." *Archives of Neurology* 42.11 (1985): 1048-1052.
Hardwig, J. "Is there a duty to die?" *Hastings Center Report* 27.2 (1997): 34-42.
Harris, J. "Are withholding and withdrawing therapy always morally equivalent? A reply to Sulmasy and Sugarman." *Journal of Medical Ethics* 20.4 (1994): 223-224.
Hassler, R. "Basal ganglia systems regulating mental activity." *International Journal of Neurology* 12.1 (1977): 53-72.
Hassler, R., G.D. Ore., A. Dieckmann., *et al.* "Behavioural and EEG arousal induced by stimulation of unspecific projection systems in a patient with post-traumatic apallic syndrome." *Electroencephalography and Clinical Neurophysiol*ogy 27.3 (1969): 306-310.
Haupt, W.F., C. Birkmann. and M. Halber. "Serial evoked potential and outcome in cerebrovascular critical care patients." *Journal of Clinical Neurophysiology* 17.3 (2000): 326-330.
Hawkes, C.H. and L. Bryan-Smyth. "The electroencephalogram in the 'locked-in' syndrome." *Neurology* 24.11 (1974): 1015-1018.

Hawton, L.A. and P.T. Ohara. "The brain of Karen Ann Quinlan." *New England Journal of Medicine* 331.20 (1994): 1378.
Hays, R.M., P.R. McHugh., and H.E. Williams. "Absence of thirst in association with hydrocephalus." *New England Journal of medicine* 269.5 (1963): 227-231.
Head, H. and G. Holmes. "Sensory disturbances from cerebral lesions." *Brain* 34.2-3 (1911): 102-254.
Heindl, U.T. and M.C. Laub. "Outcome of persistent vegetative state following hypoxic or traumatic brain injury in children and adolescents." *Neuropediatrics* 27.2 (1996): 94-100.
Heinz, E.R., J. Martinez. and A. Haenggeli. "Reversibility of cerebral atrophy in anorexia nervosa and Cushing's syndrome." *Journal of Computer Assisted Tomography* 1.4 (1977): 415-418.
Hellema, H. "'Life termination' in the Netherlands." *British Medical Journal* 302.6783 (1991): 984-985.
Hibbs, J. "'Mercy killings' court proposed." *The Daily Telegraph* (London) 10 December 1997.
Higashi, K. "Clinical analysis of patients recovered from persistent vegetative state." *Brain and Nerve. No To Shinkei* (Tokyo) 30.1 (1978): 27-35.
Higashi, K., M. Hatano. and S. Aliko. "Five year follow-up study of patients with persistent vegetative state." *Journal of Neurology, Neurosurgery and Psychiatry* 44.6 (1981): 552-554.
Higashi, K., Y. Sokata., M. Hatano., *et al*. "Epidemiological studies on patients with persistent vegetative state." *Journal of Neurology, Neurosurgery and Psychiatry* 40.9 (1977): 876-885.
Higgs, R. "Living wills and treatment refusal." *British Medical Journal* 295.6608 (1987): 1221-1222.
Himwich, H.E., K.M. Bowman., C. Daly., *et al*. "Cerebral blood flow and brain metabolism during insulin hypoglycemia." *American Journal of Physiology* 132.3 (1941): 640-647.
Himwich, W.A., E. Homburger., R. Maresca., *et al*. "Brain metabolism in man: unanesthetized and in pentothal narcosis." *American Journal of Psychiatry* 103.3 (1947): 689-696.
Hoffenberg, R. "Organ donation and permanent vegetative state." *The Lancet* 351.9097 (1998): 212-213.
Hoffenberg, R., M. Lock., N. Tilney., *et al*. "Should organs from patients in permanent vegetative state be used for transplantation?" *The Lancet* 350.9087 (1997): 1320-1321.
Hollows, K. "The lived experience of registered nurses involved in the withdrawal of nutrition and hydration in a persistent vegetative state (PVS) patient." *Nursing Praxis in New Zealand* 10.1 (1995): 28-37.
Hopkins, N. "In coma victim's eyes, the light of hope glows." *Daily Mail (London)* 27 March 1997.
Horsnell, M. and P. Foster. "Euthanasia claims sow doubt in families' minds." *The Times* (London) 6 January 1999.
House of Lords Select Committee. *Report of the select committee on medical ethics*. Vol. 1. London: H.M.S.O. 1994.
Howard, R and D.H. Miller. "The persistent vegetative state." *British Medical Journal* 310.6975 (1995): 341-342.
Howe, J.G. "Management of patients in persistent vegetative state." *British Medical Journal* 307.6904 (1993): 624.
Howsepian, A.A. "The 1994 multi-society task force consensus statement on the persistent vegetative state: A critical analysis." *Issues in Law and Medicine* 12.1 (1996): 3-29.
Hughes, J.A., L.D. Sanders., J.A. Dunne., *et al*. "The effect of suggestion during general anaesthesia on postoperative smoking habits." *Anaesthesia* 49.2 (1994): 126-128.
Hurwitz, B. *Clinical guidelines and the law. Negligence, discretion and judgement*. Oxford: Radcliffe Medical Press, 1998.
In the Matter of Jobes. 529A. 2d 434. NJ 1987.
In the Matter of a Ward of Court (1995) 2 ILRM 401
Institute of Medical Ethics Working Party on the Ethics of Prolonging Life and Assisting Death. *The Lancet* 336.8715 (1990): 610-613.
Institute of Medical Ethics Working Party on the Ethics of Prolonging Life and Assisting Death. "Withdrawal of life-support from patients in a persistent vegetative state." *The Lancet* 337.8733 (1991): 96-98.
International Working Party Report on the Vegetative State. Edited by K. Andrews. London: The Royal Hospital for Neuro-disability, West Hill, Putney, 1996.
Irish Correspondent. "Woman's life-support system can now be switched off. Irish stunned by court judgment." *The Catholic Times* (London) 6 August 1995.
Isono, M., Y. Wakabayashi., M.M. Fujiki., *et al*. "Sleep cycle in patients in a state of permanent unconsciousness." *Brain Injury* 16.8 (2002): 705-712.
Ivan, L.P. "The persistent vegetative state." *Transplantation Proceedings* 22.3 (1990): 993 –994.
Jansen, G.A. and N.M. Greene. "Morphine metabolism and morphine tolerance in goldfish." *Anaesthesiology* 32.3 (1970): 231-235.

Jarmulowicz, M. "Neuropathological findings in cases of persistent vegetative state." *Catholic Medical Quarterly* 46.1 (1995): 28-30.

Jecker, N.S. and D.J. Self. "Separating care and cure: An analysis of historical and contemporary images of nursing and medicine." *Journal of Medicine and Philosophy* 16.3 (1991): 285-306.

Jefferys, J.G.R., R.D. Traub. and M.A. Whittington. "Neuronal networks for induced '40 Hz' rhythms." *Trends in the Neurological Sciences* 19.5 (1996): 202-208.

Jelicic, M., A. De Roode., J.G. Bovill., *et al.* "Unconscious learning during anaesthesia." *Anaesthesia* 47.10 (1992): 835-837.

Jellinger, K.A. "The brain of Karen Ann Quinlan." *New England Journal of Medicine* 331.20 (1994): 1378- 1379.

Jennett, B. "Resource allocation for the severely brain damaged." *Archives of Neurology* 33.9 (1976): 595-597.

Jennett, B. "Vegetative state: causes, management, ethical dilemmas." *Current Anaesthesia and Critical Care* 2 (1991): 57-61.

Jennett, B. "Letting vegetative patients die." *British Medical Journal* 305.6865 (1992): 1305-1306.

Jennett, B. "Vegetative survival: The medical facts and ethical dilemmas." *Neuropsychological Rehabilitation* 3.2 (1993a): 99-108.

Jennett, B. "The case for letting vegetative patients die." *Ethics and Medicine* 9.3 (1993b): 40-44.

Jennett, B. "A quarter century of the vegetative state: An international perspective." *Journal of Head Trauma Rehabilitation* 12.4 (1997): 1-12.

Jennett, B. "Brain stem death defines death in law." *British Medical Journal* 318.7200 (1999): 1755.

Jennett, B. and F. Plum. "Persistent vegetative state after brain damage. A syndrome in search of a name." *The Lancet* 1.7753 (1972): 734-737.

Jennett, B. and M. Bond. "Assessment of outcome after severe brain damage. A practical scale." *The Lancet* 1.7905 (1975): 480-484.

Jennett, B., J.H. Adams., L.S. Murray., *et al.* "Neuropathology in vegetative and severely disabled patients after head injury." *Neurology* 56.4 (2001): 486-490.

Jennings, B., D. Callahan. and A.L. Caplan. "Ethical challenges of chronic illness." *Hastings Center Report, Special Supplement* 28.1 (1998): 1-16.

Jones, A.K.P., W.D. Brown., L.Y. Friston., *et al.* "Cortical and subcortical localization of response to pain in man using positron emission tomography." *Proceedings of the Royal Society* (London) B. 244.1309 (1991): 39-44.

Jones, J.G. "Memory of intra-operative events. Patients remember more than we think." *British Medical Journal* 309.6960 (1994): 967-968.

Judson, J.A., R.B. Cant. and N.A. Shaw. "Early prediction of outcome from cerebral trauma by somatosensory evoked potentials." *Critical Care Medicine* 18.4 (1990): 363-368.

Kadish, S.H. "Letting patients die: Legal and moral reflections." *California Law Review* 80.4 (1992): 857-888.

Kampfl, A., E. Schmutzhard., G. Franz., *et al.* "Prediction of recovery from post traumatic vegetative state with cerebral magnetic-resonance imaging." *The Lancet* 351.9118 (1998): 1763-1767.

Kane, N.M., T.H. Moss., S.H. Curry., *et al.* "Quantitative electroencephalographic evaluation of non-fatal and fatal traumatic coma." *Electroencephalography and Clinical Neurophysiology* 106.3 (1998): 244-250.

Kanno, T., Y. Kamel., T. Yokoyama., *et al.* "Effects of dorsal column spinal cord stimulation (DCS) on reversibility of neuronal function - experience of treatment for vegetative states." *Pacing and Clinical Electrophysiology* 12.4 (1989): 733-738.

Karlawish, J.H.T. and G.A. Sachs. "Research on the cognitively impaired: Lessons and warnings from the emergency research debate." *Journal of the American Geriatrics Society* 45.4 (1997): 474-481.

Karp, J.S. and H.I. Hurtig. "'Locked-In' state with bilateral midbrain infarcts." *Archives of Neurology* 30.2 (1974): 176-178.

Katayama, Y., T. Tsubokawa., T. Yamamoto., *et al.* "Characterization and modification of brain activity with deep brain stimulation in patients in a persistent vegetative state: Pain-related late positive component of cerebral evoked potential." *Pacing and Clinical Electrophysiology* 14.1 (1991): 116-121.

Katz, R.T., A.J. Haig., B.B. Clark., *et al.* "Long-term survival, prognosis, and life-care planning for 29 patients with chronic locked-in syndrome." *Archives of Physical Medicine and Rehabilitation* 73.5 (1992): 403-408.

Kaufman, D.M. and R.B. Lipton. "The persistent vegetative state: An analysis of clinical correlates and costs." *New York State Journal of Medicine* 92.9 (1992): 381-384.

Kaveny, C.M. "Assisted suicide, euthanasia, and the law." *Theological Studies* 58.1 (1997): 124-148.

Kearns, M. "Death of our ethics." *The Scotsman* (Edinburgh) 13 May 1996.

Kearse, L.A., C. Rosow., A. Zaslavsky., *et al.* "Bispectral analysis of the electroencephalogram predicts conscious processing of information during propofol sedation and hypnosis." *Anesthesiology* 88.1 (1998): 25-34.

Kennedy, I. "*Re R (Adult: Medical Treatment) Adult*: Order concerning future non-treatment." *Medical Law Review* 5.1 (1997): 104-108.

Kennedy, I. "Child: Terminal illness; Withdrawal of treatment." *Medical Law Review* 6.1 (1998): 99-103.

Kennedy, I. and A. Grubb. "Withdrawal of artificial hydration and nutrition: Incompetent adult. *Airedale NHS Trust v Bland*." *Medical Law Review* 1.3 (1993): 359-370.

Keown, J. "Beyond *Bland*: a critique of the B.M.A. guidance on withholding and withdrawing medical treatment." *Legal Studies* 20.1 (2000): 66-84.

King, T.T. "Organ donation and permanent vegetative state." *The Lancet* 351.9097 (1998): 211.

Kinney, H.C. and M.A. Samuels. "Neuropathology of the persistent vegetative state. A review." *Journal of Neuropathology and Experimental Neurology* 53.6 (1994): 548-558.

Kinney, H.C., J. Korein., A. Panigrahy., *et al.* "Neuropathological findings in the brain of Karen Ann Quinlan. The role of the thalamus in the persistent vegetative state." *New England Journal of Medicine* 300.21 (1994): 1469-1475.

Kitwood, T. and K. Bredin. "Towards a theory of dementia care: Personhood and well-being." *Ageing and Society* 12 (1992): 269-287.

Kohlmeyer, K., G. Lehmkuhl. and F. Poutska. "Computed tomography of anorexia nervosa." *American Journal of Neuroradiology* 4.3 (1983): 437-438.

Korein, J. "Ontogenesis of the brain in the human organism" In *Advances in bioethics* Vol 2, Edited by R.B., Edwards and E.E. Bittar, 1-74. Connecticut: JAI Press, 1998.

Korein, J. and M. Maccario. "On the diagnosis of cerebral death: A prospective study on 55 patients to define irreversible coma." *Clinical Electroencephalography* 2.4 (1971): 178-199.

Korein, J., P. Braunstein., A. George., *et al.* "Brain death. I Angiographic correlation with the radiosotopic bolus technique for evaluation of critical deficit of cerebral blood flow." *Annals of Neurology* 2.3 (1977): 195-205.

Kress, H.G., and Weigl, L. "The molecular and cellular mechanisms of general anaesthesia." In *Recent advances in anaesthesia and analgesia*, Vol. 20, edited by A.P. Adams and J.N. Cashman, 1-20. Edinburgh: Churchill Livingstone, 1998.

Krieg, J-C., C. Lauer, C. and K-M. Pirke. "Structural brain abnormalities in patients with bulimia nervosa." *Psychiatry Research* 27.1 (1988): 39-48.

La Puma, J., D.L. Schiedermayer., A.E. Gulyas., *et al.* "Talking to comatose patients." *Archives of Neurology* 45.1 (1988): 20-22.

Lakeman, G. "Girl who wouldn't die." *The Daily Mirror* (London) 11 June 1998.

Lamm, R.D. "Redrawing the ethics map." *Hastings Center Report* 29.2 (1999): 28-29.

Lamm, R.D. Cited in *The New York Times* 29 March 1984.

Lantos, J.D., P.A. Singer., R.M. Walker., *et al.* "The illusion of futility in clinical practice." *The American Journal of Medicine* 87.1 (1989): 81-84.

Larsen, P.D., N.C. Gupta., D.M. Lefkowitz., *et al.* "PET of infant in persistent vegetative state." *Pediatric Neurology* 9.4 (1993): 323-326.

Laurance, J. "Buzzer unlocks mind trapped in useless body." *The Times* (London) 5 July 1996a.

Laurance, J. "Vegetative state diagnosis wrong in many patients." *The Times* (London) 5 July 1996b.

Laurance, J. "Doctors seek new rules to let people die." *The Independent* (London) 6 July 1998.

Laureys, S., C. Lemaire., P. Maquet., *et al.* "Cerebral metabolism during vegetative state and after recovery of consciousness." *Journal of Neurology, Neurosurgery and Psychiatry* 67.1 (1999a): 121.

Laureys, S., S. Goldman., C. Phillips., *et al.* "Impaired effective cortical connectivity in vegetative state: Preliminary investigation using PET." *Neuroimage Clinics of North America* 9.4 (1999b): 377-382.

Laureys, S., M.E. Faymonville., A. Luxen., *et al.* "Restoration of thalamocortical connectivity after recovery from persistent vegetative state." *The Lancet* 355.9217 (2000a): 1790-1791.

Laureys, S., M.E. Faymonville., C. Degueldre., *et al.* "Auditory processing in the vegetative state." *Brain* 123.8 (2000b): 1589-1601.

Laureys, S., M.E. Faymonville., P. Peigneux., *et al.* "Cortical processing of noxious somatosensory stimuli in the persistent vegetative state." *Neuroimage* 17.2 (2002): 732-741.

Law Hospital NHS Trust v Lord Advocate SLT848, 1996.

Leff, B., N. Cheuvront. and W. Russell, W. "Discontinuing feeding tubes in a community nursing home." *The Gerontologist* 34.1 (1994): 130-133.

Lennard-Jones, J.E. "Giving or withholding fluid and nutrients: Ethical and legal aspects." *Journal of the Royal College of Physicians of London* 33.1 (1999): 39-45.

Levin, H.S., C. Saydjari., H.M. Eisenber., *et al.* "Vegetative state after closed-head injury. A traumatic coma data bank report." *Archives of Neurology* 48.6 (1991): 580-585.

Levinson, B.W. "States of awareness during general anaesthesia." *British Journal of Anaesthesia* 37.7 (1965): 544-546.

Levy, D.E., R.P. Knill-Jones. and F. Plum. "The vegetative state and its prognosis following non-traumatic coma." *Annals of the New York Academy of Sciences* 315 (1978): 293-306.

Levy, D.E., D. Bates., J.J. Caronna., *et al.* "Prognosis in nontraumatic coma." *Annals of Internal Medicine* 94.3 (1981): 293-301.

Levy D.E., J.J. Caronna., B.H. Singer., *et al.* "Predicting outcome from hypoxic-ischemic coma." *Journal of the American Medical Association* 253.10 (1985): 1420-1426.

Levy, D.E., J.J. Sidtis., D.A. Rottenberg., *et al.* "Differences in cerebral blood flow and glucose utilization in vegetative versus locked-in patients." *Annals of Neurology* 22.6 (1987): 673-682.

Levy, D.E., M.J. Tramo. and F. Plum. "Do positron emission tomographic scans measure quality of life?" *Annals of Neurology* 24.2 (1988): 288-289.

Libet, B. "Cortical activation in conscious and unconscious experience." *Perspectives in Biology and Medicine* 9.1 (1965): 77-86.

Libet, B., W.W. Alberts., E.W. Wright., *et al.* "Responses of human somatosensory cortex to stimuli below threshold for conscious sensation." *Science* 158.3808 (1967): 1597-1560.

Lipton, H.L. "Do-not-resuscitate decisions in a community hospital." *Journal of the American Medical Association* 256.9 (1986): 1164-1169.

Llinás, R.R. "The intrinsic electrophysiological properties of mammalian neurons: Insights into central nervous system function." *Science* 242.4886 (1988): 1654-1664.

Llinàs, R. and U. Ribary. "Coherent 40-Hz oscillation characterizes dream state in humans." *Proceedings of the National Academy of Science USA.* 90.3 (1993): 2078-2081.

Lo, B., F. Rouse, and L. Dornbrand. "Family decision making on trial. Who decides for incompetent patients?" *New England Journal of Medicine* 322.17 (1990): 1228-1232.

Lowenstein, D.H. and J.M. Parent. "Brain, heal thyself." *Science* 283.5405 (1999): 1126-1127.

Luttrell, S. "Withdrawing or withholding life prolonging treatment." *British Medical Journal* 318.7200 (1999): 1709-1710.

Lynn, J. "Why I don't have a living will." *Law, Medicine and Health Care* 19.1-2 (1991): 101-104.

MacDermid, A. "Lord Advocate clears the way for medics to make life or death judgement. Doctors to judge on right to die." *The Herald* (Glasgow) 27 April 1996.

Macdonald, V. "B.M.A. to redraw rules on brain death." *The Sunday Telegraph* (London) 17 March 1996a.

Macdonald, V. "Treatment offers hope for 'human vegetables'." *The Sunday Telegraph* (London) 17 November 1996b.

Macdonald, V. "Court hears more pleas to stop life support." *The Sunday Telegraph* (London) 23 February 1997a.

Macdonald, V. "Shock at court ruling which lets coma woman 'starve'." *The Sunday Telegraph* (London) 23 March 1997b.

Macdonald, V. "Doctors to highlight dilemma of life support." *The Sunday Telegraph* (London) 8 February, 1998.

Mackworth, J.F. "Vigilance, arousal, and habituation." *Psychological Review* 75.4 (1968): 308-322.

Maillet, J.O. "Position of The American Dietetic Association: Legal and ethical issues in feeding permanently unconscious patients." *Journal of the American Dietetic Association* 95.2 (1995): 231-234.

Maquet, P., J-M. Peters., J. Aerts., *et al.* "Functional anatomy of human rapid-eye-movement sleep and dreaming." *Nature* 383.6596 (1996): 163-166.

Martin, J.B., and S. Reichlin. "Mechanisms of thirst regulation." Pp 79-82 *in Clinical Neuroendocrinology*. Vol 28 of *Contemporary Neurology*, Philadelphia: F. A. Davis, 1987.

Mason, J.K. and D. Mulligan. "Euthanasia by stages." *The Lancet* 347.9004 (1996): 810-811.

McCann, R.M., W.J. Hall., and A. Groth-Juncker. "Comfort care for terminally ill patients. The appropriate use of nutrition and hydration." *Journal of the American Medical Association* 272.16 (1994): 1263-1266.

McCullagh, P. *Brain dead, brain absent, brain donors. Human subjects or human objects*? Chichester: John Wiley and Sons, 1993.

McDaniel, C.G. "US doctors reaffirm opposition to euthanasia." *British Medical Journal* 313.7048 (1996): 11.
McLean, S.A.M. "Legal and ethical aspects of the vegetative state." *Journal of Clinical Pathology* 52.7 (1999): 490-493.
McMahan, J. "Brain death, cortical death and persistent vegetative state." In *A companion to bioethics*, edited by H. Kuhse and P. Singer, 250-260. Oxford: Blackwell, 1998.
McMillan, T.M. "Neuropsychological assessment after extremely severe head injury in a case of life or death." *Brain Injury* 12.10 (1998): 809-816.
McMillan, T.M. and C.M. Herbert. "Neuropsychological assessment of a potential 'euthanasia' case: a 5 year follow up." *Brain Injury* 14.2 (2000): 197-203.
McQuillen, M.P. "Can people who are unconscious or in the 'vegetative state' perceive pain?" *Issues in Law and Medicine* 6.4 (1991): 373-383.
McQuillen, M.P. "The persistent vegetative state." *New England Journal of Medicine* 331.20 (1994): 1380.
Meilaender, G. "Ordinary and extraordinary treatments: when does quality of life count?" *Theological Studies* 58.3 (1997): 527-531.
Meisel, A. "The legal consensus about forgoing life-sustaining treatment: Its status and its prospects." *Kennedy Institute of Ethics Journal* 2.4 (1992): 309-345.
Meisel, A. "*The right to die*." Vol 1. 2nd Edition. New York: John Wiley and Sons, 1995.
Menon, D.K., A.M. Owen., E.J. Williams., *et al.* "Cortical processing in persistent vegetative state." *The Lancet* 352.9123 (1998): 200.
Mesulam, M.M. "A cortical network for directed attention and unilateral neglect." *Annals of Neurology* 10.4 (1981): 309-325.
Meyers, D.W. "Legal aspects of withdrawing nourishment from an incurably ill patient." *Archives of internal Medicine* 146.1 (1985): 124-128
Middleton, F.A. and P. Strick. "Anatomical evidence for cerebellar and basal ganglia involvement in higher cognitive function." *Science* 266.5184 (1994): 458-462.
Miles, S. "Death in a technological and pluralistic culture." In *The definition of death*, edited by S.J. Youngner, R.M. Arnold and R. Schapiro, 311-318. Baltimore: Johns Hopkins University Press, 1999.
Miller, P.D., R.A. Krebs., B.J. Neal., *et al.* "Hypodipsia in geriatric patients." *American Journal of Medicine* 73.3 (1982): 354-356.
Miller, R.J. "Advance directives for medical care." *New England Journal of Medicine* 325.17 (1991): 1254-1255.
Minderhoud, J.M. and R. Braakman. "Het vegeterende bestaan." *Nederlands Tijdschrift voor Geneerkunde* 129.50 (1985): 2385-2388.
Mitchell, KR., Kerridge, IH. and Lovat, TJ. "Medical futility, treatment withdrawal and the persistent vegetative state." *Journal of Medical Ethics* 19.2 (1993): 71-76
Mitchell, P.H. and N.K. Mauss. "Relationship of patient-nurse activity to intracranial pressure variations: A pilot study." *Nursing Research* 27.1 (1978): 4-10.
Molinari, G.F. "Persistent vegetative state, do not resuscitate… and still more words doctors use." *Journal of the Neurological Sciences* 102.2 (1991): 125-127.
Momose, T., T. Matsui., N. Kosaka., *et al.* "Effect of cervical spinal cord stimulation (cSCS) on cerebral glucose metabolism and blood flow in a vegetative patient assessed by positron emission tomography (PET) and single photon emission computed tomography (SPECT)." *Radiation Medicine* 7.5 (1989): 243-246.
Moray, N. "Attention." In *The Oxford companion to the mind*, Edited by R.L. Gregory, 59-61. Oxford: Oxford University Press, 1987.
Multi-Society Task Force on PVS. (M.S.T.F.) "Medical aspects of the persistent vegetative state. Part I." *New England Journal of Medicine* 330.21 (1994a): 1499-1508.
Multi-Society Task Force on PVS. (M.S.T.F.) "Medical aspects of the persistent vegetative state. Part II." *New England Journal of Medicine* 330.22 (1994b): 1572-1579.
Munby, J. "Consent to treatment: Children and the incompetent patient." In *Principles of medical law*, edited by I. Kennedy and A. Grubb, 179-282. Oxford: Oxford University Press, 1998.
Munglani, R., J. Andrade., J. Sapsford., *et al.* "A measure of consciousness and memory during isoflurane administration: The coherent frequency." *British Journal of Anaesthesia* 71.5 (1993): 633-641.
Musgrave, C.F., N. Bartal. and J. Opstad. "The sensation of thirst in dying patients receiving IV hydration." *Journal of Palliative Care* 11.4 (1995): 17-21.

Nadal, J.W., S. Pedersen., and W.G. Maddock. "A comparison between dehydration from salt loss and from water deprivation." *Journal of Clinical Investigation* 20.6 (1941): 691-703.

Najenson, T., J. Sazbon., J. Fiselzon., *et al.* "Recovery of communicative functions after prolonged traumatic coma." *Scandinavian Journal of Rehabilitation Medicine* 10.1 (1978): 15-21.

National Legal Center for the Medically Dependent and Disabled Inc. "ADA Analyses of the Oregon Health Care Plan." *Issues in Law and Medicine* 9.4 (1994): 397-424.

Nicolson, A. "A death worse than death." *The Sunday Telegraph* (London) 30 March 1997.

Nofzinger, E.A., D.J. Buysse., J.M. Miewald., *et al.* "Human regional cerebral glucose metabolism during non-rapid eye movement sleep in relation to waking." *Brain* 125.5 (2002): 1105-1115.

Norberg, A., M. Hirschfeld., B. Davidson., *et al.* "Ethical reasoning concerning the feeding of severely demented patients: An international perspective." *Nursing Ethics* 1.1 (1994): 3-13.

Nordgren, R.E., W.R. Markesbery., K. Fukuda., *et al.* "Seven cases of cerebromedullospinal disconnection: The 'locked-in' syndrome." *Neurology* 21.11 (1971): 1140-1148.

Nussbaum, M., I.R. Shenker., J. Marc., *et al.* "Cerebral atrophy in anorexia nervosa." *Journal of Pediatrics* 96.5 (1980): 867-869.

O'Connell, A.S. "The French vegetative state." *Hastings Center Report* 22.4 (1992): 36-37.

O'Connor, M., J.P. Kress., A. Pohlman., *et al.* "Pitfalls of monitoring sedation in the ICU with the bispectral index." *Anesthesiology* 89.3A (1998): 461.

O'Neill, S. "Coma victims 'could be used to test drugs'." *The Daily Telegraph* (London) 8 April 1996.

Oddy, M., M. Humphrey. and D. Uttley. "Subjective impairment and social recovery after closed head injury." *Journal of Neurology, Neurosurgery, and Psychiatry* 41.7 (1978): 611-616.

Oliver, D. "Terminal dehydration." *The Lancet* 2.8403 (1984): 631.

Overmier, J.B. and M.R. Papini. "Factors modifying the effects of teleost telencephalon ablation on retention, relearning and extinction of instrumental avoidance behaviour." *Behavioral Neuroscience* 100.2 (1986): 190-199.

Owen, A.M., D.K. Menon., I.S. Johnsrude., *et al.* "Detecting residual cognitive function in persistent vegetative state." *Neurocase* 8.5 (2002): 394-403.

Ozbudak-Demir, S., M. Akyüz., F. Güler-Uysal., *et al.* "Postacute predictors of functional and cognitive progress in traumatic brain injury: Somatosensory evoked potentials." *Archives of Physical Medicine and Rehabilitation* 80.3 (1999): 252-257.

Pallis, C. "Defining death." *British Medical Journal* 291.6496 (1985): 666-667.

Parasuraman, R. "Vigilance, arousal and the brain." In *Physiological correlates of human behaviour. Vol. II: Attention and performance*. Edited by A. Gale and JA. Edwards, 35-55. London: *Academic Press*, 1983.

Paris, J.J. "The six-million-dollar woman." *Connecticut Medicine* 45.11 (1981): 720-721

Parker, C.J.R., J.D.L. Oates., A.H. Boyd., *et al.* "Memory for auditory material presented during anaesthesia." *British Journal of Anaesthesia* 72.2 (1994): 181-184.

Passler, M.A. and R.V. Riggs. "Positive outcomes in traumatic brain injury-vegetative patients treated with bromocriptine." *Archives of Physical Medicine and Rehabilitation* 82.3 (2001): 311-315.

Patterson, J.R. and M. Grabois. "Locked-in syndrome: A review of 139 cases." *Stroke* 17.4 (1986): 758-764.

Payne, K., R.M. Taylor., C. Stocking., *et al.* "Physicians' attitudes about the care of patients in the persistent vegetative state: A national survey." *Annals of Internal Medicine* 125.2 (1996): 104-110.

Peart, N., and G. Gillett. "*Re G*: A life worth living?" *Journal of Law and Medicine* 5.3 (1998): 239-251.

Peart, N.S., A.V. Campbell., A.R. Manara., *et al.* "Maintaining a pregnancy following loss of capacity." *Medical Law Review* 8.3 (2000): 275-299.

Penfield, W. and E. Boldrey. "Somatic motor and sensory representation in the cerebral cortex of man as studied by electrical stimulation." *Brain* 60.3 (1937): 398-443.

Pernick, M.S. "Brain death in a cultural context. The reconstruction of death, (1967-1981)." In *The definition of death*, edited by S.J. Youngner, R.M. Arnold and R. Schapiro, 3-33. Baltimore: Johns Hopkins University Press, 1999.

Petty, M. "Saved by a mother's courage. A 17-year old boy, thought to be brain-dead, has survived against all odds." *The Times* (London) 23 March 1999.

Phelps, M.E., S.C. Huang., E.J. Hoffman., *et al.* "Tomographic measurement of local cerebral glucose metabolic rate in humans with (F-18)-Fluoro-2-Deoxy-D-Glucose: Validation of Method." *Annals of Neurology* 6.5 (1979): 371-388.

Phillip, P.A., B.J. Rolls., J.G.G. Ledingham., *et al.* "Reduced thirst after water deprivation in healthy men." *New England Journal of Medicine* 311.12 (1984): 753-759.

Plows, C.W. "Reconsideration of AMA opinion on anencephalic neonates as organ donors." *Journal of the American Medical Association* 275.6 (1996): 443-444.
Plum, F. "Clinical standards and technological confirmatory tests in diagnosing brain death." In *The definition of death: contemporary controversies*, edited by S.J. Youngner, R.M. Arnold and R. Schapiro, 34-65. Baltimore: Johns Hopkins University Press, 1999.
Plum, F. and J.B. Posner. *The diagnosis of stupor and coma*. Philadelphia: F.A. Davis 1966.
Plum, F., N. Schiff., U. Ribary., *et al.* "Co-ordinated expression in chronically unconscious persons." *Philosophical Transactions of the Royal Society, London (B)* 353.1377 (1998): 1929-1933.
Pollack, M.A. and P. Kellaway. "Cerebrocortical death vs. brain death: correlation of clinical, EEG, and evoked potential studies." *Electroencephalography and Clinical Neurophysiology* 49 (1980): 10p.
Pollard, B.J. "Withdrawing life-sustaining treatment from severely brain-damaged persons." *Medical Journal of Australia* 154.8 (1991): 559-561.
Polyani, M. "Scientific outlook: its sickness and cure." *Science* 125.3246 (1957): 480-484.
Pöppel, E., R. Held. and D. Frost. "Residual visual function after brain wounds involving the central visual pathways in man." *Nature* 243.5405 (1973): 295-296.
Practice Note (Official Solicitor) 4 All ER 766, 1996.
Practice Note (Official Solicitor) 2 FLR 158, 2001.
President's Commission for the Study of Ethical Problems in Medicine and Biomedical and Behavioural Research. *Deciding to forego life-sustaining treatment: a report on the ethical, medical and legal issues in treatment decisions*. Washington D.C: Government Printing Office, 1983a.
President's Commission for the Study of Ethical Problems in Medicine and Biomedical and Behavioral Research *Securing Access to Health Care*. Vol. 1. U.S. Government Printing Office, Washington DC 1983b.
Printz, L.A. "Is withholding hydration a valid comfort measure in the terminally ill?" *Geriatrics* 43.11 (1988): 84-88.
Rader, M.A. and D.W. Ellis. "The sensory stimulation assessment measure (SSAM): a tool for early evaluation of severely brain-injured patients." *Brain Injury* 8.4 (1994): 309-321.
Ramsey, P. *The ethics of fetal research*. New Haven Conn: Yale University Press, 1975.
Raps, S.P., N.R. Relkin., D.R. Labar., *et al.* "Electroencephalographic correlates of arousal in the persistent vegetative state." *Society for Neuroscience* 17.1 *Abstracts* (1991): 882.
Rawls, J. "*Collected Papers*." Ed S. Freeman. Cambridge Mass: Harvard University Press, 1999.
Re G, 2 NZLR 201, 1997.
Re Estate of Sidney Greenspan v Andrew Gelman, Guardian *ad litem*. Illinois Supreme Court. (US) 224, 1990.
Re T (Adult: Refusal of treatment) (1993) AC (Fam) 95.
Regan, R.J. "Letter to the editor". *Law and Justice* 118 (1993): 146.
Relkin, M.R., C.K. Petito. and F. Plum. "Coma and the vegetative state associated with thalamic injury after cardiac arrest." *Annals of Neurology* 28.2 (1990): 221-222.
Relman, A.S. "The Saikewicz decision: judges as physicians." *New England Journal of Medicine* 298.9 (1978): 508-509.
Report of the Swedish Committee on Defining Death *The concept of death*. Stockholm: Swedish Ministry of Health and Social Affairs, 1984.
Reynolds, B.A., and S. Weiss. "Generation of neurons and astrocytes from isolated cells of the adult mammalian central nervous system." *Science* 255.5052 (1992): 1707-1710.
Rie, M.A. "The limits of a wish." *Hastings Center Report* 21.4 (1991): 24-27
Ricci, R., B. Barbarella., P. Musi., *et al.* "Localised proton MR spectroscopy of brain metabolism changes in vegetative patients." *Neuroradiology* 39.5 (1997): 313-319.
Rice, H.K. and M.W. McDaniel. "Operant behavior in vegetative patients I." *The Psychological Record* 16.3 (1966): 279-281.
Rice, H.K., M.W. McDaniel., V.D. Stallings., *et al.* "Operant behaviour in vegetative patients II." *The Psychological Record* 17.3 (1967): 449-460.
Robertson, G.L., P. Aycinena. and R.L. Zerbe. "Neurogenic disorders of osmoregulation." *American Journal of Medicine* 72.2 (1982): 339-353.
Robertson, G.S. "Making an advance directive." *British Medical Journal* 310.6974 (1995): 236-238.
Robertson, J.A. "Cruzan and the constitutional status of nontreatment decisions for incompetent patients." *Georgia Law Review* 25.5 (1991): 1139-1202.
Rogers v Whittaker 175 CLR 479, 1992.
Rogers, L. "Brain implant revives coma victims." *The Sunday Times* (London) 1 March 1998.

Rosenberg, G.A., S.F. Johnson. and R.P. Brenner. "Recovery of cognition after prolonged vegetative state." *Annals of Neurology* 2.2 (1977): 167-168.
Rosin, A.J. and M. Sonnenblick. "Autonomy and paternalism in geriatric medicine. The Jewish ethical approach to issues of feeding terminally ill patients, and to cardiopulmonary resuscitation." *Journal of Medical Ethics* 24.1 (1988): 44-48.
Rothstein, T.L., E.M. Thomas. and S.M. Sumi. "Predicting outcomes in hypoxic-ischemic coma. A prospective clinical and electrophysiologic study." *Electroencephalography and Clinical Neurophysiology* 79.2 (1991): 101-107.
Royal College of Physicians Working Party. "Criteria for the diagnosis of brain stem death." *Journal of the Royal College of Physicians* 29.5 (1995): 381-382.
Royal College of Physicians. *The vegetative state: guidance on diagnosis and management.* R.C.P. Publications, London 2003.
Ruark, J.E., and T.A. Raffin. "Initiating and withdrawing life support. Principles and practice in adult medicine." *New England Journal of Medicine* 318.1 (1988): 25-30.
Rudolf, J., J. Sobsky., M. Grond., *et al.* "Identification by positron emission tomography of neuronal loss in acute vegetative state." *The Lancet*, 354.9198 (2000): 115-116.
Russell, J.F. "Midazolam-alfentanil: an anaesthetic? An investigation using the isolated forearm technique." *British Journal of Anaesthesia* 70.1 (1993): 42-46.
Sailly, J.C. "Economic aspects of the care of patients in the vegetative state." *Acta Neurologica Belgica* 94 (1994): 155-165.
Santo, J.L., L.M. Arias., G. Barolat., *et al.* "Bilateral cingulumotomy in the treatment of reflex sympathetic dystrophy." *Pain* 41.1 (1990): 55-59.
Sarnat, H.B. and M.G. Netsky. *Evolution of the nervous system.* Second edition. New York: Oxford University Press, 1981.
Sato, G., H. Imamura., K. Veki., *et al.* "Epidemiological study of vegetative state patients in the Tohoku District, Japan." *Neurologia Medico-Chirurgica (Tokyo)* 19.4 (1979): 327-333.
Sato, M., R. Kuroda., M. Ioku., *et al.* "Regional cerebral blood flow in the persistent vegetative state." *Neurologica Medico-Chirurgica (Tokyo)* 29.5 (1989): 389-394.
Savell, K. "Human rights in the age of technology: Can law rein in the medical juggernaut?" *Sydney Law Review* 23.3 (2001): 423-460.
Sazbon, L. and Z. Groswasser. "Medical complications and mortality of patients in the postcomatose unawareness (PC-U) state." *Acta Neurochirurgica (Wein)* 112.3-4 (1991): 110-112.
Sazbon, L., H. Costeff. and Z. Groswasser. "Epidemiological findings in traumatic post-comatose unawareness." *Brain Injury* 6.4 (1992): 359-362.
Sazbon, L., F. Zagreba., J. Ronen., *et al.* "Course and outcome of patients in vegetative state of nontraumatic aetiology." *Journal of Neurology, Neurosurgery and Psychiatry* 56.4 (1993): 407-409.
Schallert, T., T.D. Hernandez. and T.M. Barth. "Recovery of function after brain damage: severe and chronic disruption by diazepam." *Brain Research* 379.1 (1986): 104-111.
Schiedermayer, D.L. and J. La Puma. "Do positron emission tomographic scans measure quality of life?" *Annals of Neurology* 24.2 (1988): 288.
Schiedermayer, D.L., J. La Puma. and S.H. Miles, SH. "Ethics consultations masking economic dilemmas in patient care." *Archives of Internal Medicine* 149.6 (1989): 1303-1305.
Schiff, N.D., U. Ribary., D.R. Moreno., *et al.* "Residual cerebral activity and behavioural fragments can remain in the persistently vegetative brain." *Brain* 125.6 (2002): 1210-1234.
Schnaper, N. "The psychological implications of severe trauma: emotional sequelae to unconsciousness." *Journal of Trauma*, 15.2 (1975): 94-98.
Schneiderman, L.J., N.S. Jecker. and A.R. Jonsen. "Medical futility: Its meaning and ethical implications." *Annals of Internal Medicine* 112.12 (1990): 949-954.
Schuri, U. and D. von Cramon. "Electrodermal responses to auditory stimuli with different significance in neurological patients." *Psychophysiology* 18.3 (1981): 248-251.
Schwaber, E.A. "Late improvement after post-traumatic vegetative state." *New England Journal of Medicine* 334.18 (1996): 1201.
Searle, J.R. *The mystery of consciousness.* London: Granta, 1998.
Seckler, A.B., D.E. Meier., M. Mulvihill., *et al.* "Substituted judgement: How accurate are proxy predictions?" *Annals of Internal Medicine* 115.2 (1991): 92-98.
Secretary, Health and Human Services "ADA Analysis of the Oregon Health Care Plan." *Issues in Law and Medicine* 9.4 (1994): 409-412.
Sein, P., S. Searson. and A.R. Nicol. "Anorexia nervosa and pseudo-atrophy of the brain." *British Journal of Psychiatry* 139.3 (1981): 257-258.

Shalit, M.N., A.J. Beller. And M. Feinsod. "Clinical equivalents of cerebral oxygen consumption in coma." *Neurology* 22.2 (1972): 155-160.

Sharpless, S. and H. Jasper. "Habituation of the arousal reaction." *Brain* 79.3 (1958): 655-680.

Shewmon, D.A. "The probability of inevitability: the inherent impossibility of validating criteria for brain death or 'irreversibility' through clinical studies." *Statistics in Medicine* 6.5 (1987): 535-553.

Shewmon, D.A. "Recovery from 'brain death': A neurologist's apologia." *Linacre Quarterly* 64.1 (1997): 30-96.

Shewmon, D.A. and C.M. De Giorgio. "Early prognosis in anoxic coma. Reliability and rationale." *Neurologic Clinics* 7.4 (1989): 823-843.

Shiel, A., B. Wilson., S. Horn., *et al.* "Can patients in coma following traumatic head injury learn simple tasks?" *Neuropsychological Rehabilitation* 3.2 (1993): 161-175.

Shuttleworth, E. "Recovery to social and economic independence from prolonged postanoxic vegetative state." *Neurology* 33.3 (1983): 372-374.

Sibson, M. "Body and Mind. For two months a bright young student lay in a coma. 'Just you wait, I'm going to be clever again'." *The Times* (London) 25 July 1995.

Siegel, K. "Psychosocial aspects of rational suicide." *American Journal of Psychotherapy* 40.3 (1986): 405-418.

Singer, P. "Is the sanctity of life ethic terminally ill?" *Bioethics* 9.3-4 (1995): 327-343.

Smith, D.G. and R.S. Wigton. "Modeling decisions to use tube feeding in seriously ill patients." *Archives of Internal Medicine* 147.7 (1987): 1242-1245.

Smith, R. "The importance of patients' consent for publication." *British Medical Journal* 313.7048 (1996): 16.

Snyder, B.D., R.E. Cranford., A.B. Rubens., *et al.* "Delayed recovery from postanoxic persistent vegetative state." *Annals of Neurology* 14.1 (1983): 152.

Snyder, M. "Relation of nursing activities to increases in intracranial pressure." *Journal of Advanced Nursing* 8.4 (1983): 273-279.

Sobel, N., V. Prabhakaren., C.A. Hartley., et al. "Blind smell: brain activation induced by an undetected air-borne chemical." *Brain* 122.2 (1999): 209-217.

Sommerhoff, G. and K. MacDorman. "An account of consciousness in physical and functional terms: A target for research in the neurosciences." *Integrative Physiological and Behavioral Science* 29.2 (1994): 151-181.

Spiro, S.G., and J.S. Jenkins. "Adipsia and hypothermia after subarachnoid haemorrhage." *British Medical Journal* 3.5771 (1971): 411-412.

Spudis, E.V. "The persistent vegetative state – 1990." *Journal of the Neurological Sciences* 102.2 (1991): 128-136.

Stacy, T. "Death, privacy, and the free exercise of religion." *Cornell Law Review* 77.3 (1992): 490-595.

Stanley, J.M. "The Appleton Consensus: suggested international guidelines for decisions to forego medical treatment." *Journal of Medical Ethics* 15.3 (1989): 129-136.

Stanley, J.M. "The Appleton International Conference on developing guidelines for decisions for life-prolonging medical treatment." *Journal of Medical Ethics* 18 (1992): Supplement 3-21.

Stein, D.G., S. Brailowsky. and B. Will. *Brain repair*. New York: Oxford University Press, 1995.

Steinbock, B. "Recovery from persistent vegetative state?: The case of Carrie Coons." *Hastings Center Report* 19.4 (1989): 14-15.

Steinbrook, R. and B. Lo. "Artificial feeding-solid ground, not a slippery slope." *New England Journal of Medicine* 318.5 (1988): 286-290.

Stensman, R. "Severely mobility-disabled people assess the quality of their lives." *Scandinavian Journal of Rehabilitation Medicine* 17.2 (1985): 87-99.

Stoerig, P. and A. Cowey, A. "Blindsight in man and monkey." *Brain* 120.3 (1997): 535-559.

Strauss, D.J., R.M. Shavelle, and S. Ashwal. "Life expectancy and median survival time in the persistent vegetative state." *Pediatric Neurology* 21.3 (1999): 626-631.

Strich, S.J. "Diffuse degeneration of the cerebral white matter in severe dementia following head injury." *Journal of Neurology, Neurosurgery and Psychiatry* 19.3 (1956): 163-185.

Sulmasy, D.P. and J. Sugarman. "Are withholding and withdrawing therapy always morally equivalent?" *Journal of Medical Ethics* 20.4 (1994): 218-222.

Sutherland, S. *The Macmillan dictionary of psychology*. London: Macmillan, 1989.

Sweet, W.H. "Brain death." *New England Journal of Medicine* 299.8 (1978): 410-412.

Swinburn, J.M.A., S.M. Ali., D.J. Banerjee., *et al.* "Ethical dilemma: Discontinuation of ventilation after brain stem death." *British Medical Journal* 318.7200 (1999): 1753-1755.

Tanna, N.K., M.I. Kohn., D.N. Horwich., *et al.* "Analysis of brain and cerebrospinal fluid volumes with MR imaging: Impact on PET data correction for atrophy. II. Aging and Alzheimer dementia." *Radiology* 178.1 (1991): 123-130.

Taylor, M.A. "Benefits of Dehydration in Terminally Ill Patients." *Geriatric Nursing* 16.6 (1995): 271-272.

Teitelbaum, P., and J. Cytawa. "Speading depression and recovery from lateral hypothalamic damage." *Science* 147.3653 (1965): 61-63.

The Hastings Center: *Guidelines on the termination of life-sustaining treatment and the care of the dying.* Briarcliff Manor, NY, The Hastings Center 1987.

Theodore, W.H., G. DiChiro., R. Margolin., *et al.* "Barbiturates reduce human cerebral glucose metabolism." *Neurology* 36.1 (1986): 60-64.

Thomasma, D.C. and J. Brumlik. "Ethical issues in the treatment of patients with a remitting vegetative state." *American Journal of Medicine* 77.2 (1984): 373-377.

Thrasher, T.N., J.F. Nistal-Herrera., L.C. Keil., *et al.* "Satiety and inhibition of vasopressin secretion after drinking in dehydrated dogs." *American Journal of Physiology* 240.4 (1981): E394-401.

Tomkin, D. and A. McAuley. "Withdrawal of treatment." *New Law Journal* 45.6708 (1995): 1234-1235.

Tomlinson, T. and D. Czlonka. "Futility and hospital policy." *Hastings Center Report* 25.3 (1995): 28-35.

Tommasino, C., C. Grana., G. Lucignani., *et al.* "Regional cerebral metabolism of glucose in comatose and vegetative state patients." *Journal of Neurosurgical Anesthesiology* 7.2 (1995): 109-116.

Tosch, P. "Patients' recollections of their posttraumatic coma." *Journal of Neuroscience Nursing* 20.4 (1988): 223-228.

Tresch, D.D., F.H. Sims., E.H. Duthie., *et al.* "Patients in a persistent vegetative state: attitudes and reaction of family members." *Journal of the American Geriatrics Society* 39.1 (1991a): 17-21.

Tresch, D.D., F.H. Sims., E.H. Duthie., *et al.* "Clinical characteristics of patients in the persistent vegetative state." *Archives of Internal Medicine* 151.5 (1991b): 930-932.

Truog, R.D. "Is it time to abandon brain death?" *Hastings Center Report* 27.1 (1997): 29-37.

Truog, R.D., A.S. Brett. and J. Frader. "The problem with futility." *New England Journal of Medicine* 326.23 (1992): 1560-1564.

Tsubokawa, T., T. Yamamoto., Y. Katayama., *et al.* "Deep-brain stimulation in a persistent vegetative state: Follow-up results and criteria for selection of candidates." *Brain Injury* 4.4 (1990): 315-327.

Tudor, M. "Persistent vegetative state: Some clinical observations." *Ethics and Medicine* 9.3 (1993a): 37-40.

Tudor, M.A. "Give proper rehabilitation a chance." *British Medical Journal* 307.6897 (1993b): 200-201.

United States Bishops' Committee for pro-life activities. "Nutrition and hydration: Moral and pastoral reflections." *Catholic International* 3.13 (1992): 620-632.

Van Assche, F.A. "Anencephalics as organ donors." *American Journal of Obstetrics and Gynecology* 163.2 (1990): 599-600.

van den Haag, H.L.R. "The ultimate punishment: a defense." *Harvard Law Review* 99.7 (1986): 1662-1669.

van Woerkom, T.C.A.M., J.M. Minderhoud., T. Gottschal., *et al.* "Neurotransmitters in the treatment of patients with severe head injuries." *European Neurology* 21 (1982): 227-234.

Veatch, R.M. "The impending collapse of the whole brain definition of death." *Hastings Center Report* 23.4 (1993): 18-24.

Veatch, R.M. "The conscience clause: how much individual choice in defining death can our society tolerate?" In *The definition of death. Contemporary controversies*, edited by S.J. Youngner, R.M. Arnold and R. Schapiro, 137-160. Baltimore: Johns Hopkins University Press 1999.

Veatch, R.M. and C.M. Spicer. "Medically futile care: The role of the physician in setting limits." *American Journal of Law and Medicine* 18.1-2 (1992): 15-36.

Volicer, L., A. Collard., A. Hurley., *et al.* "Impact of special care unit for patients with advanced Alzheimer's disease on patients' discomfort and costs." *Journal of the American Geriatrics Society* 42.6 (1994): 597-603.

von Cramon, D. "The structure of vigilance." *Archives of Psychiatry and Neurological Sciences* 225 (1978): 201-207.

Wace, J. and M. Kai. "Anaesthesia for organ donation in the brainstem dead." *Anaesthesia* 55.6 (2000): 590.

Wade, D.T. "Misdiagnosing the persistent vegetative state." *British Medical Journal* 313.7062 (1996): 943-944.

Wade, D.T. and C. Johnston. "The permanent vegetative state: practical guidance on diagnosis and management." *British Medical Journal* 319.7213 (1999): 841-844.

Walker. A.E. "Central representation of pain." *Research Publications of the Association for Research in Nervous and Mental Disorders* 23 (1942): 63-85.

Wall, M. "Irish Supreme Court approves 'right-to-die' case." *The Lancet* 346.8971 (1995): 368.

Walshe, T.M. and C. Leonard. "Persistent vegetative state. Extension of the syndrome to include chronic disorders." *Archives of Neurology* 42.11 (1985): 1045-1047.

Wang, G-J, N.D. Volkow., A.P. Wolf., *et al.* "Intersubject variability of brain glucose metabolic measurements in young normal males." *Journal of Nuclear Medicine* 35.9 (1994): 1457-1466.

Wang, M. "Learning, memory and awareness during anaesthesia." In *Recent advances in anaesthesia and analgesia*, Vol 20, edited by A.P. Adams and J.N. Cashman, 83-106 Edinburgh: Churchill Livingstone, 1998.

Watson, M. and S. Horn. "'The ten pound note test': suggestions for eliciting improved responses in the severely brain-injured patient." *Brain Injury* 5.4 (1991): 421-424.

Weinberg, N. "Physically disabled people assess the quality of their lives." *Rehabilitation Literature* 45.1-2 (1984): 12-15.

Weir, R.F. and L. Gostin. "Decisions to abate life-sustaining treatment for nonautonomous patients." *Journal of the American Medical Association* 264.14 (1990): 1846-1853.

Weiskrantz, L., E.K. Warrington., M.D. Sanders., *et al.* "Visual capacity in the hemianopic field following a restricted occipital ablation." *Brain* 97.4 (1974): 709-728.

Werring, D.J., C.A. Clark., G.J. Barker., *et al.* "The structural and functional mechanisms of motor recovery: complementary use of diffusion tensor and functional magnetic resonance imaging in a traumatic injury of the internal capsule." *Journal of Neurology, Neurosurgery and Psychiatry* 65.6 (1998): 863-869.

Whyte, J. "Persistent vegetative state." *New England Journal of Medicine* 331.20 (1994): 1381.

Whyte, J. and M.B. Glenn. "The care and rehabilitation of the patient in a persistent vegetative state." *Journal of Head Trauma Rehabilitation* 1.1 (1986): 39-53.

Wikler, D. "Brain related criteria for the beginning and end of life." *Transplantation Proceedings* 22.3 (1990): 989-990.

Wikler, D. "Not dead, not dying? Ethical categories and persistent vegetative state." *Hastings Center Report* 18.1 (1988): 41-47.

Wikler, D. and A.J. Weisbard. "Appropriate confusion over brain death." *Journal of the American Medical Association* 261.15 (1989): 2246.

Wilson, F.C., J. Harpur., T. Watson., *et al.* "Vegetative state and minimally responsive patients – regional survey. Long-term case outcomes and service recommendations." *Neurorehabilitation* 17.3 (2002): 231-236.

Wilson, S. and H. Gill-Thwaites. "Early indication of emergence from vegetative state derived from assessments with the SMART – a preliminary report." *Brain Injury* 14.4 (2000): 319-331.

Wilson, S.L., G.E. Powell., K. Elliott., *et al.* "Sensory stimulation in prolonged coma: four single case studies." *Brain Injury* 5.4 (1991): 393-400.

Winick, M. "Malnutrition and the developing brain." In *Brain dysfunction in metabolic disorders*, Edited by F. Plum, 253-262. New York: Raven Press, (1974).

Winick, M., P. Rosso. and J. Waterlow. "Cellular growth of cerebrum, cerebellum and brain stem in normal and marasmic children." *Experimental Neurology* 26.2 (1970): 393-400.

Winkler, A.W., T.S. Danowski.,. J.R. Elkinton., *et al.* "Electrolyte and fluid studies during water deprivation and starvation in human subjects, and the effect of ingestion of fish, of carbohydrate and of salt solutions." *Journal of Clinical Investigation* 23.5 (1944): 807-815.

Winning, T. "Mercy killing - or simply an easy way out?" *The Daily Mail* (London) 27 March 1997.

Winslade, W.J. *Confronting traumatic brain injury: devastation, hope and healing*. New Haven, Conn: Yale University Press, 1998.

Winslow "One patient, 34 days in the Hospital, $7,000 syringes and a $5.2 million bill." *The Wall Street Journal* 2 August 2001.

Wood, R.L. "Critical analysis of the concept of sensory stimulation for patients in vegetative states." *Brain Injury* 5.4 (1991): 401-409.

Working Group convened by the Royal College of Physicians and endorsed by the Conference of Medical Royal Colleges and their Faculties of the United Kingdom "The permanent vegetative state." *Journal of the Royal College of Physicians of London* 30.2 (1996): 119-121.

Yamamoto, T., Y. Katayama., H. Oshima., *et al.* "Deep brain stimulation therapy for a persistent vegetative state." *Acta Neurochirurgica* Supplement 79 (2002): 79-82.

Yanagawa, T., F. Bunn., I. Roberts., *et al.* "Nutritional support for head-injured patients." In *The Cochrane Library*, Issue 3, Oxford: Update Software, 2001.

Young, N. "Don't say the W word." *British Medical Journal* 322.7296 (2001): 1243.

Young, P.J., and B.F. Matta. "Anaesthesia for organ donation in the brainstem dead – why bother?" *Anaesthesia* 55.2 (2000): 105-106.

Youngner, S.J. "Defining death. A superficial and fragile consensus." *Archives of Neurology* 49.5 (1992): 570-571.

Youngner, S.J. "Who defines futility?" *Journal of the American Medical Association* 260.14 (1988): 2094-2095.

Youngner, S.J. and E. O'Toole. "Withdrawing treatment in the persistent vegetative state." *New England Journal of Medicine* 331.20 (1994): 1382.

Youngner, S.J. and R.M. Arnold. "Ethical, psychosocial, and public policy implications of procuring organs from non-heart-beating cadaver donors." *Journal of the American Medical Association* 269.21 (1993): 2769-2774.

Youngner, S.J., C.S. Landefeld., C.J. Coulton., *et al.* "'Brain Death' and organ retrieval." *Journal of the American Medical Association* 261.15 (1989): 2205-2210.

Zeman, A. "Persistent vegetative state." *The Lancet* 350.9080 (1997): 795-799.

Zerwekh, J.V. "The dehydration question." *Nursing* 83.1 (1983): 47-51.

Zola, I.K. "Social and cultural disincentives to independent living." *Archives of Physical Medicine and Rehabilitation* 63.8 (1982): 394-397.

Zweibel, N.R. and C.K. Cassel. "Treatment choices at the end of life: A comparison of decisions by older patients and their physician-selected proxies." *The Gerontologist* 29.5 (1989): 615-621.

INDEX

International Library of Ethics, Law, and the New Medicine

1. L. Nordenfelt: *Action, Ability and Health.* Essays in the Philosophy of Action and Welfare. 2000 ISBN 0-7923-6206-3
2. J. Bergsma and D.C. Thomasma: *Autonomy and Clinical Medicine.* Renewing the Health Professional Relation with the Patient. 2000 ISBN 0-7923-6207-1
3. S. Rinken: *The AIDS Crisis and the Modern Self.* Biographical Self-Construction in the Awareness of Finitude. 2000 ISBN 0-7923-6371-X
4. M. Verweij: *Preventive Medicine Between Obligation and Aspiration.* 2000 ISBN 0-7923-6691-3
5. F. Svenaeus: *The Hermeneutics of Medicine and the Phenomenology of Health.* Steps Towards a Philosophy of Medical Practice. 2001 ISBN 0-7923-6757-X
6. D.M. Vukadinovich and S.L. Krinsky: *Ethics and Law in Modern Medicine.* Hypothetical Case Studies. 2001 ISBN 1-4020-0088-X
7. D.C. Thomasma, D.N. Weisstub and C. Hervé (eds.): *Personhood and Health Care.* 2001 ISBN 1-4020-0098-7
8. H. ten Have and B. Gordijn (eds.): *Bioethics in a European Perspective.* 2001 ISBN 1-4020-0126-6
9. P.-A. Tengland: *Mental Health.* A Philosophical Analysis. 2001 ISBN 1-4020-0179-7
10. D.N. Weisstub, D.C. Thomasma, S. Gauthier and G.F. Tomossy (eds.) : *Aging: Culture, Health, and Social Change.* 2001 ISBN 1-4020-0180-0
11. D.N. Weisstub, D.C. Thomasma, S. Gauthier and G.F. Tomossy (eds.) : *Aging: Caring for our Elders.* 2001 ISBN 1-4020-0181-9
12. D.N. Weisstub, D.C. Thomasma, S. Gauthier and G.F. Tomossy (eds.) : *Aging: Decisions at the End of Life.* 2001 ISBN 1-4020-0182-7
    (Set ISBN for Vols. 10-12: 1-4020-0183-5)
13. M.J. Commers: *Determinants of Health: Theory, Understanding, Portrayal, Policy.* 2002 ISBN 1-4020-0809-0
14. I.N. Olver: *Is Death Ever Preferable to Life?* 2002 ISBN 1-4020-1029-X
15. C. Kopp: *The New Era of AIDS.* HIV and Medicine in Times of Transition. 2003 ISBN 1-4020-1048-6
16. R.L. Sturman: *Six Lives in Jerusalem.* End-of-Life Decisions in Jerusalem - Cultural, Medical, Ethical and Legal Considerations. 2003 ISBN 1-4020-1725-1
17. D.C. Wertz and J.C. Fletcher: *Genetics and Ethics in Global Perspective.* 2004 ISBN 1-4020-1768-5
18. J.B.R. Gaie: *The Ethics of Medical Involvement in Capital Punishment.* A Philosophical Discussion. 2004 ISBN 1-4020-1764-2
19. M. Boylan (ed.): *Public Health Policy and Ethics.* 2004 ISBN 1-4020-1762-6; Pb 1-4020-1763-4
20. R. Cohen-Almagor: *Euthanasia in the Netherlands.* The Policy and Practice of Mercy Killing. 2004 ISBN 1-4020-2250-6
21. D.C. Thomasma and D.N. Weisstub (eds.): *The Variables of Moral Capacity.* 2004 ISBN 1-4020-2551-3
22. *To be published.*
23. P. McCullagh: *Conscious in a Vegetative State? A Critique of the PVS Concept.* 2004 ISBN 1-4020-2629-3

International Library of Ethics, Law, and the New Medicine

24. L. Romanucci-Ross and L.R. Tancredi: *When Law and Medicine Meet: A Cultural View*. 2004
ISBN 1-4020-2756-7

KLUWER ACADEMIC PUBLISHERS – DORDRECHT / BOSTON / LONDON